COMPREHENSIVE NEUROLOGIC REHABILITATION
Volume 2

Traumatic Brain Injury

Comprehensive Neurologic Rehabilitation

COMPREHENSIVE NEUROLOGIC REHABILITATION
Volume 2

Traumatic Brain Injury

EDITOR

Paul Bach-y-Rita, M.D.

*Professor, Department of Rehabilitation Medicine
University of Wisconsin Medical School
Madison, Wisconsin, U.S.A.*

Demos Publications, 156 Fifth Avenue, New York, New York 10010

© 1989 by Demos Publications Inc. All rights reserved. This book is protected by copyright. No part of it may be reproduced, stored in a retrieval system, or transmitted in any form or by any means, electronic, mechanical, photocopying, recording, or otherwise, without the prior written permission of the publisher.

Made in the United States of America

Great care has been taken to maintain the accuracy of the information contained in this volume. However, neither the Editor nor Demos Publications can be held responsible for errors or for any consequences arising from the use of the information contained herein.

ISBN: 0-939957-18-3
LC: 88-71751

Preface

Traumatic brain injury (TBI) is a major cause of mortality, disability, and social disruption. Yet, until recently, it has been the "silent epidemic," with virtually no formal constituency and little funding for research or for services. In recent years, patient advocacy groups, politicians, federal agencies, and medical and social service organizations have recognized its importance, and TBI is beginning to get the attention it clearly merits.

However, each of the major interest groups mentioned above is faced with the reality resulting from so many years of neglect. There is an insufficient data base for each of the aspects of TBI. This includes basic research, clinical research, epidemiology, early treatment, hospital-based rehabilitation, late rehabilitation, psychosocial factors, vocational rehabilitation, and community integration.

This volume was prepared to emphasize the unique characteristics of TBI that establish it as a separate entity, to assess the current status of each of the areas related to TBI, and to begin to develop a research agenda. It has been organized into five sections as follows.

Patient management issues. Three levels of severity are described, each presenting a specific set of management problems: the severe TBI patient—including the patient in the vegetative state—patients with moderate head injuries, and patients with mild head injuries. We have a great amount of clinical knowledge about severe head injury; it is the category that has the lowest rate of incidence and the highest rate of mortality. The advent of the Glasgow Coma Scale has helped to provide the basis for comparable studies in many institutions and countries and to standardize treatment protocols. In addition to the management issues, philosophical issues, such as the degree of aggressiveness with which very severely brain damaged patients should be treated are discussed. Guy Clifton specifically notes the need for good animal research models to guide future management advances.

John Whyte and Mel Glenn discuss the management of the patient in the persistent vegetative state, resulting from the most severe nonfatal injuries. The maintenance of good general health poses many problems, but the cognitive status is obviously the major defining feature. A number of treatment approaches are used, but the authors point out the need for research, specifically with large series of matched patients or multiple baseline designs and a variety of approaches to disentangling the various influences on cognitive recovery. The family adaptation issues are crucial, with long periods of uncertainty and a number of long-term service delivery issues to be resolved.

Moderate head injuries may require years of intervention. Sheldon Berrol notes that this category has been defined by the Glasgow Coma Scale, but the category is in fact loose, with a great diversity within it. Some of the mechanisms of the injury are discussed, including diffuse axonal injury.

Following a discussion of the factors leading to the classification of mild head injury, Steven Mattis explores the mechanisms and nature of brain damage in such cases. The two major physical mechanisms for injury are rotational dislocation (rapid angular movement of the brain) and translational dislocation related to the force and direction of impact to the skull. The pathophysiology of mild brain injury includes the results of changes in cerebral blood flow. There is an initial increase in perfusion followed a few days later by a decrease in circulation. The neuropsychological sequelae of mild brain injury vary widely, but can be grouped under the general rubric of postconcussion syndrome including memory and concentration difficulty, headache, dizziness, irritability, free-floating anxiety, and cognitive deficits.

Neuropsychological and behavioral issues. The clinical relevance of neurobehavioral findings and the clinical features that are predictive of neurobehavioral outcome are discussed in chapters by Harvey Levin and Felicia Goldstein and by Gregory O'Shanick. Levin and Goldstein point out that chronic disability after closed head injury is primarily attributed to the neurobehavioral deficits, with the motor and sensory impairments playing a less important role. Memory, attention, conceptualization, and problem-solving are affected. Gaps in the research literature that are pointed out include the need for longitudinal data and for data concerning the neurobehavioral effects of head injury in older persons. O'Shanick provides a psychiatric perspective, but notes that psychiatry has in large part ignored the effects of TBI. He emphasizes the need to work with families as well as with the patients and notes the need to reevaluate individuals in state hospitals who have been labeled as being treatment refractory.

Neural recovery. Bach-y-Rita explores the neural mechanisms of recovery and reorganization. He reviews historical concepts that have limited an appreciation of the potential for recovery that the brain exhibits. Brain plasticity can be demonstrated at all ages and extends for many years after the injury. He notes that theory-based rehabilitation programs can obtain recovery that does not occur in the absence of such programs. Theory and basic research are critical in the development of appropriate rehabilitation. Povlishock describes the morphological aspects of TBI. He notes that axons are preferentially vulnerable to the shear and tensile forces of TBI. They are not necessarily torn, but the membranes appear to be focally altered. There also appears to be diffuse synaptic damage and deafferentation. These diffuse changes may be more important than focal damage, on which traditional neurobiologic thought has focused. Following the diffuse axonal injury, rewiring and reorganization may be maladaptive; extensive research in this area is needed. Povlishock considers that TBI research is at present impeded on two fronts: the thrust of contemporary neurobiology toward the molecular level and the animal welfare movement.

A very exciting area for TBI is an emerging understanding of the role of specific neurotransmitters in recovery from brain damage. In this area, animal research studies, such as those presented here by Michael Boyeson, have provided intriguing hints on mechanisms of recovery-potentiating effects. A number of medications used at present have strong effects on neurotransmitters, and Boyeson notes that different drugs may be effective at different times in the evolution of TBI patients. Increased understanding of the roles of specific neurotransmitters should lead to the development of new drugs. Boyeson further notes that the cerebellum may have a greater role than previously thought in the development of motor dysfunction such as hemiplegia and, correspondingly, a greater role in the recovery.

Although brain regions and cells within individual brain regions are usually considered to represent a specific function, there is a great deal of sharing of function and taking over of functional representation of speech, motor control, and sensation. Andrew Papanicolaou has reviewed the data demonstrating hemispheric transfer and hemispheric sharing of the central representation of speech following damage to the left temporal cortex. This can serve as a model of brain reorganization that can be the basis of comparable studies in other systems.

Rehabilitation services are usually provided to TBI patients within a short time of the injury, as soon as they are sufficiently stable medically. However, Richard Balliet points out that appropriate rehabilitation programs beginning several or many years after injury can lead to significant increases in function. He reports studies of brain activity, including positron emission tomography (PET) and neuroelectrical studies, that are exploring the correlation between recovery of function and specific areas of activity in the late rehabilitation model. An important characteristic of this model is that, since spontaneous recovery is no longer occurring during this period of time, the functional recovery due to the specific later rehabilitation program can be measured.

Rehabilitation issues. TBI rehabilitation presents unique problems, which are reviewed by Nathaniel Mayer. He clarifies the terms *impairment, disability,* and *handicap* in order to facilitate a discussion of the goals and strategies of rehabilitation. Because of the prolonged, usually lifetime, dependency of rehabilitated TBI patients on managers or caregivers, Mayer agrees that the care and rehabilitation of the survivor becomes a social issue. He notes the need for predictive models and for systems analysis research to clarify the kinds of support that should be provided to families and social networks that serve as managers and caregivers for the TBI survivor. He considers that emphasis should be shifted to rehabilitation of the nuclear social system that includes and supports the disabled individual.

The stages of recovery and the cost-effectiveness of rehabilitation are discussed by Brigitta Rees. She emphasizes the need for research into the point in time that specific strategies would be most appropriate. Assessment issues are addressed by Leonard Diller and Yehuda Ben-Yishay, who note that specific approaches must be developed for TBI rehabilitation assessment; these include measures of frontal lobe dysfunction as well as measures of acceptance and awareness, and of generalization of what has been learned. The specific interventions in TBI are discussed by George Prigatano, who considers that research is essential in the areas of neurotransmitters combined with rehabilitation, and that it is necessary to define and evaluate the various forms of therapy such as speech and language therapy and cognitive remediation that have clear emotional appeal to the patients. Further areas for research include the basis of organic unawareness after brain injury (separating that from psychogenic denial), effective training programs for staff and for families, and the development for cost-effective ways of returning TBI patients to work.

The significance of the family in the process of TBI rehabilitation is explored by Mitchell Rosenthal. Even survivors of minor head injury can experience significant psychosocial disability for months or years, creating great stress for families. Specific deficits that have impact on the family include the loss of social support from significant others, impairments in attention and memory, executive deficits, and inappropriate social behavior. Following an initial "honeymoon" period after the return home of the TBI survivor, there are feelings of discouragement, and many families start to experience depression or despair that often reaches a stage of reorganization, usually within 18 to 24 months after the return home. Siblings are impacted dramatically, and marital relations are seriously affected. Specific interventions including family counseling and family therapy are discussed, and related research questions are developed.

At present, approaches to care delivery for TBI survivors are fragmented and lead to inefficiency. Mark Johnston and Larry Cervelli present the case for systematic care. They draw on the experience of other systems, such as the care of spinal-cord-injured persons and the developmental disability system to suggest models for the TBI population.

They suggest that cost-effectiveness research should have a high priority.

Community integration issues. These are enormous and many are unique to TBI. Ellen Lehr explores these issues; the focus of community integration is obviously not one that considers only the injured individual, but one that involves the social, educational, and vocational systems that relate to that individual. Children present a series of particular problems; Lehr emphasizes their community re-entry needs including scholastic performance assessment. Adolescent TBI survivors also present a series of community intergration considerations. These are detailed by Jeanne Fryer, while the adult issues are discussed by Harvey Jacobs. The ultimate goal of TBI rehabilitation is community integration at the highest level possible. Jacobs notes that landmark changes in public advocacy and human rights legislation since the 1950s paved the way for a concept of the TBI survivors as equal members of the society with all rights and responsibilities. Recent advances have led to programs that are designed with the unique needs of the TBI survivor in mind.

The chapters of this volume emphasize that TBI is a distinct entity, requiring specific programmatical approaches in order to obtain minimal mortality and morbidity and maximal recovery, rehabilitation, and community entry. Suggestions for research that would further these efforts have been included in each of the chapters. Thus, the framework has been established for the development of clinical programs, community programs, and research efforts directed toward TBI.

Paul Bach-y-Rita, M.D.

Acknowledgments

We acknowledge the assistance of the following persons who helped to make this book a reality: Ellen J. Liberti, of the National Institute on Disability and Rehabilitation Research (NIDRR) and Project Officer and Conference Coordinator for the National Invitational Conference on Traumatic Brain Injury Research (November 2–4, 1987); Adrienne McCollum, Ph.D., President, Angela Peebles, Contract Program Officer, and other staff of Research Assessment Management, Inc., the conference contractors; and Sheila Newman of First Editions, Inc., preliminary editor of the papers. These people ensured the success of all aspects of the conference on which this book was based.

We acknowledge Assistant Secretary Madeleine Will, Office of Special Education and Rehabilitative Services, David B. Gray, Ph.D., former Director of the National Institute on Disability and Rehabilitation Research, and Marilyn Price Spivack, President of the National Head Injury Foundation, for directing that this conference be held as part of the U.S. Department of Education's initiative on traumatic brain injury research. We were pleased that former Secretary of Education William J. Bennett underlined this effort by taking part in the conference.

We thank the OSERS Task Force for the conference, which included: J. Paul Thomas, Ph.D., Richard P. Melia, Ph.D., Naomi Karp, and the late Richard R. Leclair of NIDRR; Thelma Leenhouts, Ph.D., Office of the Assistant Secretary; Sara Conlon, Ph.D., and Sheila Friedman, Office of Special Education Programs; and Sterling Brinkley, M.D., the Rehabilitation Services Administration. This group provided clarification on the substantive issues of the paper focus areas.

In addition to the chapter authors represented here, other interested and committed people in the field contributed their time and ideas to make this conference a success and to provide a rich focus for research in traumatic brain injury.

Contents

IV. REHABILITATION ISSUES

V. COMMUNITY INTEGRATION ISSUES

Contributors

Paul Bach-y-Rita, M.D., Professor, Department of Rehabilitation Medicine, University of Wisconsin Medical School, Clinical Science Center, Madison, Wisconsin.

Richard Balliet, Ph.D., Associate Professor, Department of Rehabilitation Medicine, University of Wisconsin Medical School, and Clinical Director, NeuroMuscular Retraining Clinic, Madison, Wisconsin.

Yehuda Ben-Yishay, Ph.D., Rusk Institute of Rehabilitation Medicine, New York University Medical Center, New York, New York.

Sheldon Berrol, M.D., Associate Clinical Professor, Physical Medicine and Rehabilitation, University of California, and Chief, Rehabilitation Medicine, Rehabilitation Medicine Service, San Francisco General Hospital, San Francisco, California.

Michael G. Boyeson, Ph.D., Assistant Professor, Department of Rehabilitation Medicine, Medical Science Center, Madison, Wisconsin.

Larry Cervelli, B.S., O.T.R., Program Director, The New Medico Head Injury System, Northampton, Massachusetts.

Guy Clifton, M.D., Director of Neurosurgery, Medical College of Virginia, Richmond, Virginia.

Georg Deutsch, Ph.D., Research Associate Professor, Department of Neurology, University of Alabama, Birmingham, Birmingham, Alabama.

Leonard Diller, Ph.D., Rusk Institute of Rehabilitation Medicine, New York University Medical Center, New York, New York.

Jeanne Fryer, Ph.D., Director, Community Rehabilitation Services, Rehab Systems Co., Annapolis, Maryland.

Mel B. Glenn, M.D., Department of Rehabilitation Medicine, New England Medical Center Hospitals, Tufts University School of Medicine, and The Greenery Rehabilitation and Skilled Nursing Center, Boston, Massachusetts.

Felicia C. Goldstein, Ph.D., Division of Neurosurgery and Department of Neurology, The University of Texas Medical Branch, Galveston, Texas.

Harvey Jacobs, Ph.D., Research Psychologist, Department of Psychiatry and Biobehaviorial Sciences, Neuropsychiatric Institute, UCLA Medical Center, Los Angeles, California; Director of Behavioral Systems, Casa Colina Hospital, Pomona, California.

Mark V. Johnston, Ph.D., Office of Research, New Medico Head Injury System, Northampton, Massachusetts.

Ellen Lehr, Ph.D., Chief Pediatric Psychologist, Center for Cognitive Rehabilitation, University of Medicine and Dentistry, of New Jersey and Rutgers University, New Brunswick, New Jersey.

Harvey S. Levin, Ph.D., Associate Professor, Division of Neurosurgery and Department of Neurology, University of Texas, Medical Branch, Galveston, Texas.

Steven Mattis, Ph.D., Neuropsychology Section, New York Hospital, Cornell University Medical Center, New York, New York.

Nathaniel H. Mayer, M.D., Director, Drucker Brain Injury Center, Moss Rehabilitation Hospital, Philadelphia, Pennsylvania.

Bartlett D. Moore, Ph.D., Assistant Professor of Pediatrics, University of Texas, M.D. Anderson Cancer Center, Houston, Texas.

Gregory O'Shanick, M.D., Assistant Professor of Psychiatry and Rehabilitation Medicine, Director, Psychiatry Inpatient Services and Medical Psychiatry Service, and Director, Medical Psychiatry Service, Medical College of Virginia Hospitals, Virginia Commonwealth University, Richmond, Virginia.

Andrew C. Papanicolaou, Ph.D., Division of Neurosurgery, University of Texas Medical Branch, Galveston, Texas.

John T. Povlishock, Ph.D., Professor of Anatomy, Department of Anatomy, Medical College of Virginia, Richmond, Virginia.

George Prigatano, Ph.D., Chairman, Neuropsychology, and Clinical Director, Neurological Rehabilitation, Barrow Neurological Institute and St. Joseph's Hospital and Medical Center, Phoenix, Arizona.

Brigitta Rees, M.D., Director, Rehabilitation Research and Training Center, Emory University School of Medicine, Atlanta, Georgia.

Mitchell Rosenthal, Ph.D., Director of Psychological Medicine, Marianjoy Rehabilitation Center, Wheaton, Illinois.

John Whyte, M.D., Ph.D., Director of Research and Associate Director of Rehabilitation Medicine, New England Medical Center Hospitals, Tufts University School of Medicine, and The Greenery Rehabilitation and Skilled Nursing Center, Boston, Massachusetts.

I

Patient Management Issues

1

Advances in Management of Severe Head Injury

Guy L. Clifton, M.D.

*Division of Neurosurgery, Medical College of Virginia,
Richmond, Virginia, U.S.A.*

Head injury has been termed the "silent epidemic" by the National Head Injury Foundation. This term acknowledges that until recently, the incidence, prevalence, and socioeconomic impact of head injury have been out of proportion to the level of public awareness of the problem. Many would say that its impact has also been out of proportion to the medical efforts expended for head injury care and research. The first proof that head injury was, in fact, a national public health problem came from the National Head and Spinal Cord Injury Survey reported in 1980 (Anderson, 1980). Head injury in this study was defined as physical injury to the brain caused by an external (mechanical) force. It was found that the incidence of hospitalized patients with head injury was 200 per 100,000 population in 1974. Subsequent studies have found an incidence of 200 to 300 per 100,000 population in major metropolitan areas in the United States (Klauber, 1981; Kraus, 1984). Mortality rate from severe head injury in metropolitan areas has been found to be 20 to 30 per 100,000 population (Kraus, 1984). Thirty percent of deaths from head injury occur in the hospital; and the remaining 70%, prior to hospital admission.

Head injury severity has generally been divided into mild, moderate, and severe. Severe head injury has been defined as coma for 6 hours or longer. Mild head injury has been defined as concussion. A uniform definition for moderate head injury has not been agreed upon. It can, however, be estimated that the incidence of severe and moderately severe head injury (likely to produce lasting neurologic deficits) is between 50 to 100 per 100,000 population. The incidence of stroke in the National

3

Stroke Survey was found to be 140 per 100,000 population (Weinfeld, 1981). Spinal cord injury by contrast has an incidence of 5 per 100,000 population (Anderson, 1980). Head injury of sufficient severity to produce disability, therefore, is a major public health problem as compared to other acute neurologic disorders.

ADVANCES IN EARLY HOSPITAL MANAGEMENT

While severe head injury is relatively low in incidence compared to mild and moderate head injury, it has required attention disproportionate to its numbers. The incidence of patients with severe head injury who survive to reach the hospital and remain in coma for 6 hours or longer can be estimated to be between 10 to 30 per 100,000 population. The mortality of this group of patients is between 30% and 50%, and they usually suffer long-lasting neurologic deficits, often severe. Because of the critical illness and severe disability of these patients, they consume enormous resources. Severe head injury has been one of the most common problems seen by practicing neurosurgeons; therefore, it has been the focus of much attention by the neurosurgical community for the last 15 years.

Until 1974, relatively little was known about the frequency and the outcome of severe head injury, but major advances in care have been made since that time. The event that perhaps more than any other initiated the past years of major progress in the study of head injury was the development of the Glasgow Coma Score by Jennett and Teasdale (Teasdale, 1974). This is a numerical system that quantitates the level of consciousness using response to pain, ability to open the eyes, and ability to speak (Table 1-1). Jennett and Teasdale sought to establish a reliable neurologic grading system that would predict outcome. Data were accumulated that related the initial Glasgow Coma Score to outcome in over 1,000 patients from Glasgow, the Netherlands, and Los Angeles (Jennett, 1977, 1979). The effect of pupillary reactivity, age, and other readily quantifiable variables upon outcome was also studied. This achievement allowed surgeons to compare their management results with those of the International Data Bank and with other hospitals, since comparability of injury severity could be assessed. The Glasgow Coma Score rapidly became standard nomenclature in neurosurgery. A mortality rate of 50% was reported in the International Data Bank. Patients entered into this data bank were seen for neurosurgical care late in their course by present standards, and whether mortality could be reduced stimulated a lively and productive controversy in head injury management.

The question posed by many clinical investigators was: Could mortality be reduced without producing vegetative survivors? Becker and his

Table 1-1. *Glasgow Coma Scale*

Eye opening	
Spontaneous	4
To voice	3
To pain	2
None	1
Verbal response	
Oriented	5
Confused	4
Inappropriate words	3
Incomprehensible words	2
None	1
Motor response	
Obeys commands	6
Localizes pain	5
Withdraws	4
Flexion	3
Extension	2
None	1

associates at the Medical College of Virginia in 1977 reported a major mortality reduction with an improved number of good recoveries as compared to the International Data Bank (Becker, 1977). This improved outcome was attributed to early surgery and intracranial pressure monitoring with control of elevated intracranial pressure. A generally vigorous and highly standardized approach to the acute care of these patients had been adopted. Exactly what aspect of management resulted in improved outcome was not established. It was generally assumed that it was a combination of careful attention to the patients, early neurosurgical care, and aggressive control of elevated intracranial pressure.

Wide attention was focused on elevated intracranial pressure as a treatable cause of secondary brain injury by Miller's report in 1977 that 50% of patients with hematomas and 30% of patients without hematomas developed elevated intracranial pressure as a complication of head injury (Miller, 1978). Miller further reported a very high mortality rate in those in whom intracranial pressure could not be controlled medically. Intracranial pressure monitoring and medical treatment for elevated intracranial pressure with Mannitol, hyperventilation, and head elevation became routine in head injury centers. The question of the influence of intracranial pressure control on mortality was vigorously addressed by several centers in the ensuing years. Marshall in San Diego reported a reduction in percentage of patients dying of elevated intracranial pressure in comparison to the Richmond series with use of barbiturate coma as an adjunct to conventional therapy for elevated intracranial pressure (Marshall, 1979). Saul, in two large series of patients, reported improved outcome and decreased mortality with treatment of intracranial pressure at lower levels of elevation than had been usual (Saul, 1982). All of these studies were not randomized and there were no concurrent controls; therefore, the validity of these conclusions remained in question.

The influence of intracranial pressure control on head injury outcome has recently been studied in a multicenter trial conducted by the Comprehensive Centers for CNS Trauma. In this study, barbiturate coma was used to treat patients who did not respond to defined conventional methods. It was found that control of intracranial pressure, whether by an extension of conventional therapy with Mannitol and hyperventilation or by use of barbiturate coma, resulted in a lower mortality rate than that of patients in whom intracranial pressure was not controllable. It was also established that barbiturates were effective in decreasing intracranial pressure when other methods failed. This study would seem to have firmly established the benefit of intracranial pressure control in head injury management.

Other contributions dealt with specific aspects of management other than intracranial pressure control. Beginning in 1984 a series of publications by Clifton and Robertson on the metabolic response to head injury detailed marked nitrogen wasting and systemic hypermetabolism after severe head injury (Clifton, 1984; Robertson, 1984). Rapp and Young reported that the failure to appropriately feed patients with head injury resulted in an increased mortality rate (Rapp, 1983). The optimal caloric and protein intake for head-injured patients was established and these methods have been widely adopted in head injury care. Since half of deaths from severe head injury are the result of systemic complications and half the result of elevated ICP, improved nutritional management has probably played a role in mortality reduction. Gennarelli and Langfitt brought the heterogeneity of head injury outcome to the attention of the neurosurgical community by accumulating mortality statistics for over 1,000 patients from a number of different centers (Gennarelli, 1982). These investigators showed that mortality rates in patients in coma for 6 hours or longer varied from 15% to 80% depending upon the Glasgow Coma Score, the presence of a hematoma, and the duration of coma. This finding not only influenced the design of therapeutic studies but also led physicians to consider the outcome of patients in coma from head injury in a more individual way.

ADVANCES IN PREHOSPITAL CARE

While efforts to find better ways of managing patients with acute head injury once they reached neurosurgical care were underway, parallel efforts to improve roadside management of trauma patients have made major contributions to head injury outcome. The earliest insight into the effect of hypoxia upon patients with head injury was the work of Frost and co-workers who, in 1979, reported a high incidence of pulmonary shunting and hypoxia in comatose head-injured patients who were ventilating without airway obstruction (Frost, 1979). Frost found a high correlation between the severity of pulmonary shunt and adverse outcome. Miller reported that patients with hypoxemia or shock after head injury had a much higher mortality rate and incidence of severe disability than patients with equivalent Glasgow Coma Scores who had not sustained such systemic insults (Miller, 1978). In recent laboratory work, these clinical observations have been dramatically confirmed. In experimental head injury, a degree of hypoxia which would have no sequelae normally when superimposed upon mild head injury results in severe head injury (Ishige, 1987). For these reasons, it has generally been concluded that systemic insults in the face of head injury adversely alter outcome to an extreme degree. Delayed surgical treatment has also been reported to adversely affect outcome. Seelig reported a threefold increase in mortality from acute subdural hematomas if surgery was performed more than 4 hours after injury (Seelig, 1981). Stone also reported a major mortality reduction by early surgery (Stone, 1986).

While efforts were underway in head injury centers to establish the importance of supportive care at the roadside and early surgery, the American College of Surgeons Committee on Trauma launched an effort to improve the quality of trauma care nationally. The Committee on Trauma of the American College of Surgeons published a standards document, which proposed a method of classification of trauma centers and qualifications of hospitals that delivered trauma care (*Verification Program for Hospitals,* 1980). Many hospitals throughout the country, primarily in major metropolitan areas, sought classification as trauma centers. Data from West and Trunkey showed a high incidence of unnecessary deaths in a community without a preplanned trauma program (West, 1979). This controversial report was used as evidence to support the value of prearranged trauma care. Random delivery of trauma patients to the nearest hospital has become so unacceptable that now over 20 states require hospitals to qualify themselves for trauma care and require standardized delivery of roadside management and training of caregivers. A verification program has been established by the American College of Surgeons requiring on-site evaluation for trauma center designation. Such external certification is being increasingly sought by hospitals wishing to participate in trauma care. Legislation now before the Senate and House of Representatives would provide monies to states to support organization of trauma care if standards equivalent to those of the American College of Surgeons are adopted for that state. The impact of these efforts on the outcome of patients with severe head injury has probably been and will continue to be major. With preorganized hospital care comes early treatment of shock, oxygenation, and early removal of hematomas.

FUTURE DIRECTIONS

We are at a point of substantially new directions and of new methods in efforts to improve the outcome of patients with severe head injury. It seems unlikely that further major mortality reduction will be possible. This idea is supported by the examination of mortality rates and percentages of good outcome in comparable head injury series reported over the last 10 years (Table 1-2). These series of patients managed in different institutions have examined the effects of control of elevated intracranial pressure at lower levels than usual, control of elevated intracranial pressure with barbiturates, and the influence of improved nutritional and metabolic management on head injury outcome. Each of these series reports 50% to 60% of patients with good recovery. The mortality rate has not varied significantly from 30% among series.

Major improvement in neurologic outcome seems possible, however. From the head injury and ischemia laboratories come data that may

Table 1-2.　*Mortality Rates*

	Houston[a]	Richmond[b]	San Diego[c]	Baltimore[d]
Number	99	148	100	106
GCS 3–5	39%	46%	45%	42%
GR/MD	50%	60%	60%	50%
Death from ↑ ICP	14%	14%	8%	14%
Death from systemic and other causes	11%	16%	20%	14%
Mortality	25%	30%	28%	28%

[a]From Robertson (1984).
[b]From Becker (1977).
[c]From Marshall (1979).
[d]From Saul (1982).

influence the direction of clinical research in head injury for some time to come. During the last 7 years, extensive work in many centers with experimental cerebral ischemia has resulted in description of a profile of biochemical abnormalities thought to lead to neuronal death. A variety of pharmacologic agents have altered the production of toxic metabolites, such as lactic acid, and increased intracellular calcium, free fatty acid accumulation, prostaglandin production, and accumulation of toxic-free radicals in ischemia models. Some of these agents protect the brain from neuronal loss after ischemia. Extension of this work to experimental head injury has resulted in a biochemical profile of head injury characterized by increased levels of free radicals and prostaglandins. The finding of activation of cholinergic pathways in the brainstem as a result of experimental head injury led to investigation of excitotoxicity as a mechanism of cell death or dysfunction after head injury. Work by Hayes has shown a protective effect of anticholinergic agents administered immediately after experimental head injury (Hayes, 1987). The finding of altered biochemistry after head injury and the ability to modify outcome in animals with early drug treatment can be expected to lead to trials of early administration of pharmacologic agents in head injury.

Major development in several areas will be required as these efforts progress. The fluid percussion model of head injury represents a well-studied model of axonal injury. Cortical contusion and compressive ischemia (hematomas) are commonly seen clinically and have not been well studied experimentally. Quantifiable therapeutic endpoints in head injury models have only recently been developed. Both histologic, biochemical, and neuropsychologic endpoints will be required to fully characterize treatment effects and to study mechanisms in the laboratory. A much more extensive understanding of biochemical alterations of injury will be required to design sophisticated approaches to treatment. Finally, the Glasgow Outcome Scale, which has been used to test the effects of therapies for severe head injury, may be insensitive to significant effects, and more sophisticated neuropsychologic measures of outcome will prove necessary. It has generally been accepted that randomized trials are required to provide definitive answers to the effects of therapy. Numbers of patients are insufficient and the heterogeneity of head injury so great that few individual centers have a sufficient number of patients to conduct randomized trials within an acceptable time period. For this reason, the multicenter randomized trial of therapy can be expected to be one of the primary methods in clinical efforts to improve head injury outcome during the next 10 years.

REFERENCES

Anderson D (1980): *Report on the national head and spinal cord injury survey.* Bethesda: National Institute of Neurological and Communicative Disorders and Stroke.

Becker D (1977): The outcome from severe head injury with early diagnosis and intensive management. *Journal of Neurosurgery* 47:491.

Clifton G (1984): The metabolic response to severe head injury. *Journal of Neurosurgery* 60:687–696.

Frost E (1979): Pulmonary shunt as a prognostic indicator in head injury. *Journal of Neurosurgery* 50:768.

Gennarelli T (1982): Influence of the type of intracranial lesion on outcome from severe head injury: A multicenter study using a new classification system. *Journal of Neurosurgery,* 56:26.

Hayes R (1987): *Neurochemical mechanisms of mild and moderate head injury: Implications for treatment.* Oxford: University Press.

Ishige N (1987): XXIX-P13. Effects of hypoxia on rat brain with traumatic injury. *Journal of Cerebral Blood Flow and Metabolism* 7:S638.

Jennett B (1979): Prognosis of patients with severe head injury. *Journal of Neurosurgery* 4:283.

Jennett B (1977): Severe head injuries in three countries. *Journal of Neurology, Neurosurgery, Psychiatry* 40:291.

Klauber M (1981): The epidemiology of head injury. A prospective study of an entire community—San Diego County, California, 1978. *American Journal of Epidemiology* 113:500–509.

Kraus J (1984): The incidence of acute brain injury and serious impairment in a defined population. *American Journal of Epidemiology* 119:186–201.

Marshall L (1979): The outcome with aggressive treatment in severe head injuries. Part II: acute and chronic barbiturate administration in the management of head injury. *Journal of Neurosurgery* 50:26.

Miller J (1978): Early insults to the injured brain. *JAMA* 240:439–442.

Rapp R (1983): The favorable effect of early parenteral feeding on survival in head-injured patients. *Journal of Neurosurgery* 58:906–911.

Robertson C (1984): Oxygen utilization and cardiovascular function in head-injured patients. *Neurosurgery* 15:307–313.

Saul T (1982): Effect of intracranial pressure monitoring and aggressive treatment on mortality in severe head injury. *Journal of Neurosurgery* 56:498–503.

Seelig J (1981): Traumatic acute subdural hematoma. Major mortality reduction in comatose patients treated within four hours. *New England Journal of Medicine* 304:1511–1518.

Stone J (1986): Acute subdural hematoma: direct admission to a trauma center yields improved results. *Journal of Trauma* 26:445–450.

Teasdale G (1974): Assessment of coma and impaired consciousness—a practical scale. *Lancet* 2:81.

Verification program for hospitals (1980): Developed by the American College of Surgeons, Committee on Trauma Quality and Assurance Supplement. Chicago: Bulletin, American College of Surgeons.

Weinfeld F (1981): *The national survey of stroke*. Dallas: The American Heart Association.

West J (1979): Systems of trauma care: a study of two counties. *Archives Surgery* 114:455–460.

2

Management of the Patient in a Persistent Vegetative State: Current Status and Needed Research

John Whyte, M.D., Ph.D., and Mel B. Glenn, M.D.

Department of Rehabilitation Medicine, New England Medical Center Hospitals, Tufts University School of Medicine, and The Greenery Rehabilitation and Skilled Nursing Center, Boston, Massachusetts, U.S.A.

The majority of serious traumatic brain injuries involve coma at the onset. In most instances, coma originates through disruption of the activity of the midbrain reticular formation due to high velocity trauma (Auerbach, 1986). Low velocity trauma can also lead to coma if expanding masses cause midline shift and temporal herniation (Plum and Posner, 1972).

Survivors of acute traumatic brain injury may evolve out of coma in a matter of minutes, hours, or days. Level of consciousness gradually improves and more purposeful behavior appears. However, seriously injured patients may remain unconscious for prolonged periods. Nevertheless, coma, per se, does not last indefinitely. Rather, it evolves into the persistent vegetative state (PVS). The persistent vegetative state is described by Jennett and Bond (1975) as referring to "patients who remain unresponsive and speechless . . . after acute brain damage," but "open their eyes and have cycles of sleeping and waking . . ."; they "show an absence of function in the cerebral cortex as judged behaviorally. . . ." The appearance of such patients to those unfamiliar with their state may be misleading. Reflexive responses, grimacing to pain, etc., may be mistaken for purposeful behavior and evidence of conscious processing.

Patients in the persistent vegetative state may gradually improve in their level of consciousness. The change is slow and subtle, involving increasing consistency of responses which may initially appear random or coincidental. In general, the longer patients remain in the persistent vegetative state the lower the chance that they will make clinically significant gains in function. Significant improvement beyond 2 years in PVS is exceedingly uncommon (Berrol, 1986). Even after several weeks in PVS, a patient's chance of returning to a normal level of function is close to nil. However, clinically meaningful improvement in purposeful behavior certainly does occur. In fact, 10% of patients still in PVS at 1 month postinjury achieve a Glasgow Outcome Scale rating of moderate or good recovery (Jennett and Teasdale, 1981).

There is considerable controversy about the mechanisms responsible for recovery of neurologic function after brain damage. A variety of mechanisms have been proposed, ranging from neuroanatomical and neurochemical changes to psychological adaptation. However, in an unresponsive patient one must look to biological change as the first step to recovery (Whyte, in press).

GOALS OF CARE IN COMA AND THE PERSISTENT VEGETATIVE STATE

The goals of treatment for patients remaining unconscious after brain injury depend on the time since injury. In the early days and weeks after injury there is considerable potential for large gains in function to occur. Thus, the goals at this time involve prevention of as many types of morbidity as possible so that when recovery does occur, the patient and treatment team will not have to overcome a variety of medical problems and deformities.

These goals should begin to be addressed in the Neurosurgical Intensive Care Unit. Too often, a patient with a "poor prognosis" will not have spasticity and contractures aggressively addressed and may develop bed sores and other medical problems because survival appears unlikely. Nevertheless, many such patients do survive, and their subsequent rehabilitation is both much more expensive and much more lengthy and complex because of the preventable complications that develop acutely (Giebler, Feldman, and Gilbert, 1987). Early attention should be directed toward maintenance of range of motion, skin integrity, prevention of infection, minimization of seizure-related morbidity, avoidance of unnecessary sedating medications, and provision of adequate stimulation. Goals for the family are also important in the early period postinjury. Family members need to understand both the available knowledge and the limitations of such knowledge with regard to prognosis for the individual patient. Furthermore, this prognosis should be discussed not only with the neurosurgeon but also with the physiatrist since these two disciplines may categorize prognosis quite differently. Clinicians should avoid dogmatic predictions and should strive for an appropriate balance between hope and a realistic understanding of the likelihood of permanent disability or death.

As the duration of PVS lengthens, the goals of care and rehabilitation will be revised. For patients who make small but meaningful gains, rehabilitation goals will be defined in more circumscribed ways. For patients who fail to make any significant progress over a period of 1 to 2 years, attention should be shifted toward interventions that maintain patient comfort and facilitate care, such as treatment of contractures that interfere with bathing and positioning. At this point, attention should be shifted more toward the needs of the family. The treatment team can gradually become more definite in its prognostic predictions, and help the family adjust to what becomes an increasingly certain outcome. The family's desire to care for the patient at home or in a chronic care facility should be sensitively explored with a clear understanding of the physical and emotional requirements of home treatment.

MEDICAL ISSUES

A variety of medical complications commonly afflict the patient in the persistent vegetative state. An attempt to evaluate the current state of knowledge about these medical problems and to identify areas in need of further research follows.

Seizure Disorders

Seizures are a common consequence of severe traumatic brain injury. The likelihood of a persistent seizure disorder is increased in the face of depressed skull fracture, intracerebral hematoma, prolonged unconsciousness, and early (within the first week) seizures (Jennett and Teasdale, 1981). Thus, patients in PVS are among those at highest risk for seizure disorders.

Seizures can be associated with significant morbidity and mortality, including vomiting and aspiration, trauma against bedrails, or anoxia due to impaired air exchange from prolonged seizure activity. Frequent seizures may depress the level of consciousness on an ongoing basis. If motor manifestations are ambiguous or absent, seizures may not be diagnosed. Ironically, however, there is some evidence of a therapeutic effect of seizure activity on recovery of function (Feeney et al., 1987).

There is no firm consensus on the advisability of seizure prevention as opposed to treatment of observed seizures. However, in most institutions, some high-risk subgroup of patients is treated preventatively with phenytoin or phenobarbital. The literature is mixed about the efficacy of such preventive treatment, but much of the literature has involved outpatients with maintenance of therapeutic blood levels being difficult (Penry, 1979; Wohns, 1979; Young, 1983a, 1983b). Unfortunately the two medications available for parenteral administration in the ICU are both widely demonstrated to produce cognitive impairments (Andrews et al., 1984; Mattson and Cramer, 1982). It is likely that prolonged administration of these agents will slow cognitive recovery in PVS patients. Thus, it is prudent to switch patients from these agents to carbamezipine or valproic acid when enteral medication is feasible if continued treatment is warranted (Thompson and Trimble, 1982; Trimble and Thompson, 1984).

Further research is needed to better determine the risks and benefits of prophylactic anticonvulsant treatment versus treatment of patients after the first observed seizure. Further attempts to predict high-risk patients are also warranted. Prospective studies of the effects of sedating and nonsedating anticonvulsants on recovery of function will also be needed, but they require adequate methods of assessing pace of recovery (see below).

Hydrocephalus

Acute obstructive hydrocephalus represents a neurosurgical emergency likely to be promptly identified in the first few days after injury. At a later time, communicating hydrocephalus or normal pressure hydrocephalus will be the topics of clinical concern, but these are more difficult to diagnose (Bakay and Glasauer, 1980). Since gradual brain atrophy is common after severe injury, differentiating hydrocephalus ex vacuo from clinically significant hydrocephalus may prove challenging. Furthermore, since these patients have no purposeful behavior to deteriorate, behavioral assessment of hydrocephalus is also impossible. Patients who remain unconscious should have periodic neuroimaging studies to evaluate the course of atrophy and to screen for the possibility of hydrocephalus. If such studies are equivocal, cisternography may prove useful in diagnosis. Patients who have a shunt in place for hydrocephalus should also be screened periodically for the possibility of shunt obstruction with recurrence of hydrocephalus.

Communicating and normal pressure hydrocephalus remain enigmatic diagnoses in the general neurological population. The efficacy of shunting in improving brain function also remains controversial. These controversies are compounded in a population with severe intrinsic neurologic deficits. More research is needed to identify the appropriate frequency of screening neuroimaging studies, the useful criteria from such images for making the diagnosis of hydrocephalus, appropriate ancillary studies to assist in the diagnosis, and the appropriate selection of patients for shunting once the diagnosis is made.

Pneumonia

Vegetative patients have a number of factors that predispose them to pulmonary problems, including impaired swallowing, which leads to chronic aspiration of saliva; poor dental hygiene, which increases the bacterial flora in the mouth; poor chest mobility; periodic gastroesophageal reflux; and a tracheostomy, which provides a portal of entry for microorganisms. It is prudent to ensure that such patients are tube fed with the heads of their beds elevated to minimize aspiration. Optimal dental hygiene should be maintained. Also, attempts should be made as soon as possible to remove unnecessary tracheostomies, since they do allow colonization of the tracheobronchial tree. Prophylactic antibiotic treatment for colonization of the tracheobronchial tree is not effective.

Further research is needed to determine the efficacy of maintenance respiratory therapy in minimizing the frequency of pneumonia. In particular, it is possible that periodic chest physical therapy may offer some benefit. Furthermore, various protocols for determining the time of decannulation should be explored.

Neurogenic Bladder and Bowel

Bladder and bowel continence are disrupted through two mechanisms following brain injury. The unconscious patient cannot engage in the behaviors necessary to request help in toileting, and frontal brain structures that serve to inhibit bladder and bowel evacuation are frequently injured (Andrew and Nathan, 1964). Bladder dysfunction is most often of the uninhibited detrusor type. However, no large scale studies of brain-injured patients have been done to explore the variety of bladder dysfunctions that may be found. We have occasionally identified patients with detrusor/sphincter dyssynergia, which may be of considerable medical significance.

In the unconscious patient, continence per se is not a treatment goal. However, attempts to minimize the frequency of bladder and bowel evacuation can be of great importance to caregivers, especially family members. Furthermore, they may be useful in minimizing the frequency of skin breakdown and urinary colonization.

For males, a condom catheter may reduce the risk of skin breakdown and is less invasive than an indwelling catheter. However, injury to the skin of the penis is common, and prolonged use of a condom catheter is associated with a high rate of urinary tract infections (Johnson, 1983). Antimicrobial prophylaxis is unlikely to be effective since the organisms in the condom quickly develop resistance. For female patients, the only catheter option is an indwelling catheter, which is usually associated with unacceptably high morbidity. Urinary care must be evaluated on an individual basis, weighing the risks of infection against the risks of skin pathology and the inconvenience of frequent clothing changes. Absorbent pads and pants may be an acceptable solution for some males and females. In other cases, one may need to resort to a catheter to allow inflamed skin to heal. A decrease in the frequency of voiding may facilitate care, and this can be achieved through the administration of anticholinergic drugs. However, such drugs may produce sedation and incomplete bladder emptying (Whyte and Glenn, 1986).

Bowel management can usually be achieved through the appropriate choice of tube feedings and the addition of bulk-forming substances as necessary. Once the appropriate stool consistency has been achieved, a stimulant or glycerin suppository administered daily or every other day will usually result in evacuation of a stool only at the intended time.

Prospective studies comparing the incidence of urinary tract infection, skin pathology, and other complications under different regimens of urinary care are needed. In particular, it would be of interest to study the efficacy of the condom catheter combined with methenamine treatment, since this might suppress bacterial flora without allowing for antibiotic resistance.

Nutrition

Nutritional needs are generally increased acutely after brain injury, whether or not the patient has received steroids (Young, Ott, and Norton, et al., 1985). This may relate both to central alterations in basal metabolic rate and to the development of muscle spasticity, which consumes considerable energy. Patients are initially fed via a nasogastric tube. Pediatric feeding tubes may minimize local trauma to the nose, but their small lumen may prove to be a limiting factor in calorie intake. Initial calorie delivery should be closely monitored by obtaining frequent weights since the patient's caloric needs are highly unpredictable. Treatment usually begins with 24-hour continuous feedings.

Nocturnal feedings with the head of the bed elevated may be used when patients vomit or reflux during mobility exercises. However, daytime bolus feedings may be more rapidly absorbed and less likely to be aspirated in others. Patients who continue to require tube feeding for prolonged periods usually have the insertion of a gastrostomy, jejunostomy, or gastrojejunostomy. The latter two are more difficult to insert and reinsert but are less likely to allow aspiration (Rondeau et al., 1984).

More information is needed about the acute nutritional management of the head-injured patient. It is not clear whether aggressive attempts to prevent catabolism have any impact on outcome and recovery, and if so, how these might best be achieved. Furthermore, nocturnal feedings may have unanticipated effects on circadian biological rhythms, and the relative risk of aspiration with different feeding regimens is unknown. The appropriate timing and patient selection for the different forms of tube placements are unclear. At present, these are determined largely by the preference of the surgeon and the family's attitudes about cosmesis and the need for a long-term feeding option.

Dental Care

Dental care often seems to be a minor issue in the face of prolonged unconsciousness. However, many patients who do make significant recoveries from unconsciousness later require numerous root canals or the extraction of multiple teeth. Dental care is impeded by the inability of the patient to cooperate, spasticity in the muscles of the face and jaw, the low priority given to oral hygiene, and the significant amount of staff time needed. The use of a mouth prop, fluoride gel, and brushing and flossing performed by caregivers would be likely to improve oral hygiene. Further exploration of this problem with dentists and dental hygienists knowledgeable about the care of disabled individuals would be useful. Identification of medications such as phenytoin and some anticholinergic drugs, which may exacerbate dental problems, would also be valuable.

PHYSICAL SEQUELAE

Patients in the persistent vegetative state suffer from a variety of physical deficits that make their immediate care more difficult and that produce long-term disabilities in those who make gains in function.

Spasticity

Spasticity in dramatic proportions is the almost universal consequence of injuries that produce lasting unconsciousness. Because of the variable pattern of brain injury, the pattern of spasticity (flexor, extensor, or mixed) is also quite variable. Spasticity may be so dramatic as to make it difficult for any individual therapist to overcome the strength of contraction. In the short run, a great deal of metabolic energy is consumed, the patient may develop skin lesions or fractures through involuntary movements, and bed positioning and hygiene may be difficult. Left untreated, this spasticity will produce contractures of the affected joints. Patients who make cognitive gains will then be forced to spend a great deal of their therapy time and energy reducing these physical deformities rather than addressing cognitive and functional tasks (Giebler, Feldman, and Gilbert, 1987).

A number of physical modalities are capable of relaxing spasticity to some degree. However, none of these are capable of controlling severe spasticity for more than a few hours after the application of the modality. Spasticity may also be treated with pharmacologic agents. However, there has been no study of antispasticity medications in the head-injured population (Whyte and Robinson, in press). Extrapolations from cerebrovascular accident (CVA) patients may not be useful since much of the damage leading to spasticity in traumatic brain injury is subcortical and brain stem in nature. Dantrolene sodium is nonspecific in its relaxing effects because it acts at the level of the muscle fiber. The authors have found dantrolene to be effective in a number of patients. It is also the medication least likely to cause sedation (Young and Delwaide, 1981). However, dantrolene can be associated with severe hepatitis, and we have not found it to be effective in controlling the most severe spasticity. We have tried to avoid baclofen and, particularly, diazepam because of their more prominant sedating side effects, but have found them useful in selected patients.

Phenol nerve and motor point blocks appear to be the most effective means of controlling extreme spasticity (Glenn, 1986). However, most clinicians are reluctant to use these interventions early because they are not immediately reversible should the patient begin to improve. However, the literature in conscious patients being treated with these modalities suggests that loss of useful sensation and voluntary movement is very uncommon, so this fear may be exaggerated (Glenn, 1986). Intramuscular alcohol wash is a good alternative when prognosis is uncertain because of its shorter duration of effect (Carpenter and Seitz, 1980).

An experimental modality that holds some promise in the future is the intrathecal baclofen pump (Penn and Croin, 1985). This treatment has been used in a small number of spinal cord injured and brain-damaged patients. It appears to have more dramatic antispasticity effects and fewer adverse effects than oral medication. However, the modality has not been studied extensively enough to know whether it is universally effective and, if not, how to select appropriate candidates for this treatment.

More research is needed on the treatment of spasticity in patients who are unresponsive. Appropriate antispasticity interventions are essential both for improving the immediate care of the patient in the persistent vegetative state and for lessening the disability of those who progress. Studies on the efficacy of the three major antispasticity drugs (dantrolene, baclofen, diazepam) are needed in the traumatic brain injury population, particularly within subject drug comparisons. Such research should address not only the efficacy but also effects on alertness and cognition (see discussion below). Research is also needed on the aggressive use of phenol blocks, especially in the early postinjury period.

Heterotopic Ossification

The growth of bony tissue in periarticular soft tissues is common after severe brain injury. The etiology of the problem remains controversial. Some studies suggest that tissue trauma in an individual who lacks sensation or the ability to respond to painful stimuli may be one predisposing factor (Mitchellson, Granroth, and Andersson, 1980). Heterotopic ossification is most common in the proximal joints (shoulders, hips, elbows, knees) of spastic limbs of patients who remain severely impaired for prolonged periods. One study of the prevention of heterotopic ossification used disodium etidronate in patients who had severe brain injuries resulting in prolonged unconsciousness (Spielman et al., 1983). This study was not randomized or optimally controlled but did appear to show a lessening of heterotopic ossification in the treated group. Information is not available regarding any late occurrence of heterotopic ossification once the medication was discontinued.

Nonsteroidal anti-inflammatory drugs and radiation to the affected joints have been effective in some populations at risk for heterotopic ossification (Ritter and Gioe, 1982; Delee, Green, and Wilkins, 1984). The radiation therapy is generally given to elderly patients undergoing total hip replacement, and the long-term risks of radiation therapy in a younger population are not known. The efficacy of any of these interventions once the process of heterotopic ossification begins is less clear.

Heterotopic ossification can be removed surgically once it is "mature." This surgery is generally undertaken only for important functional goals. Patients who are unconscious for prolonged periods but then make significant gains will often have to look forward to several surgical interventions to remove their ectopic bone. Patients who remain unconscious rarely undergo such surgery, but occasionally it may be necessary to facilitate symmetrical seating or appropriate bed positioning. However, patients who remain severely impaired have a high risk of recurrence of heterotopic ossification after surgery (Garland, Hanscom, and Keenan, et al., 1985).

More research is needed on the prevention of heterotopic ossification. This should include well-controlled randomized studies of primary prevention. In addition, it would be important to know whether short-term treatment with disodium etidronate can permanently prevent or only postpone the occurrence of heterotopic bone. If the result is postponement, further research is needed to determine the long-term risks and benefits of continued treatment with such prophylactic agents. In addition, other interventions should be compared to disodium etidronate in terms of their efficacy and side effects. The role of these methods in treatment of heterotopic ossification, once it has begun, is also in need of clarification. Optimal selection of surgical candidates and timing of their surgery also needs more investigation. Additional basic science research on the etiology of heterotopic ossification may lead to other means of prevention and treatment. In particular, if a contributing factor to the formation of ectopic bone is physical therapy of spastic limbs in an unconscious patient, exploration of aggressive antispasticity treatments as a means of prevention of heterotopic ossification should also be explored. It may be, for example, that early and aggressive phenol blocks or insertion of intrathecal baclofen pumps can lower the incidence of heterotopic ossification.

Contractures

Contractures are joint deformities that result from the shortening of any of a variety of tissues surrounding the joints. Heterotopic ossification may lead to contractures on the basis of obstructing bone. Spasticity may lead to contractures by producing chronic posturing, which leads to shortening of tendons, muscles, and joint capsules. For the patient without significant spasticity or heterotopic ossification, the means are already available to prevent contractures. These would include early mobilization with passive range of motion therapy, fabrication of splints for high-risk joints, and instruction of nursing personnel and family members in patient positioning.

Once contractures have formed, however, other treatments must be sought. These may include heating of the soft tissues with ultrasound, followed by passive manual stretching; serial casting to gradually lengthen the tissues; and in selected cases, surgical release of the shortened tissues. Contracture prevention is much easier than contracture treatment. Therefore, energy should be directed toward exploration of early interventions that can control spasticity and toward dissemination of information about contracture prevention to intensive care units and acute care hospitals. It is particularly important to get the message across to the acute care facilities that even patients who remain unconscious for weeks or months should have contractures aggressively prevented, since prediction of prognosis is still far from accurate.

COGNITIVE SEQUELAE

In the persistent vegetative state, by definition, cognition is globally impaired. Cognitive recovery is also the highest priority in defining treatment outcome, since physically disabled patients with good cognitive function are capable of a great deal, whereas physically restored patients with severely impaired cognitive function remain profoundly limited. In higher level patients there are a variety of ways of assessing cognitive function, including neuropsychological testing, functional assessment, and achievement testing. In our laboratory we are developing experimental methods for assessing arousal and attention in patients who are being treated with various medications that may positively or negatively influence these functions.

All of the assessment modalities mentioned above, however, require the active participation of the patient. In patients who remain unconscious there is no objective way of determining whether a medication given to control seizures, diminish spasticity, or lower blood pressure is having any effect on arousal or attention that may prolong the patient's unconsciousness and slow his or her cognitive recovery (except in the instance where withdrawal of the drug leads to clear behavioral evidence of cortical function and reinstatement of the drug results in regression). Similarly, there are no objective means of determining whether stimulant drugs or drugs that positively alter neurotransmitter levels are having desirable effects (unless administration of a drug leads to reversible emergence from PVS).

Before one can address these critical clinical questions, means must be developed to classify unconscious patients in terms of their depth of unconsciousness. This could be similar in concept to the Glasgow Coma Scale, which has successfully predicted recovery from coma but which is not applicable to the persistent vegetative state. One strategy is to study patients who are beginning to progress out of the persistent vegetative state. Thus, when a patient begins to focus and track intermittently, assessment of the frequency and consistency of these behaviors could be done and the effects of medications on this frequency and consistency evaluated. These types of investigations would require either matched controls or ABA designs to factor out the natural recovery taking place concurrently. This strategy would not allow adequate assessment of patients who demonstrate no voluntary behavior. Here one needs to look toward neurophysiological methods. PET scanning, EEG spectrum analysis, and neurochemical studies may all turn out to have some predictive value for which patients will recover and at what pace. Various interventions such as drug treatments and stimulation programs can be studied in order to find out whether their effects on, for example, brain metabolism are also predictive of their effects on cognitive recovery.

PVS patients are a heterogeneous group. The location and extent of their neuropathology is highly variable. Thus, it is likely that some neuroanotomic subclassification may also have some important prognostic value. In particular, patients with relative preservation of cortical function who are unconscious on the basis of impairments of the systems regulating arousal and alertness probably have a better prognosis for recovery than those whose unconsciousness is due to widespread cortical pathology.

Sensorimotor Stimulation

Most treatment programs that work with patients in PVS in the first months after injury include structured sensorimotor stimulation (Whyte and Glenn, 1986). These programs expose the patient to stimuli from each sensory modality and attempt to elicit a response. Implicit in this therapy has been the hope that such stimulation would speed recovery. Although to date sensory stimulation can evoke EEG changes (Weber, 1984) no research to date has demonstrated that it promotes recovery.

Optimism about the effects of sensorimotor stimulation is based on research that shows that animals exposed to an enriched environment before or after brain injury recover more quickly (Will, Rosenzweig, and Bennett, et al., 1977). However, animals in this research are not unconscious and are able to actively interact with their environment. It is not clear how these data apply to patients passively experiencing sensory stimulation.

We believe that sensorimotor stimulation is justifiable independent of its efficacy in promoting recovery, as a structured monitoring technique. It is known that normal individuals can suffer deterioration in the face of sensory deprivation. Therefore it seems unwise and unethical to leave an unconscious patient alone in a room without any interaction. Furthermore, the ability to provide the same type of stimulation daily and observe changes in the nature of the patient's response to that stimulation can be an important way of documenting early phases of recovery, noting potential deterioration that may relate to medical complications, etc. Nevertheless, structured research on the recovery-enhancing effects of sensorimotor stimulation is critical. One would design this intervention differently if it were only a monitoring technique and would likely intensify the treatment if it were shown to have dramatic effects on recovery. At this point it would be difficult and unethical to deny a control group sensorimotor stimulation. However, different protocols for sensory stimulation, which vary in their frequency, intensity, nature of the stimuli presented, etc., could certainly be investigated. This would likely have to be done on a large multicenter scale to allow for matching or randomization of the heterogeneous patient population.

Pharmacologic Treatment

Until means are available for assessing effects of drugs on cognitive function in PVS, potentially sedating drugs should be avoided whenever possible. Psychopharmacological data from the normal geriatric population and the mentally retarded may be useful in detecting drugs least likely to impair cognition. When treating epilepsy, spasticity, hypertension, gastrointestinal dysfunction, and other disorders, the patient's cognitive deficits should guide drug selection (see Table 2-1). If a potentially sedating drug must be used, withdrawal or tapering will clarify whether the drug is masking recovery and whether it is still needed.

As mentioned previously, it is likely that unconscious patients have to depend on biological factors for their initial recovery. Research on the mechanisms of recovery of central nervous system functions suggests that alterations in neurotransmitter availability may be responsible for some behavioral deficits; and compensatory alterations in neurotransmitter sensitivity, degradation, and synthesis may be responsible for some of the recovery that is seen (Robinson, Bloom, and Battenberg, 1977; Creese, Burt, and Snyder, 1977).

Animal research has suggested that some of the noradrenergic drugs can positively effect recovery of function (Feeney et al., 1982). Many other medications have also been implicated in selected studies (Lope, 1986). Pharmacological agents hold promise for improving the recovery potential of some patients in the persistent vegetative state in the future. At present, however, there is no single drug that can be said to be demonstrably active in achieving this goal. More research is needed to define the neurochemical alterations that occur in traumatic brain injury. This may lead to a more rational choice of drug interventions for initial experimentation. However, pharmacological interventions, like all other interventions in this population, will be difficult to assess over the short run. Large-scale monitoring studies of PVS patients must be undertaken to determine whether certain drug interventions have long-

Table 2-1. *Cognitive Effects of Commonly Used Drugs*

Drug category	Sedating examples	Nonsedating examples
Anticonvulsants	Phenytoin	Carbamazepine
	Phenobarbital	Valproic acid
Antihypertensives	Propranolol	Atenolol
	Methyl-dopa	ACE inhibitors
Antispasticity agents	Diazepam	Dantrolene (may cause
	Baclofen	some sedation)
		Phenol blocks
Anti-allergics	Diphenhydramine	Terfenadine
Gastrointestinal	Cimetidine	Antacids
medications	Metochlopramide	Sucralfate

term effects on recovery. Adverse effects must also be assessed; tricyclics, for example, may provoke seizures in 20% of patients (Wroblewski, Singer, and Mooney, et al., 1987).

SOCIAL, ECONOMIC, AND POLICY ASPECTS

Patients who remain unconscious for prolonged periods consume tremendous resources in the form of nursing care, rehabilitation interventions, and various procedures intended to minimize long-term disability. They also involve their significant others in an ongoing struggle between hope for improvement and acceptance of their current status. Clearly, improvements in prognostic accuracy can have important benefits both for health care planners and for family members. However, it is unrealistic to hope that any prognostic system will accurately classify the outcome of each individual patient. Therefore, there will always be a group of patients with uncertain outcome and a need to try interventions for a period of time before a definite conclusion can be reached.

Some patients remain unconscious permanently. These patients clearly need less intensive care than those who are being actively rehabilitated. However, a well-defined model for the chronic care of patients in a persistent vegetative state who fail to make functional improvements has not been developed. The standard geriatric nursing home is often inappropriate, and the head injury rehabilitation facility is too costly as a source of lifetime care.

The care of patients in long-term PVS raises complex ethical issues. Under what circumstances should the patient be "no code" in the event an acute medical complication? Is it ever justified to remove feeding tubes from such patients? At what point following injury can one be certain enough that no improvement will occur to undertake such ethically complex decisions?

Family Adaptation

The family and significant others of the patient in coma are in a state of crisis, faced with conflicting predictions. Staff in the neurosurgical intensive care unit may tell them that the patient is very likely to die and that if he or she survives it will be in a permanently vegetative state. Television shows and occasional news reports feature patients who suddenly "wake up" from coma and begin a normal conversation. Thus, it is not surprising that family members have ambivalent feelings in this situation and sometimes have unrealistic perceptions and expectations.

A variety of resources for assisting families to adapt to this crisis are needed. The National Head Injury Foundation has shouldered most of the burden for this task but more is needed. Factual material that adequately balances the likelihood of long-term deficits or death with the possibility of significant gains in function needs to be written, assembled, and made available to acute care clinicians; but adaptation to this crisis is much more than a cognitive task. Families are often dealing with the loss of an individual that they knew and the acquisition of a quite different person. These changes redefine role relationships, legal bonds, and love relationships. In addition, this situation is often colored by issues of guilt or blame related to trauma. Thus, research on appropriate counseling and psychoeducational approaches is needed. Different family interventions designed to promote realistic adaptation to the situation and to provide useful emotional support should be developed and rigorously evaluated. The consequences to family members of taking home the patient in PVS should be assessed so that this information is available to other family members considering doing so. Including family members in needs assessments and attempts to develop such resources will also be of value.

Costs and Benefits

The patient in a persistent vegetative state consumes tremendous resources. Work is needed to better quantify these resources. Therapeutic interventions that prolong the survival of patients in PVS without improving their function add to the cost without clearly adding to the benefits. Different program designs for long-term care of such patients also will have different economic consequences. These will range from home care with some support provided to care in specialized head injury rehabilitation institutions, with many gradations in between. It is important to address the issues of costs and benefits not only through empirical gathering of cost data but also by overt discussion of values about prolonging life and enhancing recovery. The discussions that lead ultimately to health care policy decisions should not be framed in narrowly economic terms. When one speaks of rehabilitation one is always speaking of goal-oriented treatment. Implicitly, then, health care expenditures are being incurred to achieve particular functional goals. Future decisions about the appropriate organization of a health care system to address the needs of patients in PVS must speak clearly about the goals of this treatment and the appropriate use of resources in achieving these goals.

Acknowledgment: This work was supported in part by Grant G0086C3506 to Dr. Whyte from the National Institute for Disability and Rehabilitation Research, United States Department of Education.

REFERENCES

Andrew J, Nathan PW (1964): Lesions of the anterior frontal lobes and disturbances of micturation and defecation. *Brain* 87:233–262.

Andrews DG, Tomlinson L, Elwes RDC et al (1984): The influence of carbamazepine and phenytoin on memory and other aspects of cognitive function in new referrals with epilepsy. *Acta Neurol Scand* 69(Suppl 99):23–30.

Auerbach SH (1986): Neuroanatomical correlates of attention and memory disorders in traumatic brain injury: an application of neurobehavioral subtypes. *J Head Trauma Rehabil* 1(3):1–12.

Bakay LB, Glasauer FE (1980): Posttraumatic hydrocephalus. In *Head Injury*. Boston: Little, Brown, pp 377–384.

Berrol S (1986): Evolution and the persistent vegetative state. *J Head Trauma Rehabil* 1(1):7–13.

Carpenter EB, Seitz DG (1980): Intramuscular alcohol as an aid in the management of spastic cerebral palsy. *Dev Med Child Neurol* 22:497–501.

Cope DN (1986): The pharmacology of attention and memory. *J Head Trauma Rehabil* 1(3):34–42.

Creese I, Burt D, Snyder S (1977): Dopamine receptor binding enhancement accompanies lesion induced behavioral supersensitivity. *Science* 197:596–598.

Delee JC, Green DP, Wilkins KE (1984): Fractures and dislocations of the elbows. In Rockwood CA, Green DP (eds): *Fractures in Adults* (2nd ed, vol 1). Philadelphia: JB Lippincott.

Feeney DM, Gonzales A, Law WA (1982): Amphetamine, haloperidol and experience interact to affect rate of recovery after motor cortex injury. *Science* 217:855–857.

Feeney DM, Baily BY, Boyeson MG, et al (1987): The effect of seizures on recovery of function following cortical contusion in the rat. *Brain Injury* 1(1):27–32.

Garland DE, Hanscom DA, Keenan MA, et al (1985): Resection of heterotopic ossification in the adults with head trauma. *JBJS (Am)* 67:1261–1269.

Giebler K, Feldman P, Gilbert LL, et al (1987): The cost of contractures. Poster Presented at the Third Annual Houston Conference on Neurotrauma, Houston, TX.

Glenn MB (1986): Update on pharmacology: nerve blocks in the treatment of spasticity. *J Head Trauma Rehabil* 1(3):72–74.

Jennett B, Bond M (1975): Assessment of outcomes after severe brain damage: a practical scale. *Lancet* 1:480–484.

Jennett B, Teasdale G (1981): *Management of Head Injuries*. Philadelphia: FA Davis, pp 271–288.

Johnson ET (1983): The condom catheter: urinary tract infection and other complications. *South Med J* 76(5):579–582.

Mattson RH, Cramer JA (1982): Phenobarbital toxicity. In Woodbury DM, et al (eds), *Antiepileptic Drugs* (2nd ed). New York: Raven Press, pp 351–363.

Michelsson JE, Granrott G, Andersson LC (1980): Myositis ossificans following forcible manipulation of the leg. *JBJS* (Am) 62:811–815.

Penn RD, Kroin JS (1985): Continuous intrathecal baclofen for severe spasticity. *Lancet* 2:125–127.

Penry JK, White BG, Brackett CE (1979): A controlled prospective study of pharmacologic prophylaxis of post traumatic epilepsy. *Neurology* 29:600–601.

Plum F, Posner JB (1972): *Diagnosis of Stupor and Coma* (2nd ed). Philadelphia: FA Davis, pp 64–65.

Ritter MA, Gioe TJ (1982): The effect of indomethacin on para-articular ectopic ossification following total hip arthroplasty. *Clin Orthop Rel Res* 167:113–117.

Robinson RG, Bloom FE, Batenberg ELF (1977): A fluorescent histochemical study of changes in noradrenergic neurons following experimental cerebral infartion in the rat. *Brain Res* 132:259–272.

Rombeau JL, Barot LR, Low DW, et al (1984): Feeding by tube enterostomy. In Rombeau JL, Caldwell MD (eds): *Clinical Nutrition (vol 1): Enteral and Tube Feeding*. Philadelphia: WB Saunders, pp 275–291.

Spielman G, Gennarelli TA, Rogers CR (1983): Disodium etidronate: its role in preventing heterotopic ossification in severe head injury. *Arch Phys Med Rehabil* 64:539–542.

Thompson PJ, Trimble MR (1982): Anticonvulsant drugs and cognitive functions. *Epilepsia* 23:531–544.

Trimble MR, Thompson PJ (1984): Sodium valproate and cognitive function. *Epilepsia* 25(Suppl 1):60–64.

Weber PL (1984): Sensorimotor therapy: its effect on electroencephalograms of acute comatose patients. *Arch Phys Med Rehabil* 65:457–462.

Whyte J (in press): Mechanisms of recovery of function following central nervous system damage. In Griffith ER, Rosenthal M, Bond MR, et al (eds), *Rehabilitation of the Child and Adult with Traumatic Brain Injury* (2nd ed). Philadelphia: FA Davis.

Whyte J, Glenn MB (1986): The care and rehabilitation of the patient in a persistent vegetative state. *J Head Trauma Rehabil* 1(1):39–53.

Whyte J, Robinson KM (in press): Pharmacological management of spasticity. In Glenn MB, Gans GB (eds): *The Practical Management of Spasticity in Children and Adults*. Philadelphia: Lea & Febiger.

Will BE, Rosenzweig MR, Bennett EL, et al (1977): Relatively brief environmental enrichment aids recovery of learning capacity and alters brain measures after postweaning brain lesions in rats. *J Comp Physiol Psychol* 91:33–50.

Wohns NW, Wyler AR (1979): Prophylactic phenytoin in severe head injuries. *J Neurosurg* 51:507–509.

Wroblewski B, Singer WD, Mooney K, et al (1987): The incidence of seizures during tricyclic antidepressant drug treatment in a brain injured population. Paper Presented at the 6th Annual National Symposium of the National Head Injury Foundation, San Diego, December 1987.

Young B, Ott L, Norton J, et al (1985): Metabolic and nutritional sequelae in the non-steroid treated head injury patient. *Neurosurgery* 17(5):784–791.

Young PR, Delwaide PJ (1981): Drug therapy: spasticity. *N Engl J Med* 13:143–147.

Young B, Rapp RP, Norton JA, et al (1983a): Failure of prophylactically administered phenytoin to prevent early post-traumatic seizures. *J Neurosurg* 58:231–235.

Young B, Rapp RP, Norton JA, et al (1983b): Failure of prophylactically administered phenytoin to prevent late post-traumatic seizures. *J Neurosurg* 58:236–241.

3

Moderate Head Injury

Sheldon Berrol, M.D.

Physical Medicine and Rehabilitation, University of California, San Francisco, California, U.S.A.

Moderate head injury is a poorly defined category. Some have equated it with concussion, though by definition this would more appropriately fit the category of minor or mild head injury. Concussion has previously been considered a clinical entity characterized by a reversible loss of consciousness of short duration without localizing neurologic features or by patho-anatomic substrate. Animal studies in recent years, however, have clearly demonstrated considerable anatomic changes with electron microscopy, which include severe swelling of neuronal mitochondria and contra-coup extracellular edema. The most severe changes have been noted in the structures of the craniospinal junction. Transient increases in blood-brain barrier permeability have also been documented.

Since considerable data have accumulated to suggest that a patho-anatomic substrate does exist for minor head injury (Jane, Steward, and Gennarelli, 1985) it is reasonable to assume that though the sites of injury may be the same, the degree of damage is greater in the moderate category.

Moderate head injury has been defined by Frankowski, Annegars, and Whitman (1985) as that state in which loss of consciousness and/or post-traumatic amnesia (PTA) occurred for more than 30 minutes, but less than 24 hours, and/or a skull fracture was noted.

Rimel et al. (1982) have defined moderate head injury based on the Glasgow Coma Scale (GCS) as 9 to 12 at six hours after admission to hospital. The mean time from injury to admission was 2.8 hours. Bowers and Marshall (1980) have also classified moderate head injury as 9 to 12 on the Glasgow Coma Scale. Some authors, however, have included 9 in severe head injury and would, therefore, theoretically have better outcomes for severe head injury, by weighting the study toward a lesser

31

degree of damage. Collins (1985) classified moderate head injury as 8 to 10 on the GCS, further adding to the inconsistencies.

Severe head injury is considered as at least 6 hours of coma—not opening the eyes, not obeying commands, and not uttering any recognizable words. Many factors may modify the clinical picture, including patients with multiple trauma (Jennett and Teasdale, 1981, pp. 318–319).

Multiple trauma can be defined as injury to at least two of the Abbreviated Injury Scale (AIS) defined areas but does not have to include the head or brain (Gustilo, Corpuz, and Sherman, 1985). Many patients with severe multiple trauma have associated moderate to mild head injuries that go unrecognized because of the severity of other system involvement (Wilmot et al., 1985). The development of hypotension, hypoxia, or partial respiratory obstruction may lead to a classification of severe head injury, when in fact the injury to the brain may be of a lesser level. There are some in whom the neurologic status is obscured and who improve after initial resuscitation.

Drug effects, such as alcohol, barbiturates, etc., further tend to obscure the clinical picture; and in the case of a combined effect of drugs and trauma, it is impossible to calculate the degree of severity of head injury.

Although inter-rater reliability of the GCS is relatively high, a variety of factors can obscure accurate interpretation, including facial trauma, the presence of an endotracheal tube, and the position of the limbs prior to the induction of pain. Thus in spite of some clear definitions, problems exist that may interfere with accurate designation of severity.

INCIDENCE

If head injury is defined as an injury that produces a loss of consciousness, posttraumatic amnesia, confirmed brain injury, or skull fracture, then current estimates of incidence vary from 0.2% to 0.3% per year. Of the 500,000 resultant new head injuries a year in the United States, some 10% will be classified as moderate head injuries.

The etiology of the injury certainly affects the degree of brain damage that will occur; and the high incidence of motor vehicle accidents, falls, and violence yields a greater proportion of diffuse cerebral injuries than is reported in other countries (Frankowski, Annegars, and Whitman, 1985).

Studies of mortality rates from head injury suggests that 9% to 29% of all hospital admissions for head injury fall into the moderate head-injured category. There is, however, no standardization of this categorization, since severity is based upon symptoms, diagnosis, length of loss of consciousness, or GCS. In some instances severity is based on ICD codes (Kraus, 1987). Kraus has postulated that 10% of all new hospital admissions have moderate head injuries for an annual total of 40,000. He further estimates that 7% of them will die of their injuries. Since approximately 50% of severely head-injured patients will not survive, the annual survivor rate of moderate head injury is more than twice the number of the severe category.

MODERATE DISABILITY

The three survival outcomes—severe, moderate, and good recovery—though well defined, are not abruptly delineated from each other, unlike diagnostic classes (Knill-Jones, 1978). *Moderate disability,* as an outcome category of the Glasgow Outcome Scale, describes an individual who is independent but disabled. Such individuals are capable of looking after themselves and traveling by public transportation, and some are capable of work activities. Though such work may be sheltered, some types of disabilities may be compatible with return to the premorbid work activity. It is not uncommon for an individual to return to a former place of employment where a "sheltered" situation exists for some time. Because it soon becomes apparent that the disabled worker cannot function at prior levels, a limited work exposure results.

A patient's return to work in itself should not be central to classifying ultimate disability. The presence or absence of disabilities is the central issue.

Moderate disability implies independence in activities of daily living (ADLs). If not independent, a patient would be classified in *severe disability* on the GCS. The ability to perform ADLs, however, has little to do with function or independence in modern society. Furthermore, the ability to perform ADLs in a highly structured environment gives little insight into ability to function in the community.

The functional implications of cognitive sequelae may not be apparent upon discharge from the hospital, not uncommonly leading to a misclassification for a dysfunctional patient in a *good* category (Tabaddor, Mattis, and Zazula, 1984).

The Disability Rating Scale developed at Santa Clara Valley Medical Center was designed to chart the process of recovery from severe head trauma. This assessment tool compounds the problem of labeling by utilizing two categories with the term moderate—*moderately severe* and *moderate* (Rappaport, Hall, Hopkins, Belleza, and Cope, 1982).

Cognitive impairment in the moderate disability group overlaps both the severe disability and the good recovery outcome groups. Distinguishing outcomes by cognitive performance is thus difficult and, if beyond 3 months postinjury, is substantially less reliable (Brooks, Hosie, Bond, Jennett, and Aughton, 1986).

Associated injuries contribute significantly to secondary brain insults and thus the ultimate outcome. Shock is one of the major determinants of death or survival, and its presence may result in more severe brain involvement than that produced by the trauma alone. Any prognosis for moderate head injury must consider concommitant injuries and the effects of hypoxia, hypercapnia, and shock on brain integrity.

POSTCONCUSSIONAL SYNDROME

Although *postconcussional syndrome* has been reserved by some authors for the consequences of minor head injury (Lindval, Linderoth, and Norlin, 1974), others have used this terminology for the sequelae of more severe injury. Because the syndrome consists primarily of subjective complaints, some authorities have assumed a purely psychogenic basis. Considerable data have accumulated to question this conclusion in many cases of minor head injury.

Although continued use of the term postconcussional syndrome is expected in describing outcomes from moderate and severe head injury, it remains an obscure ill-defined terminology that bears little relationship to the extent of injury. Since the definition of concussion implies a lesser degree of injury, the term postconcussional syndrome should be restricted to outcomes of lesser severity. It also appears clear that a pathoanatomic basis for the symptomatology has been established (Povlishock, Becker, Sullivan, and Miller, 1978).

OUTCOME STUDIES

There are no nationally or regionally published data that provide estimates of the number of persons who sustain disability or functional limitations as a result of acute brain trauma. Prevalence estimates of some types of limitations are reported periodically (Collins, 1985).

Additionally, there is an absence of studies that have prospectively followed a clearly defined representative group for sufficient time to document limitations of all types (Kraus, Black, and Hessol, 1984). In assessing outcome, one must consider the neurologic disabilities of epilepsy, cranial nerve dysfunction, etc., as well as cognitive, physical, and psychosocial sequelae.

The detailed study of patients with moderate head injury by Rimel et al. (1982) demonstrated that as their GCS increased from 9 through 12, the incidence of suspected intracranial mass lesion decreased. Furthermore, fewer patients in this group required intracranial pressure monitoring. This, then, seems to add emphasis on the GCS as a prognostic indicator. A statistically significant increase in motor vehicle accidents (MVA) when compared to the minor head injury study by Rimel et al.

emphasizes the role of MVAs in diffuse head injury. Additionally, this group had higher alcohol blood levels than the minor group.

Subjective complaints 3 months after injury yielded an incidence of headache of 93%, memory difficulty of 90%, impaired ADLs of 87%, change in transportation (not driving) 62%, and 69% not working, an unemployment rate of twice that for minor head injury. In the small subset that were evaluated neuropsychologically, 50% scored abnormally in all 10 of the tests chosen. The frequency of cognitive impairment and, in fact, all outcome criteria evaluated in this population thus appear substantially greater than in the minor group.

Tabaddor et al. (1984) analyzed the cognitive sequelae and course of recovery during the year following moderate and severe head injury. Criterion for moderate was GCS of 9 to 11 during the 48 hours after injury. At baseline testing the moderate group performed significantly better on tests of verbal recognition, nonverbal recall, and fine motor coordination. There was also a trend toward better scores on performance I.Q. tests. Both linguistic and memory functions remained impaired throughout the study, and recognition memory did not demonstrate any statistically significant change. Unfortunately, this study did not evaluate all patients at the 1-year interval.

PTA duration of between 1 and 24 hours was used as the criteria for moderate head injury by McMillan and Glucksman (1987) in their neuropsychologic evaluation of this category. (They felt, accurately however, that their patient group would normally be classified as minor head injuries.) This study is of particular interest because of the inclusion of matched controls. The reporting of postconcussional symptoms by the head-injured group was substantially greater than in the control group. The head-injured group consistently performed at an impaired level on the rate of information processing on the Paced Auditory Serial Additional Test (PASAT). There was no statistical difference between the two groups on other neuropsychological tests. It must be restated, however, that the head injury group met the criteria for minor head injury rather than moderate head injury, in spite of the title of this chapter. Others have argued that PTA is not an adequate parameter by which to gauge the degree of head injury (MacFlynn et al., 1984).

Guilleminault, Faull, and van den Hoed (1983) evaluated a small series of patients who sustained transient loss of consciousness and brief hospitalization but regained consciousness within 24 hours. Six patients reported no loss of consciousness, 5 had a transient loss of consciousness (less than 24 hours), and 9 had a history of coma lasting at least 24 hours. The primary complaint of all was excesssive daytime sleepiness. None had locomotor difficulty, and three had objective neurologic signs stated as moderate. All 20 complained of intellectual difficulties, headaches, serious daytime sleepiness, and inability to handle their previous professional activities. Dizziness and vertigo were present in 14, headaches in 19, and mood changes in 16. The authors clearly differentiated the symptoms of this population from fatigue, a commonly reported symptom after both mild and moderate head injuries. A decline in choice reaction time performance is a useful indicator of fatigue. Fatigue is felt to be a major factor resulting in a characteristic impaired central information processing and decrease in channel capacity (MacFlynn et al., 1984).

Oddy and Humphrey (1980) evaluated patients who sustained a severe closed head injury as defined by a PTA of 24 hours or more. It is quite conceivable, therefore, that at least a small subset would be classified as moderately head injured by others. In this group, as compared to our understanding of the severely disabled group, the speed with which patients returned to work was more dependent upon physical factors than personality changes or cognitive impairment. Failure to reintegrate with former social activities, however, depended more upon the presence of cognitive deficits. They further felt that there was clear evidence that premorbid personality affects social recovery and that evidence of poor premorbid family relationships was associated with a higher incidence of subjective complaints.

Collins (1985) studied head-injured survivors 2 to 3 years postinjury. Of those studied, 10.2% sustained moderate head injury based upon a GCS of 8 to 10 on admission (severe head injury was less than 7 on the GCS, and mild head injury was 11 to 14); 48.7% were classified as having multiple trauma; 74.4% had at least one injury to other bodily areas; 61.5% were working at time of examination; and 15.5% were engaged in school plus some work.

The most significant area of dysfunction reported was in psychosocial function (social interactions), alertness behavior, and emotional behavior subscales (work, recreation, and pastimes). The greatest dysfunction was in mental alertness and work.

Little attention has been paid to the potential for multiple minor head injuries to result in the same consequences as a single moderate head injury. It has been documented that the effects of minor head injury are cumulative (Gronwall and Wrightson, 1975; Jennett and Teasdale, 1981). Thus some patients who have sustained a minor injury may develop obvious focal or diffuse neurologic sequelae and need the same level of intensity of therapeutic rehabilitation intervention as do the moderate group.

Dikman, McLean, and Temkin (1986) evaluated neuropsychologic outcome at 1 month postinjury in a group representing the spectrum of outcomes. The moderately head-injured group was impaired on all test measures. The study emphasized the need to establish a control group with the same demographic and psychosocial characteristics as the head injury subjects since there is evidence to suggest that head-injured patients differ from the general population in these respects. The performance deficits in the head-injured population then becomes far more robust. The difficulty of using retrospective PTA as a measure of severity was emphasized.

DISCUSSION

It appears quite evident from this review of the literature that the term moderate head injury lacks a clear consistent definition. By common usage, it includes severely brain-injured patients who have progressed to a moderate disability outcome, mildly brain-injured patients who demonstrate symptoms of a postconcussional syndrome, and at times, those with "traumatic neurosis." The impression that a "moderate" designation in some way suggests the degree of brain damage currently has little validity. Research proposals for study of moderate head injury have only added to the complexity by ill-defined subject criteria based upon outcomes rather than injury.

While controversy still rages regarding the legitimacy of sequelae from minor head injury, there is little question as to the organicity of moderate head injury. When, however, the moderate head injury survivor improves to a *good* outcome on the Glasgow Outcome Scale (GOS), the paucity of physical symptomatology frequently results in failure to appreciate subtle (and not so subtle) cognitive residuals. A clear distinction must be made between injury and outcome.

There exists no valid study on recovery from moderate head injury since, as yet, the definition has not been standardized.

CONCLUSIONS

The term moderate head injury lacks consistency in its definition. Studies in the literature thus far produce a confusing picture of this group, since no two studies utilize the same criteria.

Retrospective interpretation of PTA appears to be a poor indicator of the degree of brain damage.

Those studies in the literature are of insufficient numbers for drawing logical conclusions, other than that the degree of brain damage is less than in severe and more than in mild.

Associated factors of injury or the mixture of drugs and injury further compound the categorization of moderate head injury. The effect of such factors on outcome needs to be documented.

Since multiple minor head injuries can yield cumulative effects, the net result may be equivalent to the degree of injury sustained in the moderate injury category (Gerberich et al., 1983). Causes of such trauma, such as sports injuries, demand comprehensive investigation, analysis, and prophylaxis.

If moderate head injury is a result of lesser degree of brain damage than severe head injury, then the potential for improved outcome is greater and appropriate rehabilitation intervention is therefore indicated.

Psychosocial factors appear to be as significant in the recovery and rehabilitation of this group as in severe head injury. Since the integrity of the family unit appears to be a robust predictor of successful outcome, it is essential that trauma centers and rehabilitation centers address the emotional and educational needs of the families of head-injured patients.

The effect upon vocational reintegration in this group appears significant but, as yet, undefined.

Since the level of cognitive impairment resulting from moderate head injury is varied, a wide spectrum of cognitive assessment tools are needed. Standard neuropsychologic batteries may not suffice.

Just as classification of this group has varied, so has the application of intervention methodologies. Consistency is necessary for appropriate interstudy comparisons.

REFERENCES

Alves W, Jane JA (1985): Mild brain injury: damage and outcome. In: *Central nervous system trauma status report*. Becker D, Povlishock J (eds). Washington DC: National Institute of Health Publication, National Institute of Neurological and Communicative Disorders and Stroke, pp 255–270.

Annegers JF, Grabow JD, Kurland LT, et al (1980): The incidence, causes, and secular trends in head injury in Olmsted County, Minnesota. *Neurology* 30:912–919.

Bakay L, Lee JC, Lee GC, et al (1977): Experimental cerebral concussion: Part 1: an electron microscopic study. *Journal of Neurosurgery* 47:525–531.

Bowers SA, Marshall LF (1980): Outcome in 200 consecutive cases of severe head injury treated in San Diego county: A prospective analysis. *Neurosurgery* 6:237–242.

Brooks N, Hosie J, Bond MR, Jennett B, Aughton M (1986): Cognitive sequelae of severe head injury in relation to the Glasgow Outcome Scale. *Journal of Neurology, Neurosurgery, and Psychiatry* 49:549–553.

Collins JG (March 1985): Persons injured and disability days due to injuries, United States, 1980–81. *Vital and health statistics*. Washington, DC: US Government Printing Office, Series 10, No. 149 DHHS Pub No (PHS) 85-1577.

Dikman S, McLean A, Temkin NR (1986): Neuropsychologic outcome at one-month postinjury. *Archives Physical Medicine Rehabilitation* 67:507–513.

Frankowski RF, Annegars JF, Whitman S (1985): The descriptive epidemiology of head trauma in the United States. In: *Central nervous system trauma status report*, Becker D, Povlishock, J (eds). Washington DC: National Institute of

Health Publication, National Institute of Communicative Disorders and Stroke, pp 33–45.

Gerberich SG, Priest JD, Boen JR, et al (1983): Concussion incidences and severity in secondary school varsity football players. *American Journal of Public Health* (12)73:1370–1375.

Gronwall D, Wrightson P (1975): Cumulative effect of concussion. *Lancet* 2:995–997.

Guilleminault C, Faull KF, van den Hoed J (1983): Posttraumatic excessive daytime sleepiness: A review of 20 patients. *Neurology* 33:1584–1589.

Gustilo RB, Corpuz V, Sherman RE. (1985): Epidemiology, mortality and morbidity in multiple trauma patients. *Orthopedics* 8:1523–1528.

Jagger J, Levine J, Jane JA, et al (1984): Epidemiologic features of head injury in a predominantly rural population. *Journal of Trauma* 24:40–44.

Jane JA, Steward O, Gennarelli T (1985): Axonal degeneration induced by experimental noninvasive minor head injury. *Journal of Neurosurgery* 62:96–100.

Jennett B, Teasdale G (1981): *Management of head injuries*. Philadelphia: F.A. Davis Company.

Kalsbeek WD, McLaurin RL, Harris BS, et al (1980): The national head and spinal cord injury survey: Major findings. *Journal of Neurosurgery* 53:519–531.

Klauber MR, Barrett-Connor E, Marshall LF, et al (1981): The epidemiology of head injury. A prospective study of an entire community: San Diego County, California. *American Journal of Epidemiology* 113:500–509.

Klonoff PS, Snow WG, Costa LD (1986): Quality of life in patients 2 to 4 years after closed head injury. *Neurosurgery* 19(5):735–743.

Knill-Jones R (1978): New statistical approaches to prediction. *Scottish Medical Journal* 23:109–110.

Kraus JF (1987): Epidemiology of head injury. In: *Head injury*, 2nd ed. Cooper PR (ed). Baltimore: William & Wilkins, pp 14–18.

Kraus JF, Black MA, Hessol N, et al (1984): The incidence of acute brain injury and serious impairment in a defined population. *American Journal of Epidemiology* 119:186–201.

Levin HS, Grossman RG, Rose JE, Teasdale G (1979): Long term neuropsychological outcome of closed head injury. *Journal of Neurosurgery* 50:412–422.

Lindvall H, Linderoth B, Norlin B (1974): Causes of the post-concussional syndrome. *Acta Neurologica Scandinavica* 50:1–45.

MacFlynn G, Montgomery EA, Fenton GW, et al (1984): Measurement of reaction time following minor head injury. *Journal of Neurology, Neurosurgery and Psychiatry* 47:1326–1331.

McMillan TM, Gluckman EE (1987): The neuropsychology of moderate head injury. *Journal of Neurology, Neurosurgery and Psychiatry* 50:393–397.

Munday CS. Assessment of minor head injury: Assessment variables. Unpublished articles.

Oddy M, Humphrey M (1980): Social recovery during the year following severe head injury. *Journal of Neurology, Neurosurgery and Psychiatry* 43:798–802.

Parkinson D (1977): Concussion. *Mayo Clinic Proceedings* 52:492–496.

Parkinson D, Stephensen S and Philips S (1985): Head injuries: a prospective, computerized study. *The Canadian Journal of Surgery* 28:1, 79–83.

Povlishock JT, Becker DP, Sullivan HG, Miller JD (1978): Vascular permeability alterations to horseradish peroxidase in experimental brain injury. *Brain Research* 153:223–239.

Rappaport M, Hall KM, Hopkins K, Belleza T, Cope DN (1982): Disability rating scale for severe head trauma: Coma to community. *Archives of Physical Medicine and Rehabilitation* 63:118–123.

Rimel R, Giordani B, Barth J, et al (1982): Moderate head injury: Completing the clinical spectrum of brain trauma. *Neurosurgery* 11:(3), 344–351.

Tabaddor K, Mattis S, Zazula T (1984): Cognitive sequelae and recovery course after moderate and severe head injury. *Neurosurgery* 14:(6), 701–708.

Whitman S, Coonley-Hoganson R, Desai BT (1984): Comparative head trauma experiences in two socioeconomically different Chicago-area communities. A population study. *American Journal of Epidemiology* 119:570–580.

Wilmot CB, Cope N, Hall KM, et al (1985): Occult head injury: Its incidence in spinal cord injury. *Archives of Physical Medicine and Rehabilitation* 66:227–231.

4

Mild Head Trauma

Steven Mattis, Ph.D.

Neuropsychology Section, New York Hospital, Cornell University Medical Center, New York, New York, U.S.A.

Perhaps the most difficult of the problems confounding the investigation of the pathophysiology, effects, course, and treatment of mild brain injury is the lack of a widely accepted definition of the clinical entity to be studied. What criteria must an individual meet to be classified as a mild brain injury patient? While criteria establishing a clear demarcation point between patients who have sustained *mild* as contrasted with a *moderate* head injury have not been widely employed, this particular distinction is not especially controversial. It is widely accepted that patients presenting along any given arbitrary transition point from mild to moderate brain injury do seem to represent a continuum of central nervous system (CNS) impairment. All other things being equal, the single criterion measure that is generally accepted as defining the most impaired edge of the mild range is a Glasgow Coma Scale (Teasdale and Jennett, 1974) score of 12 (keeping in mind the presence of complicating factors such as skull fracture). This criterion point of 12 for the lowest edge of mild and 11 as the upper edge of moderate seems as supportable by the present literature as any other arbitrary criterion. The major controversy that exists is fought at the mildest end of the mild range of brain injuries where the possibility of discontinuity exists. At what point can investigators agree that a given event has resulted in *no* as contrasted with *some* brain injury?

In practice, most clinicians and investigators would consider an individual classifiable as a mild brain injury patient if the patient experienced a blow to the head, the length of unconsciousness was brief (usually under one hour), duration of posttraumatic amnesia was brief, presence of neurologic complications was brief (usually resolving within 24 hours), and there were no skull fracture and no known impairment

41

of brain tissue. The patient who presents no problem in classification is the one who is observed to be unconscious for about 15 minutes following a collision with a baseball bat, is unable to recall in detail the nature of the precipitating event upon awakening, and is unable to recall lists of words or drawings at normal levels of performance for another 8 hours after which he or she appears neurologically normal. Most clinicians will agree that this individual has suffered some brain injury resulting in some transient cognitive dysfunction which, compared to the patient who might be comatose for days and recover with persisting aphasia, amnesia, and apraxia, would be classified as mild. If the patient persists in complaining of memory and concentration difficulties, anxiety, dizziness, and headache several days later, most clinicians would attribute these difficulties to the head injury and assure the patient that these symptoms are very common after head injury and that the probability is very high that the symptoms will abate very shortly.

In contrast to our prototypical mild injury patient, difficulty in classification is raised by the patient who was the passenger in a car that collided with a guardrail, who sustained "whiplash" injuries without loss of consciousness, did not undergo contrast studies shortly after the accident, and whose lawyer now alleges sufficient cognitive and affective impairment to severely limited gainful employment one year after the accident. The problem with dismissing this litigation case as a frivolous example of the occurrence and effect of mild head injury is that criteria that commonly define the presence and severity of moderate and severe brain injury are often not present with mild injury.

Among the most common of criteria determining classification of brain injury are loss of consciousness and blow to the head. The literature indicates that neither of these events need occur with brain injury. Gennarelli's animal work supports his contention that the occurrence of mild head injury does not depend on concomitant loss of consciousness. Thus the index of suspicion of brain injury is raised by any physically traumatic event that results in transient neurobehavioral dysfunction. Anterograde and retrograde amnesia can occur without loss of consciousness (Yarnell and Lynch, 1973; Fisher, 1966, 1982; Levin et al., 1987). Electroencephalographic abnormalities, both diffuse and focal, can be found after mild head injury without unconsciousness (Torres and Shapiro, 1961; Bickford and Klass, 1966; Jasper et al., 1945; MacFlynn, et al., 1984). Indeed Jenkins et al. (1986) recently reported that MRI study of 50 patients within one week of head injury revealed that cortical contusion was seen irrespective of the effect of head injury on loss of consciousness. However, with any loss of consciousness, even as brief as less than 5 minutes, there was clear evidence of intracerebral lesions. In brief, maintenance of consciousness, per se, cannot be used as prima facie evidence of no brain injury.

It would also appear that a blow to the head is neither a sufficient nor necessary condition in the causation of mild brain injury. The mechanism and nature of brain damage in mild brain injury has been the subject of active animal and human investigation. In general, the nature and location of brain injury is a function of the location, speed, and direction of applied force (Nilsson and Ponten, 1977). Two major physical mechanisms for brain injury during the traumatic event have been proposed: rotational dislocation, that is, rapid angular momentum of the brain within the skull, and translational dislocation, more closely related to the force and direction of impact to the skull. Comparing the effects of rotational acceleration and translational acceleration, Gennarelli (1982) concluded that rotational acceleration is more likely to cause frontotemporal contusion and diffuse axonal injury and that translational acceleration is more likely to result in focal injury and, because of the sheer forces on brain stem, be implicated in loss of consciousness (Ommaya and Gennarelli, 1974). This does not mean that rotational acceleration cannot cause unconsciousness. In a model of whiplash injuries, rotational displacement of the head produced unconsciousness in 19 of 50 monkeys (Ommaya, Faas, and Yarnell, 1968). Mild to severe anterograde and retrograde amnesias resulting from blows that did not cause unconsciousness in man have been reported. Both delayed anterograde and retrograde amnesias are reported in the course of football injuries (Yarnell and Lynch, 1973). Fisher (1966, 1982) reports single case studies of individuals who incurred severe anterograde amnesias after whiplash.

Thus it would appear that any event that rapidly changes the position of the brain within the skull places the individual at risk for mild brain injury. The problem with classification is that not all individuals who experience such traumatic events necessarily evidence abnormalities in electroencephalographic findings, contrast studies, neurologic deficits, or abnormalities in higher cortical function and/or effect. Thus not all individuals who experience head injuries have brain injuries and not all individuals who have brain injuries have head injuries.

Toward a definition of mild brain injury: If only some individuals with head injuries have brain injuries and only some individuals who have brain injuries have head injuries, and some who have brain injuries have never lost consciousness, then the major criteria presently used in defining mild brain injury contain a sufficient number of false positives and negatives to make generalization across studies exceedingly difficult. What one needs at this juncture are research diagnostic criteria for mild brain injury. These criteria must be (a) stringent enough such that investigators and clinicians would agree that every individual demonstrating these criteria would have incurred a minor brain injury, that is, there would be no (or very few) false positives, and (b) liberal enough such that many individuals who indeed have mild brain injury are correctly detected and classified, that is, have good coverage. Both inclusionary and exclusionary criteria must be acceptable, useful, and feasible to be of heuristic value.

Submitted for discussion are the criteria for mild brain injury derived, in part, from those used by the three-center study in which I participated (Levin et al., 1987).

Suggested research diagnostic criteria are (a) history of cranial trauma with a period of unconsciousness, if present, of less than 20 minutes; or (b) whiplash injury with some period of observed unconsiousness but less than 20 minutes; and (c) lowest Glasgow Coma Scale score of 12, with a GCS score of 15 by 48 hours; (d) no focal neurologic findings; (e) no findings (or history?) indicative of toxic metabolic disorder at time of admission; (f) no findings (or history?) of psychosis at time of admission.

The above six criteria represent the patient admitted to the emergency room having been stunned by a cranial blow, who appears somewhat confused for several hours, and who then seemingly recovers over the next 24 hours, and the patient observed to be unconscious after a sports or motor vehicle accident, without clear evidence of a cranial blow, who follows a similar course. As such, the above represent the least conservative criteria that most investigators and clinicians would accept as still indicative of mild as contrasted with no brain injury and distinct from moderate injury.

The rationale for these criteria is not self-evident and requires some explication. If one uses both cranial blow *and* loss of consciousness as primary criteria for mild brain injury, then one would be fairly certain that there would be few, if any, false positives. One would lack coverage, however, because (a) not many of the mild trauma patients present with both elements and (b) of those that do, many are in the moderate range of brain injury. If one relied heavily on the recent study by Jenkins et al. (1986), which indicated that loss of consciousness for any length of time was associated with intracerebral lesions, then it would seem reasonable to use loss of consciousness, by itself, as a necessary and sufficient index of brain injury. However, report of unconsciousness, especially for brief periods, is not highly reliable and, for longer periods, encroaches upon the "moderate" edge of the mild range. Nonetheless, one might reasonably argue that reliably observed loss of consciousness and subsequent brief period of confusion, with or without head injury, must be acceptable as evidence of brain injury. Thus, whiplash injury with some period of unconsciousness might have very few false positives for brain injury and be of a sufficient rate of occurrence to provide good coverage of the mild brain injury population.

A blow to the head, while raising the index of suspicion for brain injury, would not, by itself, be sufficient evidence for such a conclusion.

However, a blow to the head paired with a period of confusion, which would satisfy Gennarelli's liberal criteria for brain injury, is generally accepted in the literature as contributing few false positives and is a common occurrence, thereby ensuring broad coverage of patients at the mildest edge of the mild range.

PATHOPHYSIOLOGY OF MILD BRAIN INJURY

Without delving very deeply into the ethics and politics of animal experimentation, it is fair to say that almost all of the current knowledge concerning the mechanics of brain injury has been derived, in large measure, from animal models. At this point, the mechanical effects of the traumatic event have not been fully explicated, nor have the secondary effects of changes in intracranial pressure, so important in the acute management of moderate to severe head trauma, been intensively investigated in the mild brain injuries.

Secondarily, there also appear to be changes in cerebral blood flow, which may be of significance in determining the nature and severity of sequelae. Peri-ictally there is an increase in perfusion, followed several days later by a decrease in circulation time (Dila et al., 1976). Both the cause and the effects of these changes in cerebral-vascular activity are unknown at this time and should be the focus of major study.

NEUROPSYCHOLOGICAL SEQUELAE OF MILD BRAIN INJURY

Given the wide range of definitions of mild brain injury, it is not surprising that the nature, severity, and incidence of neuropsychological sequelae should also vary widely. The findings and complaints, grouped under the general rubric of postconcussion syndrome, include memory and concentration difficulty, headache, dizziness, irritability, and free-floating anxiety. There is clear evidence of cognitive deficits measurable up to several days postinjury (Cronholm and Jonson, 1958; Fisher, 1966, 1982; Gronwall and Wrightson, 1974; MacFlynn et al., 1984; McLean et al., 1983; Van Zomeren and Deelman, 1978; Yarnell and Lynch, 1973; Levin et al., 1987). Anterospective studies of the acute and persisting effects of mild head injury with appropriate controls are very few (McLean et al., 1983; MacFlynn et al., 1983; Levin et al., 1987). Both the McLean et al. and Levin et al. studies measured both cognitive performance and subjective complaints. In both studies, memory and other cognitive deficits were found in the mild head injury patients within days of the injury, but significant differences between head injury patients and matched controls on cognitive measures were not found at one month postinjury. McLean et al. (1983) found persisting complaints of fatigue, headache, and memory difficulties one month postinjury. MacFlynn et al. (1983) found reaction time to be impaired immediately postinjury and to gradually improve over time but not reach normal levels for 6 months postinjury. Levin et al. (1986) found significant neurobehavioral deficits within several days of injury which remitted to levels consonant with matched controls by one month. In contrast, in the immediate postinjury phase, patient complaints of headache, decreased energy, and dizziness were the most frequent and severe of all complaints despite demonstrable cognitive deficits. These complaints, while diminished by one month, were still quite common across all three centers. While some cognitive deficits have been clearly demonstrated after brain injury, assessment of changes in cognition in the mild brain injury patient immediately after the event is still relatively uncharted territory. Moreover, the incidence of postconcussion symptomatology, for example, headache, dizziness, anxiety, and so forth, its prevalence in matched controls, and the relationship between the cognitive deficits and complaints have not been sufficiently clarified.

PREDISPOSING FACTORS

Alcohol and controlled substance abusers and individuals with prior head injuries are overly represented in a sample of consecutively enrolled head injury patients (Field, 1976; Rimel et al., 1981). Thus the severity and nature of the postinjury deficits are confounded by the possible cumulative effects of repeated head injuries (Gronwall and Wrightson, 1975) and by acute and persisting effects of toxic metabolic disorders.

THE NECESSITY FOR CAREFULLY SELECTED CONTROLS

Because one is dealing with criteria for the presence of brain injury that are not too far removed from criteria for normal functioning, any study that attempts to assess the effects of mild brain injury on performance and complaints must take extraordinary pains to obtain appropriate control subjects. The necessity for appropriate controls is not, as one might suppose, to obtain the necessary power to be able to demonstrate significant differences between normal controls and the subtle dysfunction obtained in patients with mild brain injury. Quite the contrary, the recent literature suggests that if one is not careful, one is quite readily able to find statistically significant differences between mild head injury patients and published norms which dissipate as one contrasts the findings with appropriately matched controls. Who are the mild head injury patients? What must we control for in order to demonstrate that behavior and complaints subsequent to the traumatic event were indeed secondary to that event? Head trauma patients, as a group, are, in all likelihood, not drawn from the general population. As compared to the general population, the brain-injured patient is likely to be male, in his mid-20s, to have high likelihood of a history of alcohol or substance abuse (indeed is likely to be intoxicated at the time of injury), is likely to have had a previous head injury, and is likely to have come to the attention of the mental health worker or the law. Indeed the prevalence of such factors as well as site-specific demographic factors make the necessity of site-specific control groups critical to the acceptance of a given study's conclusions.

THE NATURE, ETIOLOGY, AND REMEDIATION OF PERSISTING COMPLAINTS

Recently, Laurence Binder (1986) conducted an extensive and carefully considered review of the literature concerning persisting symptoms following mild head injury. Binder concludes, in part, that the studies indicating persisting cognitive deficits were methodologically flawed by the absence of appropriate controls, account of premorbid history, or statistical analysis. Only two studies, to date, appear to be sufficiently sound methodologically to reach some generalizable conclusions. In both studies, head injury patients were seen within days of the injury and, at least once again, at one month. Both studies assessed cognitive functioning and subjective complaints and used appropriate site specific matched controls. Unfortunately, each study contained a significant methodologic flaw; fortunately, not the same one. The study by McLean et al. (1983) failed to obtain repeated measures on cognitive tasks by controls, and the Levin et al. study failed to obtain repeated measures on subjective complaints from controls. Taken together, however, it would appear that patients with mild brain injury (a) demonstrate significant cognitive deficits shortly after the event, (b) make significant gains in cognitive functioning in the first month such that performance on repeated measures by head injury patients do not differ significantly from performance on repeated measures by control subjects, and (c) classic postconcussion syndrome complaints (especially headache, dizziness, and fatigue) may persist past one month and vary somewhat independently from cognitive performance. A quarter to a third of the normal controls admit to symptoms consonant with postconcussion syndrome. It is not clear, therefore, whether the persisting complaints of some mild brain injury patients represent new symptoms or an elaboration of old symptoms experienced before the traumatic event.

CONCLUSIONS

Most of the serious biomedical and neuropsychological efforts have been focused on the problems confronting the patient incurring moderate to severe brain injuries—still an issue of immense import. However, recently, some attention has been focused on the problems presented by the patient incurring mild brain injury, the incidence of which is presumed to be quite high. Since the event is generally unreported, the incidence and prevalence are unknown. It is clear, however, that serious, at times incapacitating, deficits in higher cortical functions and physical discomfort are frequent sequelae to the traumatic event. The field appears to be on the threshold of a major commitment to the study of mild brain injury. The following are questions raised by the studies to date:

1. What are reasonable and useful research diagnostic criteria for mild brain injury?
2. What is the incidence and prevalence of this disorder?
3. What are the demographic characteristics of the mild brain injury patient?
4. What prognostic factors are associated with the incidence and severity of and recovery from mild brain injury?
5. What do high technology imaging and metabolic monitoring procedures tell us about the pathophysiology of mild brain injury and recovery of function?
6. What will a comprehensive neuropsychological investigation of cognitive and affective processes reveal as the primary postinjury deficits? Are there differing clusters of deficits producing differing postconcussion syndromes?
7. What is the nature and rate of recovery of function?
8. What is the relationship between cognitive deficits and subjective complaints? Are there differing etiologic factors affecting the occurrence and recovery of cognitive deficits and postconcussive complaints?
9. What are the etiologic factors underlying persisting deficits and complaints? What are the interactive effects (if any) of psychogenic and neurogenic factors in producing persisting symptoms and findings?
10. What are the effects of personal history factors (e.g., prior head injury, alcoholism, psychopathology) on the incidence and severity of and recovery from mild brain injury?
11. What medical rehabilitative procedures effectively influence the rate of recovery (and incidence of persisting deficits and complaints)?

At present, the patient who has incurred a mild brain injury and who persists in complaining that the cognitive deficits and personal discomfort he or she is experiencing have significantly impaired his or her social and vocational abilities is looked upon with some suspicion as either a malingerer or an individual who clearly admits to some serious character flaws. While in some instances these hypotheses may, indeed, be true, there are sufficient data to strongly suggest that the medical rehabilitative community must take seriously such complaints. Unfortunately, to date, we have not sufficient data to reliably "rule out" alternative hypotheses and tend to make alternate diagnosis and treatment plans by exclusion rather than by positive indications. Progress in answering the above questions will significantly diminish the personal distress of the individual who has incurred a mild brain injury and reduce the personal and societal cost of maintaining his or her patient status.

REFERENCES

Bickford RG, Klass DW (1966): Acute and chronic EEG findings after head injury. In Caveness WF, Walker AE (eds.), *Head Injury Conference Proceedings* (pp. 63–88). Philadelphia: JB Lippincott.

Binder LE (1986): Persisting symptoms after mild head injury: A review of the post concussive syndrome. *Journal of Clinical and Experimental Neuropsychology* 8(4):323–346.

Cronholm B, Jonson I (1958): Memory functions after cerebral conscussion. *Acta Chirurgica Scandinavica* 113:263–271.

Dila C, Bouchard L, Myer E, Yamamoto L, Feindel W (1976): Microvascular response to minimal brain trauma. In McLaurin RL (ed.), *Head injuries* (pp. 213–215). New York: Grune & Stratton.

Field JH (1976): *A study of the epidemiology of head injury in England and Wales, with particular application to rehabilitation.* London: HMSO.

Fisher CM (1966): Concussion amnesia. *Neurology* 16:826–830.

Fisher CM (1982): Whiplash amnesia. *Neurology* 32:667–668.

Gennarelli TA (1982): Cerebral concussion and diffuse brain injuries. In Cooper PR (ed.), *Head injury* (pp. 83–97). Baltimore: Williams and Wilkins.

Gronwall D, Wrightson P (1974): Delayed recovery of intellectual function after minor head injury. *Lancet* 2, 605–609.

Gronwall D, Wrightson P (1975): Cumulative effects of concussion. *Lancet* 2, 995–997.

Jasper H, Kershman J, Elvidge A (1945): Electroencephalography in head injury. *Research Publications Association for Research in Nervous and Mental Disease* 24, 388–420.

Jenkins A, Teasdale G, Hadley MDM, MacPherson P, Rowan SO (1986): Brain lesions detected by magnetic resonance imaging in mild and severe head injuries. *Lancet* 2, 445–446.

Levin HS, Mattis S, Ruff RM, Eisenberg HM, Marshall LF, Tabaddor K, High WM, Frankowski RF (1987): Neurobehavioral outcome following minor head injury: a three-center study. *Journal of Neurosurgery* 66:234–243.

MacFlynn G, Montgomery EA, Fenton GW, Rutherford W (1984): Measurement of reaction time following minor head injury. *Journal of Neurology, Neurosurgery, and Psychiatry* 47, 1326–1331.

McLean A, Temkin NR, Dikman S, Wyler AR (1983): The behavioral sequelae of head injury. *Journal of Clinical Neuropsychology* 5:361–376.

Nilsson B, Ponten U (1977): Experimental head injury in the rat. Part 2: Regional brain metabolism in concussive trauma. *Journal of Neurosurgery* 47, 252–261.

Ommaya AK, Fass, Yarnell P (1968): Whiplash injury and brain damage. *Journal of the American Medical Association* 204, 285–289.

Ommaya AK, Gennarelli TA (1974): Cerebral concussion and traumatic unconsciousness. *Brain* 97, 633–654.

Rimel RW, Giordani B, Barth JT, Boll TJ, Jane JA (1981): Disability caused by minor head injury. *Neurosurgery* 9, 221–228.

Teasdale G, Jennett B (1974): Assessment of coma and impaired consciousness: A practical scale. *Lancet* 1:1–5.

Torres F, Shapiro SK (1961): Electroencephalograms in whiplash injury. *Archives of Neurology* 5:40–47.

Van Zomeren AH, Deelman BG (1978): Long-term recovery of visual reaction time after closed head injury. *Journal of Neurology, Neurosurgery, and Psychiatry* 41:452–457.

Yarnell PR, Lynch S (1973): The "ding": Amnestic states in football trauma. *Neurology* 23:196–197.

II

Neuropsychological and Behavioral Issues

5

Neurobehavioral Aspects of Traumatic Brain Injury

Harvey S. Levin, Ph.D.,
and Felicia C. Goldstein, Ph.D.

Division of Neurosurgery and Department of Neurology,
University of Texas Medical Branch, Galveston, Texas, U.S.A.

Outcome studies of severe closed head injury (CHI) have indicated that chronic disability is primarily related to neurobehavioral sequelae, whereas motor and sensory impairments contribute less to the overall level of functioning in most patients (Jennett et al., 1981). Investigations of patients following mild and moderate CHI further support a dissociation between neurologic findings that are typically normal or likely to resolve and the persistence of neurobehavioral deficits (Levin et al., 1987b; Rimel et al., 1981). The neurobehavioral effects of head injury involve cognition, memory, language, and psychosocial functioning. Our appreciation of the impact of CHI on psychosocial adjustment has been greatly advanced through systematic studies using interview techniques and measures of global outcome such as return to work (McKinlay et al., 1981; Oddy and Humphrey, 1980; Van Zomeren and Van Den Burg, 1985).

The following sections review the most prominent subacute and chronic cognitive sequelae that have been implicated in adult CHI patients. The reader is referred to reviews by O'Shanick (this volume), Prigatano (1987), and Rosenthal (1983) for discussions of personality and behavioral changes. Pediatric head injury will not be covered in view of the additional methodological and maturational considerations and differences in neuropsychological assessment techniques (see Goldstein and Levin, 1986; Shapiro, 1983).

CLINICAL RELEVANCE OF NEUROBEHAVIORAL FINDINGS

Neuropsychological research and assessment combines methodologies from clinical and experimental psychology in the analysis of cognitive and behavioral disturbances (Levin and Benton, 1984). One caveat for interpreting neurobehavioral outcome involves an appreciation of premorbid patient characteristics. The British neurologist Sir Charles Symonds (1937) noted that "it is not only the kind of injury that matters, but the kind of head." A high level of preinjury education and occupation is generally related to improved prognosis for resumption of employment (Gilchrist and Wilkinson, 1979; Rimel et al., 1981). Careful screening of preinjury conditions that potentially compromise cognitive function is also necessary for interpretation of neurobehavioral outcome. Antecedent neuropsychiatric conditions such as alcoholism, drug abuse, previous head injury, behavioral disorder, and cognitive problems are generally overrepresented in the head injury population (Rimel et al., 1981; Tsuang, Boor, and Fleming, 1985). In addition to pertinent historical information, the clinician should consider the social support system in assessing potential for recovery and rehabilitation.

A second caveat is that evaluation of neurobehavioral outcome should include the "executive functions" (i.e., the capacity to schedule, initiate, and perform activities of daily living) as well as the potential for achieving psychosocial adjustment (Goldstein and Levin, 1987; Levin et al., 1987a; Oddy, Humphrey, and Uttley, 1978; Prigatano et al., 1984). Extrapolation from test scores obtained in the laboratory without information about the patient's behavior in daily situations can be misleading. Consequently, follow-up assessment should include an interview with a family member to characterize the patient's everyday performance.

Finally, it is important to evaluate changes that might determine eligibility for rehabilitative programs and employment. Due to impressive gains in cognitive function during the first year after injury (Mandleberg and Brooks, 1975; Tabaddor, Mattis, and Zazula, 1984), frequent monitoring of recovery is indicated initially; follow-up assessments can then be spaced farther apart. In contrast to the relative advances in early prognosis of survival based on variables such as age, the Glasgow Coma Scale (GCS) scores (Teasdale and Jennett, 1974), and type of lesion (Gennarelli et al., 1982; Narayan et al., 1981), prediction of long-term neurobehavioral functioning remains a more complex task.

SUBACUTE NEUROBEHAVIORAL MANIFESTATIONS OF CLOSED HEAD INJURY

Posttraumatic Amnesia

Russell (1932) proposed that the loss of full consciousness be utilized as an index of the severity of CHI. Russell and Nathan (1946) introduced the term "posttraumatic amnesia" (PTA) and modified the original criterion to include the patient's capacity to become "sufficiently aware of his surroundings to commit them to memory." The definition of PTA was revised by Russell and Smith (1961) as "the length of the interval during which information has not been stored." Accordingly, PTA is used synonymously with anterograde amnesia, i.e., inability to consolidate daily events. These early studies included the period of coma in estimating the duration of PTA. Investigators have recently differentiated the duration of coma as measured by the Glasgow Coma Scale (GCS) developed by Teasdale and Jennett (1974) from the ensuing period of gross confusion and amnesia. Prior to the introduction of the GCS, the duration of PTA was probably the most widely used index of severity.

Figure 5-1 depicts the stages of recovery from a severe CHI, i.e., an injury that produces coma. After resolution of disorientation and confusion, the interval of PTA remains a gap in the patient's memory apart from preserved "islands" (i.e., fragments) of memory. Although injuries

EARLY STAGES OF RECOVERY FROM CLOSED HEAD INJURY

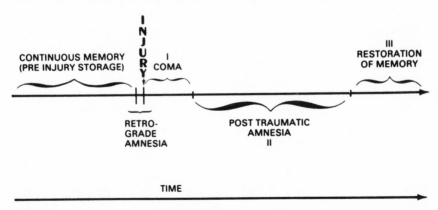

FIG. 5-1. Sequences of subacute disturbance of memory after closed head injury. The periods of coma (I) and posttraumatic amnesia (II) have been traditionally combined to yield a total interval of impaired consciousness that extends until continuous memory for ongoing events (III) is restored. (Reprinted with permission from Levin HS, et al., 1982.)

that produce periods of coma tend to result in longer periods of PTA than less severe head trauma, a subgroup of patients with mild to moderate head injuries exhibit disproportionately long periods of disorientation, confusion, and anterograde amnesia.

Posttraumatic amnesia, unlike the anterograde amnesia arising from other etiologies, is frequently characterized by a concomitant attentional deficit. Failure to selectively focus attention on the examiner, difficulty in sustaining attention, and excessive distractibility undoubtedly contribute to this gross amnesic disorder. Behavioral manifestations include agitation, inappropriate speech, and disinhibitory behavior such as screaming or combativeness. In addition, patients may confabulate concerning the circumstances of their injuries. These subacute behavioral manifestations may raise the question of a preexisting psychiatric disorder, but head-injured patients without a history of emotional disturbance can exhibit this early clinical picture (Levin, Benton, and Grossman, 1982).

Retrograde Amnesia

Retrograde amnesia (RA) (i.e., the period prior to the injury for which the patient has no recollection) is usually briefer than the period of PTA. Russell and Nathan (1946) reported that the duration of RA was less than 30 minutes in over 80% of their total series of 1029 patients at the Military Hospital for Head Injuries in Oxford; in 50% of those patients with PTA, duration was 7 days or longer. Russell (1935) described a CHI patient who initially exhibited an RA that extended 9 years into his past. Over a period of 10 weeks the patient gradually recalled events from the remote past, beginning with the earliest event and later filling in more recent events that had occurred within a few minutes of his accident. In most cases, the shrinkage of RA parallels the resolution of PTA and may reflect restoration of memory retrieval from long-term storage (Benson, Gardner, and Meadows, 1976). The more frequent finding of a brief (e.g., 30-second), irreversible period of RA may reflect interference with consolidation of memory for events immediately before the impact.

Using a quantitative technique to assess remote memory, we have shown that residual impairment (but not necessarily abolition) of retention for public events antedating the injury is common even after resolution of PTA (Levin et al., 1985). In contrast, retention of autobiographical information is relatively intact, especially for material from childhood.

Measurement Techniques

Daily monitoring of disorientation, amnesia, and confusion during PTA by a brief standardized scale provides a measure of the temporal course of recovery. The Galveston Orientation and Amnesia Test (GOAT) (Levin, O'Donnell, and Grossman, 1979), which measures daily changes in orientation and memory, is used in the ongoing main phase of the Traumatic Coma Data Bank of the National Institute of Neurologic and Communicative Disorders and Stroke (NINCDS). Serial GOAT scores of a 28-year-old foreman who sustained a severe CHI (GCS score of 5) complicated by left frontal contusions in a motor vehicle accident on August 16, 1984, are shown in Figure 5-2. Although the patient's level of consciousness improved during the first five days after injury, he exhibited temporal and geographic disorientation for more than three weeks after

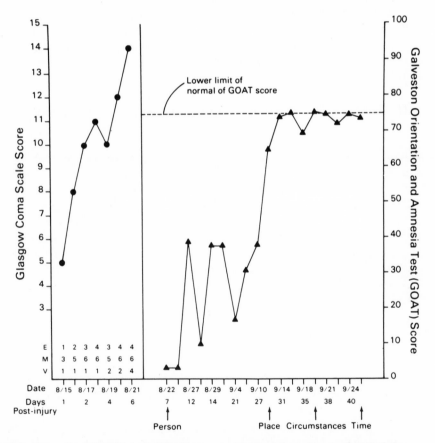

FIG. 5-2. Serial GCS and GOAT scores obtained in patient admitted for a severe nonmissile head injury (GCS score of 5) after a motor vehicle accident. Note the delay of three weeks before the patient's confusion and disorientation resolved to a marginal level after impressive gains in his GCS score. Despite orientation to person, his geographic and temporal disorientation persisted as well as confusion regarding the circumstances of his hospitalization.

his GCS score approached a normal level. Restoration of his orientation followed the sequence of person, place, circumstances of injury, and time.

Daily administration of the GOAT to consecutive admissions for CHI has disclosed that patients with mild head injury (i.e., initial GCS score of 13 to 15, normal neurological findings, and no extracranial injuries requiring surgery or hospitalization longer than 48 hours) typically improved to the normal range within 48 hours. In contrast, Levin and Eisenberg (1986) analyzed the GOAT data from 50 survivors of severe CHI (initial GCS score ≤8), who were entered in the Pilot Phase of the NINCDS Traumatic Coma Data Bank, and found a median PTA duration (excluding coma) of nine days. Individual variation in the duration of PTA (one to 132 days) was impressive, but there was no consistent difference between patients with mass lesions and those with diffuse injury. Maintenance of the GOAT score in the normal range (≥75) for 2 consecutive days indicates that cognitive functioning has improved sufficiently to consider discharge or at least transfer to a unit providing less intensive supervision.

RESIDUAL NEUROBEHAVIORAL EFFECTS OF CLOSED HEAD INJURY

Levin, Benton, and Grossman (1982) have reviewed the methodological problems that hinder interpretation of residual cognitive impairments including (1) lack of information concerning preinjury cognitive ability and neuropsychiatric functioning; (2) the absence of appropriate control groups; (3) inadequate and nonuniform documentation of acute injury severity; (4) variable injury-test intervals and lack of serial testings to depict the time-course of recovery; and (5) variation in neuropsychological measurement techniques. Consequently, caution is advised in generalizing from any single published study of cognitive function after CHI.

Recovery of Cognitive Functioning

Investigations of cognitive functioning after moderate and severe head injury have primarily employed the WAIS or WAIS-R (Wechsler, 1955; 1981). Initial research completed in Glasgow (Mandleberg, 1975; 1976; Mandleberg and Brooks, 1975) suggested that the severity of CHI primarily affects the rate of rather than the eventual return to an average intellectual level. However, later research has shown that residual cognitive impairment is directly related to indices of acute severity (Alexandre et al., 1983; Levin et al., 1979). As indicated in Table 5-1, the presence and degree of cognitive impairment two years after head injury were strongly related to the initial GCS score. A similar relationship

Table 5-1. *Cognitive Outcome Two Years after Injury (Excluding Fatal Cases) in Relation to Glasgow Coma Scale (GCS) Score on Admission*

Cognitive outcome	15–8	7–5	4–3	Total cases
Minimal/no deficit	21 (84%)	16 (34%)	3 (10%)	40 (39%)
Mild deficit	4 (16%)	19 (40%)	7 (23%)	30 (29%)
Severe deficit		12 (26%)	18 (60%)	30 (29%)
Vegetative			2 (7%)	2 (3%)
Total cases	25	47	30	102

The percentages have been recomputed after excluding fatal cases.
Reprinted with permission from Colombo et al. (1983).

was present for the 24-hour GCS score and for the integrity of eye movements.

During the first 6 to 12 months after moderate or severe CHI, there is rapid improvement in cognitive function on the WAIS that begins to plateau after one year (Figure 5-3) (Mandleberg and Brooks, 1975). This asymptote is reached early, particularly for the Verbal Scale, and may reflect relative sparing of semantic knowledge such as range of vocabulary, judgment in practical situations, and abstract reasoning. As shown in Figure 5-3, the Performance Scale of the Wechsler Test indicates that visuospatial and visuomotor functions recover more gradually than verbal skills after head injury. However, the presence of a large hemispheric mass lesion can contribute to the degree and persistence of impairment in verbal or visuospatial skills, depending on its size and lateralization (Uzzell et al., 1979). In addition, an overall score within the normal range on the Verbal or Performance Scale might obscure specific cognitive defects.

The evaluation of cognitive recovery raises the issue of whether the current findings represent a decline from estimated premorbid level. Wilson and colleagues (1979) have derived regression equations to estimate premorbid intellectual functioning on the Wechsler Adult Intelligence Scale (WAIS). These formulas utilize demographic variables (age, sex, race, education, and occupation) and provide a reasonable approximation to actual IQs in neurologically intact individuals (Goldstein, Gary, and Levin, 1986). More recently, regression equations for prediction of IQs on the WAIS-R have also appeared in the literature (Barona, Reynolds, and Chastain, 1984). The application of these formulas may be important to evaluate preinjury characteristics and clinical indices related to degree of recovery.

Although recovery to an average intellectual level may be necessary

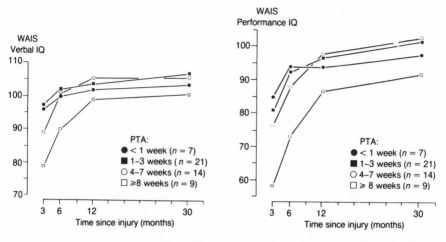

FIG. 5-3 Recovery of WAIS Verbal IQ (left) and Performance IQ (right) in 51 patients who underwent serial cognitive assessment at the Institute of Neurological Sciences, Glasgow, after a nonmissile head injury. (Reprinted with permission from Mandleberg IA and Brooks DN, 1975.)

for a good overall outcome, it is clearly not a sufficient condition. CHI often produces frontal lobe contusions and hematomas (Jennett and Teasdale, 1981). Damage to the frontal lobes, particularly the orbitofrontal region, may result in alterations of behavior characterized by disinhibition, emotional lability, impaired impulse control, and agitation; whereas lesions to the frontal convexities can lead to behaviors consisting of indifference, apathy, and loss of initiative (Massey and Coffey, 1983). Patients may recover to a normal range of intelligence on standard IQ tests while evidencing marked disability in social/occupational functioning, flexibility of problem solving, modulation of behavior, and capacity for planning and scheduling activities (Eslinger and Damasio, 1985; Stuss and Benson, 1986).

Recently, Levin et al. (1987a) developed the Neurobehavioral Rating Scale, an adaptation of the Brief Psychiatric Rating Scale (Overall and Gorham, 1962), which includes 27 dimensions rated by the clinician following a structured interview and a brief mental status examination. In a study involving 101 survivors of CHI, a principal components analysis identified a number of factors underlying neurobehavioral sequelae such as cognition/energy (coherence of cognition, efficiency of memory, behavioral slowing), metacognition (inaccurate self-appraisal, unrealistic planning, and disinhibition), somatic concern/anxiety (physical complaints, anxiety, depression, and irritability), and language (expressive and receptive language deficits). Disturbances involving self-appraisal (e.g., exaggerated self-opinion, overrating ability or underrating personality change in comparison to family and clinicians) and planning (e.g., poor formulation of future goals) were characteristic of patients sustaining severe injuries (GCS≤8). There were suggestions that disturbances in metacognition were common in patients with frontal lobe damage.

Administration of the Modified Wisconsin Card Sorting Test (Nelson, 1976), which emphasizes shifts in the principle of sorting according to color, number, and shape, is one of the procedures used in the NINCDS Traumatic Coma Data Bank to assess residual cognitive impairment after severe head injury. This type of relatively unstructured procedure, which is sensitive to deficits resulting from frontal lobe injury, is a useful adjunct to conventional tests of intelligence. The original version of the Wisconsin Card Sorting Test (Grant and Berg, 1948), which is longer and more difficult, is especially appropriate for evaluating the relatively subtle deficits in mild to moderate head-injured patients. Tests of fluency involving the capacity to generate words beginning with a particular letter (Benton, 1968) or nonsense designs (Jones-Gottman and Milner, 1977) may also be useful for detecting frontal lobe impairments.

Recovery of Memory

Memory impairment is one of the sequelae on which objective tests and subjective complaints by patients are in relatively close agreement. Van Zomeren and Van Den Berg (1985) found that 54% of severely injured patients complained of forgetfulness when interviewed two years after injury. Oddy and colleagues (1985) described memory disturbance as the most frequent complaint by patients and relatives seven years postinjury.

Short-term memory. Psychologists distinguish short-term memory (STM), which has a capacity of approximately seven chunks of information for less than one minute, from long-term memory (LTM), which has a relatively unlimited capacity for storing material over extended periods. Researchers have used forward digit span (i.e., repetition of digits in the same order as they are presented) to assess STM. In general, STM has been found to be relatively resistant to the effects of head trauma and improves more rapidly than LTM.

Consistent with studies showing preservation of immediate recall in alcoholic Korsakoff's syndrome (Butters and Cermak, 1980), CHI patients exhibit a transient impairment of auditory digit span during PTA with rapid improvement after clearing of disorientation and confusion (Mandleberg, 1975; Mandleberg and Brooks, 1975). Brooks (1972) found that forward digit span was relatively preserved in oriented patients tested at varying intervals after injury, whereas backward span was impaired. This disparity may be attributed to the necessity for engaging

LTM while reversing the order of digits before recall in backward span. However, reduction in forward auditory digit span may persist in severely injured patients who exhibit residual linguistic disturbance (Thomsen, 1977). Levin, Grossman, and Kelly (1976) investigated visual STM by employing irregularly shaped designs which the patient had to match to a target stimulus after a brief delay. Impaired visual STM persisted on this task in severely injured patients tested at long intervals after injury.

Long-term memory. Deficient LTM on verbal tasks such as recall of word lists, paired associate learning, and retention of paragraphs is a common finding after severe CHI. In a longitudinal investigation of long-term verbal recall of word lists, Parker and Serrats (1976) reported that one-half of severely injured patients exhibited residual impairment as compared to a control group two years after injury. In contrast, the investigators found that more than 90% of patients sustaining mild head injuries had improved to the normal range on this task during the same time period. Employing a verbal LTM procedure (Buschke and Fuld, 1974) in which the examiner reminds the patient on each trial of only those words that were forgotten on the preceding trial, we have shown that impairment of LTM persists after severe CHI despite adequate recovery of intellectual ability (Levin, Benton, and Grossman, 1982). More recently, we have characterized the presence of an amnesic disturbance (disproportionate impairment of memory with relatively intact IQ) in approximately 25% of survivors of moderate or severe CHI. Manifestation of amnesia appears related to acute neurologic indices, including the presence of nonreactive pupils (Levin, Goldstein, & High, 1987).

Semantic memory, i.e., memory for general principles, associations, and rules (Cermak, 1984; Tulving, 1972) has been relatively neglected in studies of CHI as compared to the extensive research concerning other neurologic and psychiatric conditions such as Korsakoff's syndrome (Cermak, Butters, and Gerrein, 1973), progressive degenerative dementia (Weingartner et al., 1981a), and depression (Weingartner et al., 1981b). Semantic memory is necessary for understanding relationships among events and for processing and organizing these events to aid future recall. In a study examining semantic memory (Levin and Goldstein, 1986), we asked survivors of severe CHI enrolled in a rehabilitation facility to learn and remember unrelated words, words that belonged to conceptual categories (i.e., animals, fruits, parts of a house) but were unclustered at input, and words that belonged to conceptual categories, but were presented in an organized fashion. Relative to control performance, we found that head-injured patients showed evidence for partially preserved semantic memory, i.e., their ability to remember more words presented in an organized manner (see Figure 5-4). However, recall by the

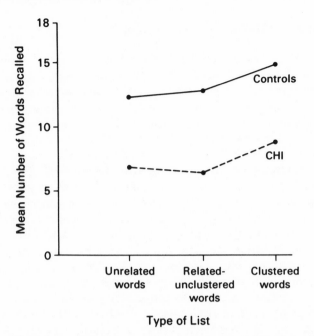

FIG. 5-4. Mean recall of words as a function of type of list for patients with severe closed head injuries and for controls. (Reprinted with permission from Levin HS and Goldstein FC, 1986.)

CHI patients was characterized by low levels of subjective organization and clustering, demonstrating inactive retrieval patterns. Semantic strategies (e.g., clustering, exhaustive category search) could be explored in cognitive rehabilitation programs.

Long-term memory for relatively nonverbal information has also been studied after CHI. In these procedures, recurring target pictures are interspersed with distractor pictures that are shown only once during continuous presentation of a series of 100 or more pictures. These recognition memory tasks, which engage LTM, can be administered to children or adults and offer the advantages of requiring no verbal response and forcing a choice between responses of old (a picture seen before) and new (a picture seen for the first time).

The pattern of recognition memory deficit after moderate head injury is characterized primarily by excessive false positive errors, that is, incorrectly identifying a new picture as one previously seen (Hannay, Levin, and Grossman, 1979). However, patients with durations of impaired consciousness for 24 hours or more after injury also exhibit difficulty in recognizing recurring pictures, as reflected by their reduced number of hits.

Attention and Information Processing

Head-injured patients are frequently distractible and have difficulty in sustaining attention. Geschwind (1982) postulated that these impairments contribute to the apparent memory disorder exhibited by many patients. Although survivors may eventually regain the capacity to solve complex problems, they often require a much longer period of time to reach the solution as compared to control subjects.

Reaction time. Diminished capacity for processing information under time pressure is a prominent finding after severe CHI. Slowing of reaction time is most noticeable under conditions that require a decision concerning selection of the correct response key that corresponds to the onset of a particular light (Van Zomeren and Deelman, 1978). In contrast, the degree of psychomotor slowing is less marked under a simple reaction time condition (i.e., the same key is pressed at the onset of the same light on each trial). Van Zomeren and Deelman (1978) found that the degree of residual psychomotor retardation on a complex reaction time task is commensurate with the severity of acute injury. Although the relevance of reaction time tasks to real-life activities may be questioned, there are frequent situations such as driving and occupations such as commercial flying that depend on rapid decision making.

Information processing speed. To investigate information processing speed after nonmissile head injury, Gronwall and her colleagues (Gronwall and Sampson, 1974; Gronwall and Wrightson, 1974) developed the Paced Auditory Serial Addition Test (PASAT) which involves addition of tape-recorded, single-digit numbers that are presented at progressively faster pacing rates. Performance of the PASAT requires auditory processing of each number, holding it in STM for addition to the next digit, and inhibiting a tendency to add numbers to the previous sum. The pace of information processing is driven by the intervals between the tape-recorded numbers. Gronwall and Sampson (1974) found that a severe concussion group (PTA of one hour to seven days) showed improvement on a final retest four weeks after discharge but still performed below the level of mild concussion (PTA less than one hour) and control groups. In contrast, the initial impairment exhibited by the mildly injured patients (consecutively treated) was resolved by 35 days postinjury. However, other patients with minor head injury who were referred to the investigators after a delay because of residual postconcussional complaints required a longer period to improve their performance.

We have reported that relatively permanent reductions in information processing rate are related to the severity of diffuse brain injury (Meyers, Levin, and Eisenberg, 1983). Figure 5-5 depicts the serial PASAT scores in a 24-year-old woman who recovered to the average level of intellectual functioning on the WAIS after a severe, apparently diffuse

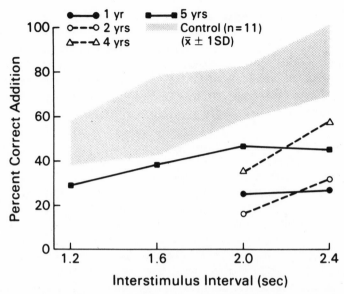

FIG. 5-5. Percent correct addition plotted against the pacing intervals separating successive numbers on the PASAT administered to patient C.H. five years after severe head injury that was considered to be diffuse. The hatched area corresponds to the mean ±1 S.D. for 11 women of comparable age and education. As shown, the patient was unable to add numbers at the fastest rates of presentation until the most recent examination five years after injury, which disclosed persistent slowing of information processing speed. (Reprinted with permission from Levin HS, et al., 1983.)

head injury that she sustained five years earlier. MRI at the time of the five-year follow-up examination revealed bilateral, parasagittal frontal lobe, and occipitotemporal lesions that primarily involved the white matter. Residual slowing of information processing was paralleled by difficulty in maintaining gainful employment because of her slow performance, particularly under stressful conditions. As shown in Figure 5-5, she was unable to even complete the PASAT at the more rapid pacing rate until the fifth year after injury.

Vigilance and distractibility. Investigations of other components of attention have yielded variable results in head-injured patients. Ewing et al. (1980) found that college students who sustained a mild head injury one to three years earlier showed a residual impairment on a vigilance test when they were examined in a hyperbaric chamber under a simulated altitude of 3,800 meters that produced mild hypoxia. In comparison with a matched control group, the injured students exhibited difficulty in discriminating long versus short intervals of tape-recorded digits played over a 30-minute period.

The previous studies have demonstrated persistent deficits on attention and information processing tasks that stress performance under time pressure or emphasize maintenance of vigilance over relatively long intervals. In contrast, the presence of irrelevant, potentially distracting information does not disproportionately perturb the performance of head-injured patients (after resolution of PTA) in comparison with control subjects (Miller and Cruzat, 1981).

Recovery of Speech and Language

Frank aphasic disorder is relatively rare after CHI, whereas linguistic disturbance, as reflected by performance on standardized tests of expressive and receptive language, is a frequent sequel during the early stages. Studies of consecutive admissions for CHI have indicated that about 2% of patients are unequivocally aphasic, a finding that is influenced by the occurrence of mass lesions involving the dominant hemisphere. Levin and co-workers (1979) investigated the long-term outcome (approximately one year) of acute, unequivocal aphasia in 21 CHI patients and found that nine (43%) had full recovery of language. The remaining patients were divided nearly equally between those who exhibited a specific defect (usually anomia or generally decreased word finding) and those with residual impairment of both expressive and receptive skills with concurrent cognitive impairment. Subtle, persisting linguistic defects include paucity of verbal description and spontaneous speech and difficulty in the use of antonyms, synonyms, and metaphors (Thomsen, 1975).

In head-injured patients who are clinically nonaphasic, residual defects in word finding (fluency), naming, writing to dictation, and comprehension of complex, multistage commands are common in survivors of severe CHI, including patients with putative "diffuse" injury (Levin, Grossman, and Kelly, 1976; Sarno, 1980). Anomic disturbance and/or difficulty in word finding were present during the initial hospitalization in nearly one-half of 50 consecutive admissions for head injury studied after resolution of PTA (Levin et al., 1976). Dysarthria, which can range from minor articulation problems to nearly unintelligible, linguistically correct speech, is the most common nonaphasic speech disturbance.

The intrahemispheric locus of left hemisphere mass lesions is an important determinant of acute linguistic deficit, whereas the duration of coma (and by inference, the severity of diffuse cerebral insult) is related to linguistic functioning in the later stages of recovery. As depicted in Figure 5-6, Levin et al. (1981) found a nearly linear relationship between naming performance evaluated about one year after injury and duration of coma in CHI patients who had been acutely aphasic, whereas the lateralization of mass lesion had only a minor effect.

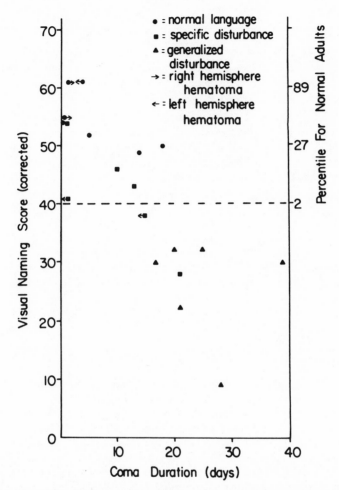

FIG. 5-6. Visual naming scores corrected for age and education plotted against duration of coma for patients with specific linguistic defect, generalized aphasia, and normal language examined at least six months postinjury. (Reprinted with permission from Levin HS, et al., 1981.)

CONCLUSIONS

Indices of widespread brain insult such as the GCS and durations of coma and PTA currently provide the most useful prognostic information for neurobehavioral outcome. Advances in neuroimaging techniques (e.g., magnetic resonance imaging, positron emission tomography) will also contribute to our understanding of the relationships between the presence and localization of intracranial mass lesions, alterations in regional brain metabolism, and recovery. The course and recovery of intellectual function over the first 6 to 12 months after head injury is one of impressive gain with more gradual improvement during later stages. However, subtle changes in memory, attention, and behavioral adaptation may continue for two years or more after injury. Memory deficit, reduced speed of information processing, inflexibility in problem solving, and language disturbance impose major constraints on the quality of life, even in cases with seemingly adequate intelligence on standardized tests. The emergence of rehabilitation programs dedicated to traumatic brain injury presents a challenge for investigators to determine the most effective techniques for remediating these neurobehavioral sequelae and developing compensatory strategies.

REFERENCES

Alexandre A, Colombo F, Nertempi P, Benedetti A (1983): Cognitive outcome and early indices of severity of head injury. *Journal of Neurosurgery* 59:751–761.

Barona A, Reynolds CR, Chastain R (1984): A demographically based index of premorbid intelligence for the WAIS-R. *Journal of Consulting and Clinical Psychology* 52:885–887.

Benson DF, Gardner H, Meadows JC (1976): Reduplicative paramnesia. *Neurology* 26:147–151.

Benson DF, Geschwind N (1967): Shrinking retrograde amnesia. *Journal of Neurology, Neurosurgery, and Psychiatry* 30:539–544.

Benton AL (1968): Differential behavioral effects in frontal lobe disease. *Neuropsychologia* 6:53–60.

Brooks DN (1972): Memory and head injury. *Journal of Nervous and Mental Disease* 155:350–355.

Buschke H, Fuld PA (1974): Evaluating storage, retention, and retrieval in disordered memory and learning. *Neurology* 24:1019–1025.

Butters N, Cermak LS (1980): *Alcoholic Korsakoff's syndrome: An information-processing approach to amnesia.* New York: Academic Press.

Cermak LS (1984): The episodic-semantic distinction in amnesia. In Squire LR, Butters N (eds.), *Neuropsychology of memory.* New York: The Guilford Press.

Cermak LS, Butters N, Gerrein J (1973): The extent of the verbal encoding ability of Korsakoff patients. *Neuropsychologia* 11:85–94.

Eslinger PJ, Damasio AF (1985): Severe disturbance of higher cognition following bilateral frontal ablation: Patient EVR. *Neurology* 38:1731–1741.

Ewing R, McCarthy D, Gronwall D, Wrightson P (1980): Persisting effects of minor head injury observable during hypoxic stress. *Journal of Clinical Neuropsychology* 2:147–155.

Gennarelli TA, Spielman GM, Langfitt TW, Gildenberg PL, Harrington T, Jane JA, Marshall LF, Miller TD, Pitts LH (1982): Influence of the type of intracranial lesion on outcome from severe head injury. A multicenter study using a new classification system. *Journal of Neurosurgery* 56:26–32.

Geschwind N (1982): Disorders of attention: A frontier in neuropsychology. *Philosophical Transactions of the Royal Society of London* 298:173–185.

Gilchrist E, Wilkinson M (1979): Some factors determining prognosis in young people with severe head injuries. *Archives of Neurology* 36:355–358.

Goldstein FC, Gary Jr. HE, Levin HS (1986): Assessment of the accuracy of regression equations proposed for estimating premorbid intellectual functioning on the Wechsler Adult Intelligence Scale. *Journal of Clinical and Experimental Neuropsychology* 8:405–412.

Goldstein FC, Levin HS (1987): Disorders of reasoning and problem-solving ability. In Meier M, Diller L, Benton A (eds.). *Neuropsychological rehabilitation*. New York: The Guilford Press.

Goldstein FC, Levin HS (1986): Intellectual and academic recovery in closed head injured children and adolescents. *Developmental Neuropsychology* 1:195–214.

Grant DA, Berg EA (1948): A behavioral analysis of degree of reinforcement and ease of shifting to new responses in a Weigl-type card sorting problem. *Journal of Experimental Psychology* 38:404–411.

Gronwall D, Sampson H (1974): *The psychological effects of concussion*. Auckland: Auckland University Press.

Gronwall D, Wrightson P (1974): Delayed recovery of intellectual function after minor head injury. *Lancet* 2:605–609.

Hannay HJ, Levin HS, Grossman RG (1979): Impaired recognition memory after head injury. *Cortex* 15:269–283.

Jennett B, Snoek J, Bond MR, Brooks N (1981): Disability after severe head injury: Observations on the use of the Glasgow Outcome Scale. *Journal of Neurology, Neurosurgery, and Psychiatry* 44:285–293.

Jennett B, Teasdale G (1981): *Management of head injuries*. Philadelphia: F.A. Davis Company.

Jones-Gottman M, Milner B (1977): Design fluency: The invention of nonsense drawings after focal cortical lesions. *Neuropsychologia* 15:653–674.

Levin HS, Benton AL (1984): Neuropsychologic assessment. In Baker AB (ed.), *Clinical Neurology*. Philadelphia: Harper & Row.

Levin HS, Benton AL, Grossman RG (1982): *Neurobehavioral consequences of closed head injury*. New York: Oxford University Press.

Levin HS, Eisenberg HM (1986): The relative durations of coma and posttraumatic amnesia after severe non-missile head injury: Findings from the pilot phase of the National Traumatic Coma Data Bank. In Miner M, Wagner K (eds.), *Neural trauma: Treatment, monitoring and rehabilitation issues*. Stoneham, MA: Butterworth Publishers.

Levin HS, Goldstein FC (1986): Organization of verbal memory after severe closed-head injury. *Journal of Clinical and Experimental Neuropsychology* 8:643–656.

Levin HS, Goldstein FC, High Jr. WM (1987): Distinction of amnesic disorder versus general cognitive impairment after closed head injury. Presented at the Tenth Annual European Meeting of the International Neuropsychological Society, Barcelona, Spain, July, 1987.

Levin HS, Grossman RG, Kelly PJ (1976): Short-term recognition memory in relation to severity of head injury. *Cortex* 12:175–182.

Levin HS, Grossman RG, Rose JE, Teasdale G (1979): Long-term neuropsychological outcome of closed head injury. *Journal of Neurosurgery* 50:412–422.

Levin HS, Grossman RG, Sarwar M, Meyers CA (1981): Linguistic recovery after closed head injury. *Brain and Language* 12:360–374.

Levin HS, Handel SF, Goldman AM, Eisenberg HM, Guinto Jr. FC (1983): Magnetic resonance imaging after "diffuse" nonmissile head injury: A neurobehavioral study. *Archives of Neurology* 42:963–968.

Levin HS, High Jr. WM, Goethe KE, Sisson RA, Overall JE, Rhoades HM, Eisenberg HM, Kalisky Z, Gary Jr. HE (1987a): The Neurobehavioral Rating Scale: Assessment of the behavioral sequelae of head injury by the clinician. *Journal of Neurology, Neurosurgery, and Psychiatry* 50:183–193.

Levin HS, High WM, Meyers CA, Von Laufen A, Hayden MD, Eisenberg HM (1985): Impairment of remote memory after closed head injury. *Journal of Neurology, Neurosurgery, and Psychiatry* 48:556–563.

Levin HS, Mattis S, Ruff RM, Eisenberg HM, Marshall LF, Tabaddor K, High Jr. WM, Frankowski RF (1987b): Neurobehavioral outcome following minor head injury: A three-center study. *Journal of Neurosurgery* 66:234–243.

Levin HS, O'Donnell VM, Grossman RG (1979): The Galveston orientation and amnesia test: A practical scale to assess cognition after head injury. *Journal of Nervous and Mental Disease* 167:675–684.

Mandleberg IA (1975): Cognitive recovery after severe head injury. 2. Wechsler Adult Intelligence Scale during post-traumatic amnesia. *Journal of Neurology, Neurosurgery, and Psychiatry* 38:1127–1132.

Mandleberg IA (1976): Cognitive recovery after severe head injury. 3. WAIS verbal and performance IQs as a function of post-traumatic amnesia duration and time from injury. *Journal of Neurology, Neurosurgery, and Psychiatry* 39:1001–1007.

Mandleberg IA, Brooks DN (1975): Cognitive recovery after severe head injury. I. Serial testing on the Wechsler Adult Intelligence Scale. *Journal of Neurology, Neurosurgery, and Psychiatry* 38:1121–1126.

Massey EW, Coffey CE (1983): Frontal lobe personality syndromes: Ominous sequelae of head trauma. *Postgraduate Medicine* 73:99–106.

McKinlay WW, Brooks DN, Bond MR, Martinage DP, Marsall MM (1981): The short-term outcome of severe blunt head injury as reported by relatives of the injured persons. *Journal of Neurology, Neurosurgery, and Psychiatry* 44:527–533.

Meyers CA, Levin HS, Eisenberg HM (1983): Early versus late ventricular enlargement following closed head injury. *Journal of Neurology, Neurosurgery, and Psychiatry* 46:1092–1097.

Miller E, Cruzat A (1981): A note on the effects of irrelevant information on task performance after mild and severe head injury. *British Journal of Clinical Psychology* 20:69–70.

Narayan RK, Greenberg RP, Miller JD, Enas GG, Choi SC, Kishore PRS, Selhorst JB, Lutz HA, Becker DP (1981): Improved confidence of outcome in severe head injury. *Journal of Neurosurgery* 54:751–762.

Nelson HE (1976): A modified card sorting test sensitive to frontal lobe defects. *Cortex* 12:313–324.

Oddy M, Coughlan T, Tyerman A, Jenkins D (1985): Social adjustment after closed head injury: A further follow-up seven years after injury. *Journal of Neurology, Neurosurgery, and Psychiatry* 48:564–568.

Oddy M, Humphrey M (1980): Social recovery during the year following severe head injury. *Journal of Neurology, Neurosurgery, and Psychiatry* 43:798–802.

Oddy M, Humphrey M, Uttley D (1978): Subjective impairment and social recovery after closed head injury. *Journal of Neurology, Neurosurgery, and Psychiatry* 41:611–616.

Overall JE, Gorham DR (1962): The brief psychiatric rating scale. *Psychological Reports* 10:799–812.

Parker SA, Serrats AF (1976): Memory recovery after traumatic coma. *Acta Neurochirurgica* 34:71–77.

Prigatano GP (1987): Personality and psychosocial consequences after brain injury. In Meier MJ, Benton AL, Diller L (eds.). *Neuropsychological Rehabilitation*. New York: Churchill Livingstone.

Prigatano GP, Fordyce DJ, Zeiner HK, Roueche JR, Pepping M, Wood BC (1984): Neuropsychological rehabilitation after closed head injury in young adults. *Journal of Neurology, Neurosurgery, and Psychiatry* 47:505–513.

Rimel RW, Giordani B, Barth JT, Boll TJ, Jane JA (1981): Disability caused by minor head injury. *Neurosurgery* 9:221–229.

Rosenthal M (1983): Behavioral sequelae. In Rosenthal M, Griffith ER, Bond MB, Miller JD (eds.). *Rehabilitation of the head injured adult*. Philadelphia: F.A. Davis Company.

Russell WR (1932): Cerebral involvement in head injury. *Brain* 55:549–603.

Russell WR (1935): Amnesia following head injuries. *Lancet* 2:762–763.

Russell WR, Nathan PW (1946): Traumatic amnesia. *Brain* 69:183–187.

Russell WR, Smith A (1961): Post-traumatic amnesia in closed head injury. *Archives of Neurology* 5:4–17.

Sarno MT (1980): The nature of verbal impairment after closed head injury. *Journal of Nervous and Mental Disease* 168:685–692.

Shapiro K (ed.). (1983): *Pediatric Head Trauma*. New York: Futura Publishing Co., Inc.

Stuss DT, Benson DF (1986): *The frontal lobes*. New York: Raven Press.

Symonds C (1937): Mental disorder following head injury. *Proceedings of the Royal Society of Medicine* 20: 1081–1094.

Tabaddor K, Mattis S, Zazula T (1984): Cognitive sequelae and recovery course after moderate and severe head injury. *Neurosurgery* 14:701–708.

Teasdale G, Jennett B (1974): Assessment of coma and impaired consciousness: A practical scale. *Lancet* 2:81–84.

Thomsen IV (1975): Evaluation and outcome of aphasia in patients with severe closed head trauma. *Journal of Neurology, Neurosurgery, and Psychiatry* 38:713–718.

Thomsen IV (1977): Verbal learning in aphasic and non-aphasic patients with severe head injuries. *Scandinavian Journal of Rehabilitation Medicine* 9:73–77.

Tsuang MT, Boor M, Fleming JA (1985): Psychiatric aspects of traffic accidents. *American Journal of Psychiatry* 142:538–546.

Tulving E (1972): Episodic and semantic memory. In Tulving E, Donaldson W (eds.). *Organization of Memory*. New York: Academic Press.

Uzzell BP, Zimmerman RA, Dolinskas CA, Obrist WD (1979): Lateralized psychological impairment associated with CT lesions in head injured patients. *Cortex* 15:391–401.

Van Zomeren AH, Deelman BG (1978): Long-term recovery of visual reaction time after closed head injury. *Journal of Neurology, Neurosurgery, and Psychiatry* 41:452–457.

Van Zomeren AH, Van Den Burg W (1985): Residual complaints of patients two years after severe head injury. *Journal of Neurology, Neurosurgery, and Psychiatry* 48:21–28.

Wechsler D (1955): *Manual for the Wechsler Adult Intelligence Scale.* New York: Psychological Corporation.

Wechsler D (1981): *Manual for the Wechsler Adult Intelligence Scale—Revised.* New York: Psychological Corporation.

Weingartner H, Cohen RM, Murphy DL, Martello J, Gerdt C (1981b): Cognitive processes in depression. *Archives of General Psychiatry* 38:42–47.

Weingartner H, Kaye W, Smallberg S, Ebert MH, Gillin JC, Sitram N (1981a): Memory failures in progressive idiopathic dementia. *Journal of Abnormal Psychology* 90:187–196.

Wilson RS, Rosenbaum G, Brown G (1979): The problem of premorbid intelligence in neuropsychological assessment. *Journal of Clinical Neuropsychology* 1:49–53.

6

Behavioral Dimensions of Traumatic Brain Injury

Gregory O'Shanick, M.D.

Departments of Psychiatry and Rehabilitation Medicine, Medical College of Virginia Hospitals, Virginia Commonwealth University, Richmond, Virginia, U.S.A.

Without question, behavioral changes that arise following traumatic brain injury (TBI) are the most enduring consequences of this event (Thomsen, 1984). The full range of one's individual "style" resides in the brain. Here, neurochemical and neurophysiological events provide the biologic substrate for those coping strategies (mechanisms of defense) that are of interest to behavioral scientists. Integration of these coping strategies into more elaborate, predictable patterns of behavior, given certain consistent provocation, results in the observable social interaction of the individual. This triad of biologic, psychologic, and social determinants of behavior is underscored in traumatic brain injury. Stated simply, alterations in behavior could result from changes in any of these areas. Damage to that portion of the brain responsible for understanding and expressing emotion in speech (aprosodia) would impact upon communication of stress to the environment. The profound psychologic trauma encountered in the catastrophic event which culminated in TBI could result in Post-Traumatic Stress Disorder (PTSD), which would complicate the recovery process. Profound social changes that occur as a result of loss of vocational productivity impact upon the patient and family following traumatic brain injury.

Development of research strategies to assess the behavioral dimension of traumatic brain injury requires the cooperation of psychiatrists, neuropsychologists, psychologists, neuropathologists, basic neuroscientists, epidemiologists, and other behavioral specialists to adequately address the behavioral components of traumatic brain injury. The interagency agreement now in place among the National Institute of Mental Health (NIMH), the National Institute on Disability and Rehabilitation Research (NIDRR), and the National Institute of Neurologic and Communicative Diseases and Stroke (NINCDS) is one such example of the high level of integration needed to address these issues. Given the heterogeneity of individuals who sustain TBI, large multicentered series will most likely be required to validate findings of evaluation, treatment, or outcome studies.

What, then, is the best strategy for defining these behavioral changes? As these changes evolve over time, a longitudinal understanding of the entire TBI spectrum is essential. This spectrum includes evaluation of premorbid factors; injury type; postinjury complications; treatment received during medical attention; environmental factors before, during, and after injury; and toxic exposure of the central nervous system to abusable substances, environmental toxins, or other biologic agents.

PREMORBID/DEVELOPMENTAL FACTORS

Ample evidence indicates that TBI is not a random event among humans (Frankowski, 1986). Age factors, risk-taking factors, and impulsivity factors have been identified as premorbid traits of large groups of TBI victims. Further definition of premorbid psychobehavioral profiles of high-risk groups would permit the elaboration of more specific intervention strategies. Such specificity would render these interventions more cost-effective. Studies addressing compliance with these intervention strategies would aid in the large-scale application of these in a broader public health program. Traumatic brain injury presents in a most clear and compelling fashion one of the first preventive psychiatry paradigms. There are potential health behavior and health education studies for TBI prevention. Other psychiatric disorders that have an element of "predictability" (e.g., bereavement, catastrophic loss, PTSD) would receive direct and indirect benefits from such TBI studies. Assessment of the impact of TBI upon a family's development is essential (Romano, 1974). Studies of the spouses and children of TBI victims may provide important insights regarding vulnerability to psychiatric disturbances.

PATHOPHYSIOLOGIC STUDIES

While pathophysiologic studies may technically be the more appropriate province of neuroscientists and neurosurgeons, the *applied behavioral studies* of pathophysiologic alteration *must involve psychiatry.* Psychiatry's previous experience with the definition of neurochemical and neuroanatomic changes in syndromes, such as schizophrenia, that were previously considered to be "functional" in origin permit the application of these strategies to behavior change following TBI. Evidence is accumulating regarding profound neurochemical, neurophysiologic, and neuroanatomical changes, which are seen with great regularity among neurobehavioral syndromes after TBI (Bakay, Sweeney, Wood, 1986; O'Shanick, 1987). The use of invasive and noninvasive techniques to define these physiologic alterations is essential. Positron emission tomography with appropriate chemical markers to define structural correlates of behavioral syndromes has demonstrated utility in defining brain-behavior relationships (Phelps, Mazziotta, and Huang, 1982). Other technologies that have demonstrated regional changes in psychiatric syndromes include regional cerebral blood flow (Barclay, Zemcov, Reichert, et al., 1985; Gur, Gur, Obrist, et al., 1987), evoked potentials (Morstyn, Duffy, McCarley, 1983; Kutcher, Blackwood, St. Clair, et al., 1987), brain electrical activity mapping (BEAM) (Morihisa, Duffy, and Wyatt, 1983), and polysomnography (Reynolds and Kupfer, in press). Studies such as these can and should be combined with specific and nonspecific pharmacological challenges to clarify not only resting but also activated central nervous system response following TBI. Expansion of research regarding changes that evolve over time must define those occurring spontaneously as well as those that change with therapeutic intervention. Such an understanding will define "treatment windows" and key intervention points following TBI. The use of complex, familiar sensory stimulation would also provide invaluable data regarding the developmental acquisition of primary interpersonal attachments, environmental attachments, and group attachments.

The complicating or enhancing effects of drugs present at injury must be explored. Evidence that correlates more ultimate impairments with preexisting substance abuse exists (Reilly, Kelley, and Faillace, 1986). Conversely, presence of certain chemicals that impede cholinergic activity has been shown to be beneficial regarding long-term outcome following experimentally induced TBI (Hayes, Stonnington, Lyeth, et al., 1986). Linkage of active and passive evaluative methods is essential and could be accomplished through combinations of drug studies and electrophysiologic studies, drug studies and behavioral challenges, behavioral challenges and electrophysiologic studies, etc.

To date, no definitive evaluation has been promulgated for mild, moderate, or severe TBI from a behavioral standpoint. Clearly, the generation of such an evaluative standard would assist with the wide-scale accumulation of data from large multicenter population studies and provide statistical strength.

Critical assessment of the epidemiology of TBI in "treatment resistant" chronically mentally ill patients and in those individuals currently residing in state mental health, mental retardation, and substance abuse facilities is imperative to permit more appropriate and cost-effective interventions for these individuals. While the rehabilitation cost and ordeal for the "average" TBI patient are extreme, one can only imagine the added duress of preinjury psychiatric illness (e.g., schizophrenia, bipolar disorder, mental retardation) upon the ultimate outcome of the individual.

INTERVENTION STUDIES

While the above studies will provide insight into the natural history of TBI-induced behavioral changes, the ultimate question remains: What, if any, intervention or combination of interventions will alter the behavioral outcome in a positive direction? The devastation wrought by traumatic brain injury has left many TBI patients and their families desperate for any intervention, whether well substantiated or flagrantly fraudulant. It becomes essential that high-quality intervention studies be conducted under the auspices of scientifically neutral research organizations to permit scientifically valid conclusions to be reached.

Few standardized treatment protocols have been critically studied regarding TBI-induced behavior change. Small case studies and anecdotal reports create the preponderance of the current scientific literature (O'Shanick, Parmelee, in press). Standardized treatment protocols to ascertain the efficacy of psychotropic agents in the treatment of aggressive behavior, memory impairment, affective/sleep disturbances, and attention/concentration impairment following TBI would add substantially to the existing body of knowledge and yield direct patient benefits. Once again, given the heterogeneity of the population studied, large-scale assessment studies (similar to the NINCDS Barbiturate Coma Study) would be required. Psychotherapeutic interventions for behavior problems following TBI would also require such large-scale proportions to validate findings. The use of neuropsychological testing and neurophysiologic studies as outcome measures for these psychotherapeutic interventions is encouraged. Evaluation of individual, group, and family psychotherapeutic techniques in dealing with behavior change following TBI is indicated (Forssmann-Falck, Christian, in press). Assessment of behavioral methods versus pharmacologic methods for substance abuse treatment in patients following TBI is critical given the high correlation between substance use/abuse and TBI (Bond, 1984; Reilly, Kelley, Faillace, 1986).

As brain topographical mapping becomes more refined, investigation into methods of regional pharmacotherapy through the use of reservoirs or site-specific cannula would be in order. Definition of precursor treatment strategies for behavior syndromes following TBI would also yield potential benefit. Basic methodologic issues relating to tissue availability of these compounds must first be addressed and overcome.

FINANCING BEHAVIORAL TREATMENT

While not the ultimate consideration in health care, certainly one of the more current problems resides with the escalating cost of "cutting edge" services. This cost escalation can be readily observed in the proliferation of private sector treatment facilities for traumatic brain injury over the past ten years (Vogenthaler, 1987). As the burden of financing this treatment can readily exhaust even the most extensive reserves, ascertainment of cost-efficacy of intervention versus nonintervention at various points in time following TBI may have merit. The need for natural history studies of TBI-induced behavior change will provide insight regarding spontaneous remissions versus intervention-induced change in either a positive or negative fashion. The education of clinical personnel regarding TBI behavioral sequelae is also indicated given the dearth of such material appearing in current professional education. The financing of these educational endeavors again must be borne by someone. Strategies for assessing educational competence in this area could be patterned after other consultation liaison endeavors as conducted in the past by NIMH.

CONCLUSIONS

Behavior change following traumatic brain injury is an untapped area of research in biologic, psychologic, and social aspects of this phenomenon. Psychiatrists, given their medical training combined with their appreciation for psychosocial variables in behavior, become the best professionals for directing assessment and intervention of the behavior changes following traumatic brain injury. Now that psychiatry has once again revived its identity as a medical subspecialty, and has rediscovered its roots in neurobehavioral evaluation, the contemporary psychiatrist will bring an appreciation of the multiple determinants of behavior. This understanding will greatly aid in intervention and assessment of the behavioral aspects of traumatic brain injury. Prevention of unnecessary psychiatric morbidity and mortality will be the ultimate outcome of such a national research initiative.

REFERENCES

Bakay RAE, Sweeney KM, Wood JH (1986): Pathophysiology of cerebrospinal fluid in head injury: Part I. *Neurosurgery* 18:234–243.

Barclay L, Zemcov A, Reichert W, Blass JP (1985): Cerebral blood flow decrements in chronic head injury syndrome. *Biologic Psychiatry* 20:146–157.

Bond M (1984): The psychiatry of closed head injury. In Brooks N (ed.). *Closed Head Injury: Psychological, Social, and Family Consequences.* Oxford: Oxford University Press.

Forssmann-Falck R, Christian F (in press): The use of group therapy as a treatment modality for behavioral change following head injury. *Psychiatric Medicine.*

Frankowski, RF (1986): Descriptive epidemiologic studies of head injury in the United States: 1974–1984. *Advances in Psychosomatic Medicine* 16:153–172.

Gur RC, Gur RE, Obrist WD, Skolnick BE, Reivich M (1987): Age and regional cerebral blood flow at rest and during cognitive activity. *Archives of General Psychiatry* 44:617–621.

Hayes RL, Stonnington HH, Lyeth BG, Dixon CE, Yamamoto T (1986): Metabolic and neurophysiologic sequelae of brain injury: A cholinergic hypothesis. *Central Nervous System Trauma* 3:163–173.

Kutcher SP, Blackwood DHR, St. Clair D, Gaskell DF, Muir WJ (1987): Auditory P300 in borderline personality disorder and schizophrenia. *Archives of General Psychiatry* 44:645–650.

Morihisa JM, Duffy FH, Wyatt RJ (1983): Brain electrical activity mapping (BEAM) in schizophrenic patients. *Archives of General Psychiatry* 40:719–728.

Morstyn R, Duffy FH, McCarley RW (1983): Altered P300 topography in schizophrenia. *Archives of General Psychiatry* 40:729–734.

O'Shanick GJ (1987): Closed head injuries. In Michels, RM (ed.). *Psychiatry.* Philadelphia: Lippincott.

O'Shanick GJ, Parmelee, DX (in press): Psychopharmacologic agents in the treatment of brain injury. In Christensen AL, Ellis DW (eds.). *Neuropsychologic Treatment of Head Injury.* Boston: Martinus Nijhoff.

Phelps, ME, Mazziotta JC, Huang S (1982): Review: Study of cerebral function with positron computed tomography. *Journal of Cerebral Blood Flood and Metabolism* 2:113–162.

Reilly EL, Kelley JT, Faillace LA (1986): Role of alcohol use and abuse in trauma. *Advances in Psychosomatic Medicine* 16:17–30.

Reynolds CF, Kupfer DJ (in press): Sleep research in affective illness: State-of-the-art circa 1987. *Sleep.*

Romano MD (1974): Family response to traumatic head injury. *Scandinavian Journal of Rehabilitation Medicine* 6:1–4.

Thomsen IV (1984): Late outcome of very severe blunt head trauma: A 10–15 year second follow-up. *Journal of Neurology, Neurosurgery, and Psychiatry* 47:260–268.

Vogenthaler DR (1987): An overview of head injury: Its consequences and rehabilitation. *Brain Injury* 1:113–127.

III

Neural Recovery

7

A Conceptual Approach to Neural Recovery

Paul Bach-y-Rita, M.D.

Department of Rehabilitation Medicine, University of Wisconsin Medical School, Madison, Wisconsin, U.S.A.

Following brain damage, some recovery usually takes place. But what are the mechanisms of the recovery and how can maximum recovery be obtained? To date there has been little attention paid to the theoretical basis of recovery, and most rehabilitation procedures are not based on scientific findings.

A scientific body of knowledge has been gathering over the last 30 years that is particularly pertinent to brain rehabilitation. Appropriate studies are required to bring this knowledge into the clinic in the form of new rehabilitation procedures in areas such as physical, behavioral, educational, and pharmacological therapy. In this chapter I will briefly review some of the historical factors that have delayed the development of scientifically based rehabilitation, and will discuss some of the scientific findings that are particularly pertinent to brain rehabilitation.

HISTORICAL CONCEPTS OF RECOVERY POTENTIAL

The evolution of neuroscience has had significant influence on the field of brain rehabilitation. For about 100 years, following Broca's (1861) demonstration of a specific area in the left temporal cortex related to speech, neuroscience was dominated by concepts of strict point-to-point localization of function. The rigid concepts excluded recovery or reorganization potential, and thus no recovery was expected following brain damage (except for some recovery due to the resolution of local factors such as edema and tissue debris). Thus, rehabilitation was not in the mainstream of neurological sciences. These issues have been discussed further elsewhere (Bach-y-Rita, 1988).

Rehabilitation was relegated to being primarily a practitioner's art, generally aiming to obtain compensatory function rather than neural reorganization or recovery. Methodologies were developed by trial and error and by clinical observations rather than by scientific studies. The problems of developing scientifically validated rehabilitation procedures have been compounded by the difficulty of undertaking good rehabilitation research. Among the problems are the following: inaccurate lesion localization and the matching of research groups; inaccurate quantification and measurement of functional improvement; inappropriate application of statistical methods; long time-course of recovery; high cost of the labor-intensive procedures; rehabilitation usually occurring during the first year when some "spontaneous" recovery is occurring with the result that no accurate baseline is present against which the value of the specific procedure can be measured (but see below, section on late rehabilitation, and chapter in this volume by Balliet); a large number of factors, such as environmental and psychosocial, influencing outcome. Some of these have been discussed elsewhere (e.g., Bach-y-Rita, 1980, 1981).

All during the "dark ages" (from the perspective of a rehabilitation neuroscientist!) of neuroscience, there were a few scientists interested in the capacity of the brain to reorganize following damage, and a few of them were interested in rehabilitation (discussed in Bach-y-Rita, 1988). However, in the last 30 years, interest in the potential for recovery has led to scientific studies (cf. Finger and Stein, 1982; Cotman and Nieto-Sampedro, 1985; Bach-y-Rita, 1980, 1981, 1988) revealing the capacity for recovery of function and exploring the mechanisms of the recovery. Brain plasticity studies have now come of age, and exciting results are appearing continuously (see also chapters in this volume by Balliet, by Papanicolaou, and by Boyeson).

BRAIN PLASTICITY

Brain plasticity has been defined very broadly, in which case all learning would be included in the concept, or very narrowly, requiring evidence of morphological changes such as neuronal sprouting. I consider a middle position to be approrpiate, and have defined it as ". . . the adaptive capacities of the central nervous system—its ability to modify its own structural organization and functioning" (Bach-y-Rita, 1980). It permits an adaptive (or a maladaptive) response to functional demand. Konorski (1961) considered plasticity to be one of the two fundamental properites of the nervous system: it permits enduring functional changes to take place. Konorski considered the other fundamental property to be excitability, which relates to rapid changes leaving no trace in the nervous system. Mechanisms of brain plasticity can include neurochemical, endplate, receptor, and neuronal structural changes.

Some Mechanisms Underlying Brain Plasticity

We have recently reviewed the literature on mechanisms of recovery (Bach-y-Rita et al., 1988), and it has been discussed extensively elsewhere (e.g., Bach-y-Rita, 1980, 1981; Finger and Stein, 1982). Therefore, only a brief summary will be provided here.

Sprouting. Sprouting is the growth from a cell body to another cell as a consequence of normal growth, a vacancy at a particular site, or a return to a particular site. Collateral sprouts are new axonal processes that have budded off an uninjured axon and grown to a vacated synaptic site. It has been shown to occur in the central nervous system. However, sprouting can be adaptive or maladaptive, and its role in recovery from brain damage is still uncertain.

Denervation supersensitivity. Denervation supersensitivity results in a permanent increase in neuronal responsivity to diminished input. The receptor site may become more sensitive to a neurotransmitter, or the receptors may increase in numbers. This may be a factor in the central nervous system reorganization.

Behavior compensation. Following brain damage, new combinations of behaviors can develop. For example, a patient may use different groups of muscles or cognitive strategies.

Unmasking. Quiescent neuronal connections that are inhibited in the normal state may be unmasked following brain damage. This may be an important mechanism of recovery of function. Negative effects of unmasking may also occur. For example, reflexes that were normal in infancy but had become inhibited during development, such as the Babinski reflex, are considered pathological when they reappear, having been unmasked by the lesion.

Models of Brain Plasticity

Animal models of brain plasticity are numerous and many have been discussed in the publications above. These include the demonstration by Chow and Steward (1972) that following lid suture of one eye of a kitten during the few critical months of vision development (which usually leads to permanent blindness in that eye), appropriate rehabilitation not only led to some functional recovery but also produced morphological changes in the lateral geniculate body and physiological changes in the visual cortex. Other studies have shown the role of appropriate environments in recovery from brain damage (Rosenzweig, 1980) and the effect on the recovery of function of specific neurotransmitters following brain damage when combined with appropriate physical rehabilitation (see Chapter 9 in this volume).

Human models include the demonstration that following the loss of a major sensory input (e.g., vision), a tactile sensory substitution system can deliver information from a TV camera which the brain can be taught to interpret as "visual" information. Blind persons not only develop the ability to perceive visual information but use visual means of analysis (parallax, looming and zooming, monocular clues of depth and perspective, and subjective spatial localization). This model has served to provide a considerable amount of information on brain plasticity, perceptual mechanisms, the coordination of sensory and motor factors in the development of a *perceptual organ,* and other data (cf. Bach-y-Rita, 1972; Bach-y-Rita and Hughes, 1985). It is also being used as a means to develop visual spatial concepts in congenitally blind children. Tactile sensory substitution systems are under development for persons with other sensory losses (e.g., deafness; insensate feet and hands) as well as for sensory augmentation (e.g., for space suit gloves for extravehicular space activities of astronauts) (Bach-y-Rita et al., 1987).

The intensive study of the recovery of brain-damaged persons with an appropriate rehabilitation procedure several years following the lesion provides an excellent model of brain plasticity. In such cases, since the brain-damaged persons are no longer recovering spontaneously (as demonstrated by an appropriate battery of studies delivered several times over a period of a year), an accurate baseline can be obtained from which to measure the effects of the rehabilitation. This model is further discussed by Balliet in this volume.

THE IMPLICATIONS FOR CLINICAL MANAGEMENT OF BRAIN-DAMAGED PERSONS

Well-designed studies related to brain plasticity and recovery of function will undoubtedly lead to the evaluation and refinement of present rehabilitation methodologies and the development of new rehabilitation techniques. Such studies are not only needed in regard to the mechanisms of recovery from brain damage but in all aspects of rehabilitation. These include learning theory (discussed in Bach-y-Rita, 1980, 1981); specific neurotransmitters and neurotrophic factors to minimize the damage immediately following the lesion and in the later management of the patient; environmental, behavioral, and psychosocial aspects of the rehabilitation program as well as the prevention of brain damage (this latter is undoubtedly the most important aspect epidemiologically). Furthermore, the availability of scientifically sound results will lead clinicians to order and apply the validated methodologies and the third party payors to appropriately reimburse the therapy. It will also lead to more scientifically literate rehabilitation clinicians with a greater understanding of the means to obtain recovery of function. It is, however, important that in the process of developing rehabilitation into a more scientifically sound field, we do not lose the human values and the caring that are such important parts of this field.

REFERENCES

Bachy-y-Rita P. *Brain mechanisms in sensory substitution.* New York: Academic Press, 1972, p. 192.

Bach-y-Rita P. (ed). *Recovery of function: theoretical considerations for brain injury rehabilitation.* Bern: Hans Huber, 1980.

Bach-y-Rita P. Brain plasticity as a basis for the development of rehabilitation procedures for hemiplegia. *Scand J Rehabil Med* 13:73, 1981a.

Bach-y-Rita P. Brain plasticity. In: *Rehabilitation medicine.* J Goodgold (ed.), New York: C.V. Mosby Co., 1988, pp. 113–118.

Bach-y-Rita P, Lazarus JC, Boyeson MG, Balliet R, Myers T. Neural aspects of motor function as a basis of early and post-acute rehabilitation. In: *Rehabilitation medicine: principles and practice.* DeLisa J, Currie D, Gatens P, Leonard J, McPhee M (eds.), Philadelphia: J.B. Lippincott Pub., 1988, pp. 175–195.

Bach-y-Rita P, Hughes B. Tactile vision substitution: some instrumentation and perceptual considerations. In: *Electronic spatial sensing for the blind.* Warren C, Strelow E (eds.), Dordrecht, The Netherlands: Martinus-Nijhoff Pub., 1985.

Bach-y-Rita P, Webster J, Tompkins W, Crabb T. Sensory substitution for space gloves and for space robotics. In: *Proceedings of 1986 Space Telerobotics Workshop.* G. Rodriquez (ed.), Pasadena: Jet Propulsion Laboratories, pub. 87–13, Vol. II, 1987, pp. 51–57.

Broca P. Nouvelle observation d'aphemie produite par une lesion de la 3ᵉᵐᵉ circonvolution frontale. *Bull Soc Anat* 6 (2ᵉᵐᵉ Serie), 1861, pp. 398–407.

Chow KL, Steward DL. Reversal of structural and functional effects of long-term visual deprivation in cats. *Exp Neurol* 34:409, 1972.

Cotman CW, Nieto-Sampedro M. Progress in facilitating the recovery of function after central nervous system trauma. Hope for a new neurology. *Ann NY Acad Sci* 457:83–104, 1985.

Finger S, Stein DG. *Brain damage and recovery: research and clinical perspectives.* Orlando, FL: Academic Press, 1982.

Konorski J. *The physiological approach to the problem of recent memory. Brain mechanisms and learning.* Oxford: Blackwell Press, 1961, pp. 115–132.

Rosenzweig M. Animal models for effects of brain lesions and for rehabilitation. In: *Recovery of function: theoretical considerations for brain injury rehabilitation.* Bach-y-Rita P (ed.), Bern: Hans Huber, 1980, pp. 127–172.

8

Structural Aspects
of Brain Injury

J.T. Povlishock, Ph.D.

*Department of Anatomy, Medical College of Virginia,
Richmond, Virginia, U.S.A.*

Until recently the basic understanding of the brain's morphopathologic response to traumatic brain injury was limited and, in fact, sometimes biased by various popular yet unproved assumptions. In general, it has been assumed that when the brain is insulted by a traumatic insult, such as typically occurs with either vehicular accidents or falls, an avalanche of structural changes ensue. Most clinicians have assumed that all structural damage seen with traumatic brain injury occurs immediately and involves an irreversible series of changes, most of which are refractile to therapeutic intervention. Overall, in view of these factors, the clinical impression of traumatic brain injury has been rather grim with little hope existing for any significant rehabilitation/recovery of brain-injured individuals, particularly those sustaining severe traumatic insults. It is well known that when traumatic brain injury occurs, focal areas of the brain which impact upon the bony cranial cavity become contused. Similarly, it is known that the intracranial vessels, physically tethered and fixed in their course, are vulnerable to the shear and tensile forces of injury and thus tear, leading to the formation of large hematomas and/or more discrete forms of intraparenchymal hemorrhage. Such hemorrhage, in concert with other traumatically induced perturbations of the blood-brain barrier, obviously contributes to the genesis of local tissue damage. In severe cases, edema develops and results in increased intracranial pressure, which exerts a devastating impact upon the brain parenchyma by further impeding cerebral blood flow. Furthermore, should the patient sustain a secondary insult associated with hypotension and/or hypoxia, the brain parenchyma can be damaged further by diffuse hypoxic/ischemic change. Together with all the above described changes, direct traumatically induced damage to the brain parenchyma also has been observed. Typically, the presence of axon retraction balls (reactive axonal swellings), scattered throughout the brain, has suggested to many that the shear and tensile forces of injury immediately tear axons, causing them to retract and expel a ball of axoplasm. Evidence of such traumatically induced axonal damage also has been supported by the finding of Wallerian degeneration and gliosis. Collectively, then, traumatic brain injury has been envisioned to entail focal contusion, hemorrhage, and diffuse brain parenchymal disruption, all of which contribute to the morbidity and mortality associated with the injury. Such structural changes have been believed to occur in severe, moderate, and even minor injury, with the overall magnitude and extent of distribution of such changes decreasing with the severity of injury. As all these events have been assumed to occur immediately upon impact, little consideration has been given to the potential for evolving and therefore therapeutically amenable change. Additionally, since most injuries have been thought to involve focal tissue damage as well as hemorrhage, which in itself would cause additional tissue destruction, the conditions and environment appropriate for neuroplastic change/reorganization, described in the experimental literature, simply did not seem operant in the case of head-injured man. Therefore, in view of these rather negative impressions, the rationale for pursuing rigorous rehabilitative efforts appeared rather poorly grounded. Although contemporary thought on the general nature of those brain parenchymal and vascular changes which occur with traumatic brain injury has remained unaltered from that described above, considerable change has occurred in the contemporary appreciation of the genesis, temporal progression, and reorganization of the traumatically induced damage. Such change has been influenced primarily by findings obtained in studies of experimental animal models of traumatic brain injury. However, new information gleaned from the postmortem examination of head-injured humans as well as new data obtained from imaging studies also have helped reshape our appreciation of the morphopathological consequences of head injury.

Consistent with both the goals and format of this volume, I will address, in the following passages, those issues which have recently altered thought on the morphological consequences of traumatic brain injury. Following a consideration of these features, the focus of the chapter will shift to provide insight into new research needed to resolve many of the key questions in this area.

NEW FINDINGS IN TRAUMATIC BRAIN INJURY

As noted in the above passages, traumatic brain injury, in addition to contusion and hemorrhage, has long been associated with occurrence of direct brain parenchymal damage reflected primarily in damage to axons. Varying degrees of traumatically induced axonal damage have been described in cases of severe, moderate, and even minor brain injury (Strich, 1961; Adams, 1977; Pilz, 1983). In general, it has been assumed that the shear and tensile forces associated with the traumatic event physically tear axons throughout the neuraxis. In the past, most clinicians have considered that such axonal damage always occurred in concert with various forms of vascular damage. Thus, little enthusiasm could be generated for the importance of any observed axonal damage when it seemed reasonable to conclude that any concomitant vascular damage would have the most adverse impact upon outcome. Within the last 5 years, however, many began to question the overall correctness of this assumption. Due, in part, to the experimental animal model work of Gennarelli et al. (1982) and the detailed human postmortem evaluations conducted by Adams et al. (1982), it became apparent that axonal damge in itself was a significant consequence of trauma and, as such, appeared to bear a direct relationship to the patients' and/or experimental animals' functional status (Gennarelli et al., 1982; Adams et al., 1982). Importantly, as such axonal injury could occur without concomitant significant vascular damage, it was inferred that the overall number of axons damaged was the determining factor in predicting the severity of the ensuing functional abnormalities (Adams et al., 1982; Gennarelli et al., 1982). In general, diffuse axonal damage was visualized in the corpus callosum, the subcortical white matter, and the cerebellar peduncles as well as dispersed throughout the midbrain, pons, and medulla. Within these fiber systems, damaged axons could be recognized adjacent to other intact axons as well as unaltered intraparenchymal vessels. Although the functional status of these related axons, which appeared morphologically intact, is not known, it is reasonable to speculate that even they could have been at least transiently perturbed with injury, thereby also contributing to the initially observed functional abnormalities. Although little speculation was given to explain the genesis of the observed axonal damage, most clinicians have ascribed to the hypothesis that all damaged axons were immediately torn at the time of injury (Gennarelli et al., 1982; Strich, 1961).

At the same time that the above studies were performed in humans and animals receiving relatively severe head injuries, our laboratory demonstrated the occurrence of axonal damage even in the case of minor injury, wherein concomitant vascular damage was not a consideration (Povlishock et al., 1983). Such studies confirmed the finding that varying amounts of axonal damage are a consistent feature of traumatic brain injury. Importantly, however, our studies also conclusively rejected the hypothesis that axons are immediately torn by the traumatic insult and then retract expelling a ball of axoplasm, the retraction ball. Rather, our studies, through the evaluation of anterograde axoplasmic transport, coupled with ultrastructural analyses, revealed that the traumatic event initially perturbed the axolemma at a singular focus along its length. The physical source of such axolemmal perturbation has not been critically evaluated; however, our working hypothesis suggests that traumatically induced stretch is a factor pivotal in its genesis. As, in both animals and man, long-tract decussating fibers appear to have a predilection for injury and as such fibers would appear the most likely to be stretched with injury, this argument appears compelling. Following the observed axolemmal perturbation, a local impairment in axoplasmic transport occurred and, over a course of several hours postinjury, this resulted in a local accumulation of organelles and axoplasm. With continued survival, the locus of axonal injury demonstrated a continued accumulation of organelles accompanied by dramatic focal axonal swelling. Such swelling progressed to focal lobulation with ultimate separation of the damaged axon into a locally swollen axon forming a reactive swelling, the retraction ball, in continuity with the cell body and a distally swollen and detached axonal segment that rapidly manifested Wallerian change. In general, 12 to 24 hours were required for this sequence of evolving axonal change; and when observed, this sequence of events occurred in axons interspersed among other axons or cell bodies displaying no sign of abnormality. Collectively, these findings challenge the concept that tissue tearing with immediate frank axonal disruption is the necessary consequence of traumatic brain injury. Recently, in a series of unpublished observations, we have reevaluated these axonal phenomena in animals subjected to either moderate or severe traumatic brain injury. In these animals, similar patterns of axonal change were observed. Although their rate of progression was somewhat accelerated in comparison to the minor traumatic state, the fact remains that no evidence for immediate traumatically induced axonal tearing could be found, once again suggesting a reevaluation of traditional thought on this issue. Interestingly, limited reports in the human literature suggest that in traumatically injured man, many hours must elapse postinjury before any evidence of reactive axonal swellings, retraction balls, can be found (Pilz, 1983); and therefore, this delayed appearance of axonal swellings in man would suggest that the same conditions described in experimental animals are also operant in humans.

Although this sequence of traumatically induced change must be considered fascinating, the key question from the rehabilitation/recovery perspective would obviously center on the fate of such damaged axons and their target structures. When axons are damaged with traumatic brain injury, they generally occur in clusters coursing within otherwise unaltered tracts and/or nuclear groups (Povlishock, 1986). With injuries of increasing severity, the overall proportion of damaged axons per tract or nuclei increases; yet, the damaged axons still coexist with other unaltered axonal and neuronal elements. Due to the more limited and diffuse nature of the axonal damage, gliosis is minimal; and as intraparenchymal hemorrhage is not commonly associated with the axon damage, it does not pose a confounding problem. Thus, in the case of traumatic brain injury, particularly minor and moderate, one encounters damaged axons positioned in a relatively intact brain microenvironment, which from the theoretical perspective should be ideal for supporting posttraumatic neuronal connectivity.

To explore the fate of the damaged axons in such an environment, we have followed them over 3 months posttrauma (Povlishock and Becker, 1985; Povlishock and Kontos, 1985). As noted above, those axonal segments in continuity with the cell body initially display local dramatic swelling, the reactive swelling or retraction ball, while the more distal, detached segment undergoes Wallerian change. The ensuing degeneration of the distal segment elicits deafferentation of the respective target sites, which due to the clustering of such axonal damage can, in some cases, be rather extensive in specific loci (unpublished findings). In fact, within some identified target sites dramatic focal dendritic restructuring most likely linked to deafferentation can be observed within several weeks of the traumatic event. Typically, in specific areas of the target nuclei, dendrites become varicose and laden with autophagic vacuoles and myelin figures, all of which appear consistent with a deafferentation-induced response. While these dendritic changes are occurring, both damaged and intact axons mount a sustained and dramatic regenerative response. Within the first week posttrauma, many of the reactive axonal swellings give rise to numerous sprouts. Over time, these same axonal swellings give rise to growth cone processes. With the appearance of both growth cones and sprouts, the reactive swellings decrease in size as their axoplasmic volume is redirected into the new outgrowths. With continued survival, both the sprouts and growth cones are found to enter the substance of the adjacent brain parenchyma and, frequently, they are recognized to course within the collapsed distal axonal segments undergoing Wallerian change. To date, these reactive/regenerative changes have been followed over a 3-month period. By all standards such persistent regenerative effects within the mammalian central nervous system (CNS) must be considered truly unique, as all have previously adhered to the belief that CNS regeneration proves rapidly abortive. It is intriguing that the regenerative effort seen in the brain-injured animals appears remarkably similar to that described for regenerating peripheral nerves (Friede and Bischhausen, 1983) and regenerating amphibian spinal cord (Stensaas, 1983). The reason for this sustained regeneration in brain-injured animals is unclear; but perhaps the diffuse pattern of axonal injury seen with brain injury, coupled with the retention of a relatively normal brain environment, allows this unprecedented regenerative effort. Concomitant with these events, many intact axons near the deafferentated sites manifest reactive synaptogenesis (sprouting), which obviously leads to the return of synaptic input into the previously deafferentated site. Thus, traumatic brain injury can be recognized to involve considerable posttraumatic neuronal rearrangement. Perhaps, with minor and moderate injury, this reactive/regenerative effort is associated with an adaptive restructuring consistent with recovery; whereas with severe injury, these efforts are maladaptive in nature.

SYNTHESIS AND NEW PERSPECTIVES FOR RESEARCH ENDEAVORS

We believe that a convincing case has been made for the predilection for axonal injury with various forms of traumatic brain injury. Based upon the above cited animal and human studies, it is apparent that axonal damage is perhaps the most consistent feature of minor and moderate traumatic brain injury and, clearly, widespread axonal damage is a consistent feature of severe traumatic brain injury. In case of minor and moderate injury, it would appear reasonable to conclude that the initial posttraumatic morbidity associated with these insults is linked to the overall magnitude of the traumatically induced axonal damage, while in the case of severe injury, large-scale axonal damage also must contribute to the ensuing functional abnormalities. This is not to say that neither contusion, petechial hemorrhage, nor mass lesions play any role in influencing the resulting functional abnormalities; yet, at the risk of being pedagogical, we would caution that it appears tenuous to assume that all the sequelae of traumatic brain injury represent the sum of the resulting focal lesions. Obviously, when mass lesions occur with severe head injury, they exert a major role in influencing outcome; yet, when mass lesions are not present, a case can be made that axonal damage constitutes the most consistent feature linked with functional outcome. Perhaps, the overall consistency of axonal damage in human traumatic brain injury can be gleaned from a critical analysis of the previously cited work of Pilz (1983). In this study, Pilz histologically examined the brains of 324 unselected cases of severe head injury, excluding all brain foci that revealed any evidence of focal lesions. Through such an approach Pilz identified reactive axonal swellings and retraction balls in various brain loci in 100 of 324 cases evaluated. Although this finding seems inconsistent with the concept that axonal damage is a consistent feature of brain injury, reevaluation of his data suggests otherwise. It is noteworthy that in 107 cases in which axonal damage was not observed the patients had survived for less than 12 hours. As our experimental work (Povlishock et al., 1983) suggests that at least 12 hours of survival are required for the genesis of the reactive swellings, Pilz's findings appear all the more consistent with our basic beliefs. Additionally, since Pilz's study also failed to observe reactive axonal swellings in an additional 13 patients who survived more than 4 weeks, this negative finding is entirely consistent with our experimental data which demonstrate that as the swellings give rise to both sprouts and growth cones, their volume is significantly reduced. Thus, it is easy to appreciate why large histologically identifiable reactive swellings were not seen with increased survival. Assuming, then, that an additional 120 individuals in Pilz's study sustained axonal damage, this would argue strongly that axonal damage is a consistent feature of traumatic brain injury.

Although the above findings are of interest, the ultimate question, as noted earlier, still centers on the issue of the overall meaning of this finding for the rehabilitation of brain-injured humans. The finding that such axonal damage requires a several-hour period for the development of frank axonal detachment and swelling indicates that a temporal therapeutic window exists during which one perhaps can intervene to blunt the progression of the axonal damage and thereby improve the outcome. Admittedly, due to our fragmentary knowledge of the precise subcellular events causing this progressive reactive axonal change, it is difficult to speculate on a specific therapeutic strategy, at this point. Yet, as our knowledge evolves in this area, it is an obvious issue for detailed evaluation in well-controlled animal models.

Another issue of particular merit from the rehabilitation/recovery perspective centers on both the further characterization and potential augmentation of the sustained regenerative response manifested by reactive swellings and the reactive synaptogenesis (sprouting) displayed by intact fibers. In our estimation, the sustained regenerative efforts seen in experimental studies of minor and moderate injury are neurobiologically unprecedented and suggest that in brain injury, conditions may exist which make it unique from other forms of brain insult. The observation of damaged axons interspersed in a relatively unaltered brain environment poses a biologically unique situation. Would it not seem appropriate to follow in such regenerating fibers the potential beneficial effects of a myriad of drugs purported to expedite neural growth and elongation? Although the criticism may be raised that innumerable investigators have tried such drugs in various experimental paradigms, with limited success at best, we would argue that the situation of brain injury presents such a totally new and different experimental situation as to mandate their reevaluation. Traditionally, such drug studies have entailed the production of focal lesions which generally have involved tissue sectioning with resulting frank tissue disruption, hemorrhage, gliosis, and collagen ingrowth. As these overt tissue responses are not typically related to the axonal damage seen with traumatic brain injury, a reevaluation appears warranted. It would be of considerable interest to determine if continued and targeted neurite outgrowth can be achieved following brain injury.

In relation to the issue of reactive synaptogensis (sprouting) involving undamaged fibers, we would also submit that there is need for its continued investigation in the situation of traumatic brain injury. Although the issue of reactive synaptogenesis (sprouting) and neural plasticity has been evaluated over the past 25 years (for reviews see Davis, 1985; Marshall, 1985), once again most information related to this issue has been gleaned from animal model systems in which relatively large invasive focal lesions were the primary method of deafferentation for the induction of sprouting. As previously observed, the rather widespread nonfocal axonal damage seen with traumatic brain injury may also create a situation somewhat different from the past experimental approaches. With minor injury, wherein relatively few damaged fibers are interspersed among undamaged fibers of similar type, it is easy to conceive how sprouts from the anatomically and functionally related intact fibers could reinnervate a region to restore appropriate connections and function. To carefully evaluate this issue, immunocytochemical studies examining the loss and return of various neurotransmitter populations within a specific target site would appear to constitute a meaningful approach and, at present, preliminary work in our laboratory has suggested the correctness of this assumption. With moderate traumatic brain injury, the more widespread axonal damage could result in the situation whereby sprouts from anatomically yet nonfunctionally related fibers enter the target nuclei, causing some maladaptive reinnervation. Lastly, with severe head injury this situation would appear to become all the more exacerbated and thereby partially explain the relatively poor recovery. Although all these hypotheses require extensive evaluation in the experimental setting, they obviously do appear to constitute areas worthy of aggressive research.

In summary, this chapter has attempted to dispel the notion that the anatomical response of the brain to trauma is but a collection of focal parenchymal and vascular lesions. Emphasis has been placed on the consistency of widespread axonal damage in cases of severe, moderate, and minor traumatic brain injury. Moreover, considerable import has been attached to the fact that the ultimate traumatically induced axonal detachment requires at least 12 hours for its genesis. The observation of the sustained and dramatic regenerative attempts that occur following traumatic brain injury suggests that a template for recovery exists. Perhaps, as more information is gathered regarding the anatomical and functional connectivity of both the regenerating axons and the sprouting intact fibers, strategies can be devised to manipulate, influence, and direct their targeted growth. Admittedly, this is not a trivial task; yet, the very description of such phenomena in traumatic brain injury offers the hope for recovery and the potential beneficial effect thereupon of various rehabilitative efforts.

Acknowledgment: The experimental work reported herein was supported by NIH grant NS-20193.

REFERENCES

Adams JH, Michell DE, Graham DI, Doyle D (1977): Diffuse brain damage of immediate impact type. *Brain* 100:489–502.

Adams JH, Graham DI, Murray LS, Scott G (1982): Diffuse axonal injury due to non-missile head injury in humans: An analysis of 45 cases. *Annals of Neurology* 12:557–563.

Davis JN (1985): Neuronal rearrangements after brain injury: A proposal classification. In: *Central nervous system traumatic status report—1985,* Povlishock JT, Becker DP, eds. Richmond: William Byrd Press, pp. 491–501.

Friede RL, Bischhausen R (1980): The five structures of stumps of transected nerve fibers in subserial sections. *Journal of Neurological Science* 44:181–192.

Gennarelli JA, Thibault LE, Adams JH, Graham DI, Thompson CS, Marcincin RP (1982): Diffuse axonal injury and traumatic coma in the primate. *Annals of Neurology* 12:564–575.

Marshal JF (1985): Neural plasticity and recovery of function after brain injury. *International Review of Neurobiology* 26:201–247.

Pilz P (1983): Axonal injury in head injury. *Acta Neurochirgica Supplement* 32:119–124.

Povlishock JT, Becker DP, Cheng CLY, Vaughan GW (1983): Axonal change in minor head injury. *Journal of Neuropathology and Experimental Neurology* 42:225–242.

Povlishock JT, Becker DP (1985): Fate of reactive axonal swellings induced by head injury. *Laboratory Investigation* 52:540–552.

Povlishock JT, Kontos HA (1985): Continuing axonal and vascular change following experimental brain trauma. *Central Nervous System Trauma* 2:285–298.

Povlishock JT (1986): Traumatically induced axonal damage without concomitant change in focally related neuronal somata and dendrites. *Acta Neuropathologica* 70:53–59.

Stensaas LJ (1983): Regeneration in the spinal cord of the newt notophalmus

(Triturus) pyrrhogaster. In: *Spinal cord reconstruction.* Kao CC, Bunge RP, Rier PH (eds.) New York: Raven Press.

Strich SJ (1961): Shearing of nerve fibers as a cause of brain damage due to head injury. *Lancet* 2:443–448.

9

Neurotransmitter Aspects of Traumatic Brain Injury

Michael G. Boyeson, Ph.D.

Department of Rehabilitation Medicine, Medical Science Center, Madison, Wisconsin, U.S.A.

In recent years, considerably more attention has been focused on the mechanisms of recovery from traumatic brain injury. In part, this resurgence is due to scientific developments that allow for more refined analyses of brain processes, e.g., positron emission tomography (PET) and nuclear magnetic resonance (NMR) scans and electrophysiological and neurohistochemical techniques. Nevertheless, the brain remains the most exquisitely complex of all human structures and will probably be the last structure to be thoroughly understood. The number of theoretical mechanisms proposed to explain recovery of function, e.g., sprouting, denervation supersensitivity, compensation, reorganization, vicariation, diaschisis, etc., reflects the basic complexity of the brain. Since empirical evidence has been given for all of the theoretical mechanisms, it is probably the case that the recovery of function represents a process that relates, to some degree, all of the proposed mechanisms.

The importance of understanding the mechanisms of recovery of function following traumatic brain injury is not trivial. Over 500,000 brain-injured patients are admitted annually to hospitals in the United States, and the economic and emotional burden is staggering on all people touched by brain injury (Anderson and McLauren, 1980; Langfitt and Gennarelli, 1981). Any intervention that can be shown to facilitate recovery of function from brain injury, and thereby reduce the emotional and economic impact of the injury, would be welcomed by those involved in the rehabilitation.

However, while much of medicine concerns itself with pharmacological treatments to alleviate symptoms from disease conditions, it is surprising how little attention has been directed toward alleviating functional deficits of traumatic brain injury through pharmacological means. Rehabilitation rarely utilizes pharmacological intervention to facilitate recovery from brain injury. Generally only secondary consequences of brain injury, e.g., bleeding, edema, and metabolic perturbations (Langfitt and Gennarelli, 1982; Kotila et al., 1984), are treated to limit the spread of brain damage, although not without some controversy (Hossman, 1983; Marshall, 1974). It might be noted also that some drugs administered to brain-injured patients for symptomatic reasons may have detrimental effects on later recovery (Feeney et al., 1982; Porch and Feeney, 1986; Schallert et al., 1986). The resistance to a neuropharmacological treatment of traumatic brain injury probably has multiple reasons, beginning with a common root of a rigid structure/function conceptualization of the brain. Another branch of this resistance relates to the many empirical observations on the lack of significant and functionally relevant regrowth of tissue following traumatic brain injury in adults. Still another branch of resistance relates to the rapidity of developments in relevant basic science compared to the slowness encountered in the application of the findings in a clinical setting. In some respects this reflects methodological difficulties and/or a lack of desire or training among clinicians to experimentally extend the findings to a clinical setting. In other respects it reflects a general inertia to change the status quo, which is common to all fields.

ACETYLCHOLINE AND BRAIN INJURY

Despite the above limitations, I would like to present evidence (some of which has been around for a good number of years) indicating that beneficial effects may be achieved with pharmacological manipulation of neurotransmitters in brain-injured patients.

Sciclounoff, in the 1930s, was one of the first scientists to attempt pharmacologically to alleviate some of the functional deficits of brain injury by administering a drug that effected cholinergic transmission in the brain. Acetylcholine, the first neurotransmitter to be characterized, when stimulated, produced marked improvements in the prognosis for stroke recovery and reductions in mortality rates. The improvement was particularly enhanced for patients who were given concomitant physical therapy with the drug treatment. This important physical therapy by drug interaction will be addressed more fully in a later section, since it appears to represent a critical element in facilitating (or retarding) recovery from traumatic brain injury.

In a more controlled laboratory setting, Ward and Kennard (1942) attempted to replicate the improvement in motor function findings in monkeys with motor cortex injuries. By administering drugs that block the breakdown of acetylcholine, thereby leaving more available to brain tissue, the investigators found some motor improvement compared to undrugged control animals. This lack of a strong effect may be due to methodological problems in the study or may relate to the time or duration of the drug administration (immediately after injury in the case of Ward and Kennard). A drug may not have the same effect immediately after an injury as it would later; e.g., the stimulant drug amphetamine, if given to cats too early after traumatic brain injury, results in death, yet later administration promotes recovery (Hovda and Feeney, 1984). For various reasons, an injury to neurons may produce the release of the stored neurotransmitter in excess amounts, which later may return to normal or subnormal amounts. This may help explain why pretreatment with antagonists to the cholinergic system prior to a brain injury may improve neurological outcome in animals if given close to the time of injury (Lyeth et al., 1985; Dixon et al., 1984). Additionally, recent evidence has suggested that the increased excitatory neurotransmission during the "acute" phase of an injury may produce deleterious effects on later recovery (Simon et al., 1984).

Finally, some mention should be made of Luria's work on facilitating recovery from brain-injured patients that was conducted in Russia. Luria and his colleagues (Luria, 1963; Luria et al., 1969) have reported beneficial effects of treating patients with neostigmine for motor recovery and galanthamine for aphasia. It is difficult to fully evaluate Luria's claims since methodological information is inaccessible, but his claims have been supported in general by other investigators (see above) and warrant further investigation. In interpreting the data, Luria made the distinction between primary damage (actual neuronal loss) and a secondary inhibition of intact neurons at some distance from the primary injured site, a conceptual stance similar to that of Von Monakow in 1914. Luria indicated that the cholinergic drugs were presumably acting to "de-block" the secondary inhibitor and allowing for functional recovery. The pharmacological removal of remote functional depressions of intact structures (a diaschisis-like effect) as a basis for recovery of function following brain injury has recently been resurrected and placed on firmer experimental grounds by Feeney and his collaborators (Feeney et al., 1982; Hovda and Feeney, 1984; Feeney et al., 1985; Boyeson et al., 1986).

CATECHOLAMINES AND BRAIN INJURY

Under a variety of conditions, behaviors, and brain injuries, pharmacological manipulations of the catecholamine transmitters (norepinephrine and dopamine) have been shown to affect recovery outcomes following or prior to brain injury. Due to the vast data base, I refer the reader to several comprehensive reviews (Finger and Stein, 1982; Feeney and

Sutton, 1987; Marshall, 1985) on the role of catecholamines in recovery of function. This section will concentrate on the role of norepinephrine (NE) in recovery from sensorimotor cortex injury. It has been shown that drugs that stimulate NE systems promote recovery of motor function in animals (Feeney et al., 1982; Boyeson and Feeney, 1984; Boyeson et al., 1986; Feeney and Sutton, 1987) and humans (Davis et al., 1987). Moreover, drugs that antagonize the NE system have been shown to retard recovery of motor function when given early after injury (Boyeson, 1983; Feeney et al., 1982; Porch and Feeney, 1986) and reinstate deficits in animals long since recovered from sensorimotor cortex injuries (Hovda et al., 1983). The drug-dependent ability to pharmacologically reinstate deficits in recovered animals suggests that the brain remains in a vulnerable state. It is noteworthy that in accelerating or retarding functional recovery, a single dose of the drug can permanently affect recovery if the animal is given appropriate motor experience while under the influence of the drug (Feeney et al., 1982). If the drug is given and the animal immobilized for an 8-hour period, NE antagonists and agonists neither retard nor accelerate functional recovery from motor cortex injuries. Extrapolated to a rehabilitation setting, intense physical therapy and drug administration have resulted in accelerated recovery of motor function in stroke patients (Davis et al., 1987).

Recent research has indicated that injury to the sensorimotor cortex may not be directly involved in hemplegia. Following the finding that intraventricular infusion of NE, but not dopamine, facilitated motor recovery (Boyeson and Feeney, 1984), it was found that localized microinfusions of the neurotransmitter into the cerebellum contralateral to the injury were even more effective in acceleration of motor recovery (Boyeson et al., 1986). Significant acceleration of motor recovery was noted within 5 minutes after a single infusion of NE and the improvement in motor function was permanent. To understand this phenomenon, one must consider the vast ramifications of the intensively studied locus cereleus (LC), the major ascending NE pathway. A single cell in the LC simultaneously communicates with the contralateral cerebellum and the sensorimotor cortex on one side of the brain (Nagai et al., 1981). When brain injury impacts on the sensorimotor cortex, the terminal projecting fibers of the LC are also damaged, causing a shift from neurotransmitter production to protein synthesis for repair (Ross et al., 1975). The shift results in disturbances in NE functioning in the contralateral cerebellum due to the simultaneous innervation of both areas by single cells of the LC. If it is the case that motor disturbances are being mediated by depressive actions on the terminal LC projections to the cerebellum, then prior depletion of only cortical NE (which does not affect motor performance) to a sensorimotor cortex injury should provide protection from hemiplegia. Animals given a unilateral lesion of the dorsal bundle of the LC (which supplies cortical NE) leaves the cerebellum LC input intact. If in two weeks the animal is given a unilateral sensorimotor cortex injury, the animal is remarkably protected from the hemiplegia (Boyeson et al., 1987). On a theoretical level, these findings provide strong support for a diaschisis-like effect (remote disturbances in tissue following injury) in the hemiplegia observed after sensorimotor cortex injury. The results also provide a scientific rationale for the possible rapid alleviation of hemiplegia in patients with injuries to these areas through appropriate therapy and drug protocols.

EFFECTS OF GABA AND SEROTONIN ON BRAIN INJURY

The effects of the inhibitory neurotransmitter GABA on recovery of function from traumatic brain injury suggests that elevated levels of this transmitter are deleterious to the recovery process. Brailowsky (1986) found that infusion of the neurotransmitter into sensorimotor cortex resulted in marked motor deficits in animals. Consistent with these findings is that diazepam administered three times a day for 3 days and twice a day for 19 days after cortical injuries in a rat results in a permanent sensory neglect compared to the one-week recovery period for control animals (Schallert et al., 1986). These findings suggest that the benzodiazapines may be contraindicated in the acute phase of traumatic brain injury. Serotonin, like GABA, is an inhibitory neurotransmitter and has been found to be elevated in the plasma of stroke patients (Costa et al., 1974; Weintraub, 1985), and methysergide (a serotonin blocker) treatment has been suggested to be effective in ameliorating stroke symptoms, although the latter study was difficult to evaluate on methodological grounds (Weintraub, 1985).

CONCLUSIONS

Although it was not to be the subject of review for this chapter, the hopeful prospects of nerve grafting techniques (Bjorklund and Stenevi, 1985) may provide a way for constant infusions of neurotransmitters to patients with suspected specific needs, as is the case for the neurotransmitter dopamine in Parkinson's disease and acetylcholine in Alzheimer's disease (Friedman et al., 1981). Additionally, with the advent of new neurohistochemical techniques using monoclonal antibodies and recombinant DNA methods, considerable specificity of markers for neurotransmitters was enhanced compared to older techniques, leading to improved anatomical maps.

There are a number of factors that should be considered when utilizing pharmacological agents in the treatment of traumatic brain-injured patients. Following a traumatic brain injury, the drug may have different effects than prior to the injury. This phenomenon may take the form of altered sensitivity to the drug, either through a change in responsivity of brain tissue to denervation or through increased availability of the drug due to a compromised blood brain barrier (Edvinsson et al., 1976). Other variables that may affect outcome and can be pharmacologically manipulated include, but are not limited to, the psychological and physical state of the patient (Weber and Stelzner, 1977; Richey and Bender, 1977; Reinberg and Halberg, 1971), genetic variability in responsiveness to drugs (Bennett et al., 1973; Kalow, 1962), and environmental conditions (Sahlins, 1977; Seigel, 1976). In the final analysis, pharmacological treatment of brain-injured patients represents a multifactorial process and therapy may have to be tailored to each brain-injured individual.

In the foregoing sections, one is correctly left with the impression that multiple neurotransmitter disturbances occur after a traumatic brain injury. In the future, it will be necessary to tease out those neurochemical events that are correlated with traumatic brain injury from casual events involved in recovery processes. It is also important to realize that all of the neurotransmitter systems communicate with each other to varying degrees. The understanding of the anatomical and functional relationships between these neurotransmitters and the many other putative neurotransmitters not covered in this chapter is a task of staggering proportions, yet such an understanding will eventually be necessary for designing the most effective therapeutic protocols. Nevertheless, significantly effective neurotransmitter protocols for the treatment of brain injury are beginning to be developed in this country and elsewhere.

REFERENCES

Anderson DW, McLauren RL (1980): Report on the national head and spinal cord injury survey. *Journal of Neurosurgery* 53:S1.

Beller SA, Overall JE, Swann AC (1985): Effiacy of oral physostigmine in primary degenerative dementia. *Psychopharmacology* 87:147.

Bennett EL, Rosenzweig MR, Wu SYC (1973): Excitant and depressant drugs modulate effects of environment on brain weight and cholinesterase. *Psychopharmacologia (Berl.)* 33:309–328.

Boyeson MG (1983): *The role of norepinephrine in recovery of function following unilateral sensorimotor or neocortical cerebellar lesions in the rat.* Unpublished doctoral dissertation, University of New Mexico, Albuquerque.

Boyeson MG, Feeney DM (1984): The role of norepinephrine in recovery from brain injury. *Society for Neuroscience Abstracts* 10:68.

Boyeson MG, Krobert KA, Grade CM (in press): Cortical norepinephrine depletion protects animals from hemiparesis induced by sensorimotor cortex injury. *Society for Neuroscience Abstracts* 13:1665.

Boyeson MG, Krobert KA, Boyeson MG, Krobert KA, Hughes JM (1986): Norepinephrine infusions into cerebellum facilitate recovery from sensorimotor cortex injury in the rat. *Society for Neuroscience Abstracts* 12:1120.

Brailowsky S, Knight, RT, Blood K, Scabini D (1986): y-Aminobutyric acid-induced potentiation of cortical hemiplegia. *Brain Research* 362:322.

Costa JL, Ito U, Spatz M, Klatzo I, Demiriian C (1974): 5-Hydroxytryptamine accumulation in cerebrovascular injury, *Nature (Lond)* 248:135.

Davis JN, Crisostomo EA, Duncan PW, Propst M, Feeney DM (in press). Amphetamine and physical therapy facilitate recovery from stroke: Correlative animal and human studies. In *The 15th Princeton Conference on Cerebrovascular Disease.* New York: Raven Press.

Dixon CE, Lyeth BG, Giebel ML, Yamamoto T, Stonnington HH, Becker DP, Hayes RL (1985): Pretreatment with scopolamine accelerates recovery of locomotor functioning following cerebral concussion in the rat. *Society for Neuroscience Abstracts* 11:432.

Edvinsson L, Sercombe R (1976): Influence of pH and PCO2 on alpha-receptor mediated contractions in brain vessels. *Acta Physiologica Scandinavica* 97:325.

Feeney DM, Gonzalez A, Law WA (1982): Amphetamine, haloperidol and experience interact to affect rate of recovery after motor cortex injury. *Science* 217:855.

Feeney DM, Sutton RL (1987): Pharmacotherapy for recovery of function after brain injury. *CRC Critical Reviews in Neurobiology* 13:135–197.

Feeney, DM, Sutton RL, Boyeson MG, Hovda DA, Dail WG (1985): The locus coeruleus and cerebral metabolism: recovery of function after cortical injury. *Physiol Psychol* 13:197.

Finger S, Stein DG (1982): *Brain damage and recovery: Research and clinical perspectives.* New York: Academic Press.

Friedman E, Sherman KA, Ferris SH, Reisberg B, Bartus RT, Shenick MK (1981): Clinical response to choline plus piracetam in senile dementia: Relation to red cell choline levels. *New England Journal of Medicine* 304:1490.

Hossman KA (1983): Experimental aspects of stroke. In RW Ross Russel (ed.), *Vascular disease of the central nervous system* 73. Edinburgh: Churchill Livingston.

Hovda DA, Feeney DM (1984): Amphetamine with experience promotes recovery of locomotor function after unilateral frontal cortex injury in the cat. *Brain Research* 298:358.

Hovda DA, Feeney DM, Salo AA, Boyeson MG (1983): Phenoxybenzamine but not haloperidol reinstates all motor and sensory deficits in cats fully recovered from sensorimotor cortex ablations. *Society for Neuroscience Abstracts* 9:1001.

Kalow, W. (1962): *Pharmacogenetics: heredity and the response to drugs.* Philadelphia: WB Saunders.

Kotila M, Waltimo O, Niemi ML, Laaksonen R, Lempinen M (1984): The profile of recovery from stroke and factors influencing outcome. *Stroke* 15:1039.

Langfitt TW, Gennarelli TA (1982): Can the outcome from head injury be improved? *Journal of Neurosurgery* 53:11.

Luria AR (1963): *Restoration of function after brain injury* (B. Haigh, Trans.). New York: Macmillan.

Luria AR, Naydin VL, Tretkova LS, Vinarskaya EN (1969): Restoration of higher cortical functions following local brain damage. In PJ Vinken, GW Bruyn (eds.), *Handbook of clinical neurology 3* (Vol 3, p. 368). Amsterdam: North-Holland.

Lyeth BG, Dixon CE, Hamm RJ, Yamamoto T, Giebel ML, Stonnington HH, Becker DP, Hayes RL (1985): Neurological deficits following experimental cerebral concussion in the rat attenuated by scopolamine pretreatment. *Society for Neuroscience Abstracts* 11:432.

Marshall JF (1985): Neural plasticity and recovery after brain injury. In JP Smythies, RJ Bradley (eds.), *International review neurobiology* (Vol. 26, p. 201). New York: Academic Press.

Marshall JF (1985): Wonder drugs: fact or fiction? In RG Dacey, Jr., HR Winn, RW Rimel, JA Jane (eds.), *Trauma of the central nervous system* (p. 215). New York: Raven Press.

Nagai T, Satoh K, Imamoto K, Maeda T (1981): Divergent projections of catecholamine neurons of the locus coeruleus as revealed by fluorescent retrograde double labeling technique. *Neuroscience Letters* 23:117–123.

Porch BE, Feeney DM (in press): Effects of antihypertensive drugs on recovery from aphasia. *Clinical Aphasiology,* Minneapolis: BKR Publishers.

Reinberg A, Halberg F (1971): Circadian chronopharmacology. *Annual Review of Pharmacology* 11:445–492.

Richey DP, Bender AD (1977): Pharmacokinetic consequences of aging, *Annual Review of Pharmacology* 17:49–65.

Ross, RA, Joh TH, Reis DJ (1975). Reversible changes in the accumulation and activities of tyrosine hydroxylase and dopamine-beta-hydroxylase in neurons of nucleus locus coeruleus during the retrograde reaction. *Brain Research* 92:57–72.

Schallert T, Hernandez TD, Barth TM (1986): Recovery of function after brain damage: Severe and chronic disruption by diazepam. *Brain Research* 379:104.

Sciclounoff F (1934): L'acetylcholine dans le traitement de l'ictus hemiplegique. *Presse Medicine* 42:1140.

Simon RP, Swain JH, Griffiths T, Meldrum BJ (1984): Blockade of NMDA receptors may protect against ischemic damage in the brain. *Science* 226:850–852.

Von Monakow C (1969): 'Diaschisis,' the localization in the cerebrum and functional impairment by cortical loci, G Harris (Trans.). In KH Pribam (ed.), *Brain and behavior* vol 1: *Mood states and mind.* Baltimore: Penguin, p. 27.

Ward AA, Kennard MA (1942): Effect of cholinergic drugs on recovery of function following lesions of the central nervous system in monkeys. *Yale Journal of Biological Medicine* 15:189.

Weber ED, Stelzner DJ (1977): Behavioral effects of spinal cord transection in the developing rat. *Brain Research* 125:241–255.

Weintraub MI (1985): Methysergide (Sansert) treatment in acute stroke, community pilot study. *Angiology* 36:137.

10

Reorganization of Cerebral Function Following Lesions in the Left Hemisphere

Andrew C. Papanicolaou, Ph.D.,
Bartlett D. Moore, Ph.D., and
Georg Deutsch, Ph.D.

Division of Neurosurgery, The University of Texas Medical Branch, Galveston, Texas, U.S.A.

The most debilitating consequence of focal traumatic injury or stroke to the left, language-dominant hemisphere is aphasia. In the majority of aphasic patients, however, at least partial spontaneous recovery of language may occur within about a year. Although this phenomenon is quite common and occurs with all types of aphasia, its neurophysiological basis is poorly understood. One of the mechanisms that have been proposed to account for spontaneous recovery of language is functional reorganization of the brain involving a hemispheric dominance shift or increasing involvement of the relatively intact right hemisphere in mediating linguistic operations.

This chapter presents the results of our efforts to explore this hypothesis and determine the extent to which hemispheric dominance shift underlies linguistic recovery. Aside from the theoretical motives, serious practical considerations prompted us to undertake the studies to be summarized here. Specifically, at the present time, several types of language rehabilitation procedures are used. Some of those emphasize retraining of skills such as articulation that are mediated normally by the left hemisphere. Others are aimed at facilitation of language recovery via retraining of language-related operations, such as melodic intonation and imagery, which are most likely mediated by the right hemisphere. Consequently, we felt that information regarding the role of the right hemisphere in spontaneous restitution of language would be of value in the design of the appropriate rehabilitation strategies for individual trauma or stroke patients.

To assess patterns of hemispheric asymmetries and the relative degree of involvement of each hemisphere in language and language-related tasks we have used two physiological measures of cerebral activation, evoked potentials (EPs) and regional cerebral blood (rCBF), along with a measure of shift in ear advantage using a dichotic listening task. In the following sections I will (1) summarize some of the clinical and experimental evidence which indicates that following left hemisphere lesions, the relatively intact right hemisphere may assume some of the left hemisphere function; (2) describe the EP method used to assess the degree of hemispheric involvement in language and the results of its application to normal subjects and recovering aphasic patients; and (3) summarize dichotic listening and rCBF evidence of increasing right hemisphere participation in recovery from aphasia.

EVIDENCE SUGGESTING HEMISPHERIC DOMINANCE SHIFT

The idea that spontaneous restitution of function originally subserved by the compromised left hemisphere may be due to increasing proficiency of the right hemisphere in mediating that function is a specific case of the more general concept of neural plasticity and has been explored experimentally in animals in which functions are lateralized in one hemisphere. An exemplary series of studies of this kind has been carried out by Nottebohm and his associates using canaries. First, they demonstrated left hemisphere dominance for vocalization in these birds, and second, they found some evidence that restitution of singing behavior may involve a hemispheric dominance shift. They lesioned the tracheosyringealis branch of the right and left hypoglossus nerve and found differential effects on sound-spectrographic studies of canaries' song (Nottebohm and Nottebohm, 1976). Lesions involving the right hypoglossus modified or eliminated only one tenth of the syllables in the song repertoire of the canaries. However, lesions in the left tracheosyringealis nerve affected dramatically all syllables in the birds' vocal repertoire. These studies suggested an asymmetry for efferent control of vocalization in the canary. Central asymmetries were also demonstrated. Nottebohm, Strokes, and Leonard (1976) made unilateral lesions in the hyperstriatum ventricle that also showed differential effects: Left-sided lesions disturbed the quality of canary song, whereas right-sided lesions did not. These data indicate that the left hemisphere is specialized for song control.

Song recovery in these unilaterally lesioned animals showed that the song repertoire of right-hyperstriatum ventral-lesioned birds was equivalent to or superior to premorbid song characteristics. Left-lesioned animals' song included only a small number of syllables from premorbid song and the repertoire was, in general, smaller than that observed before the surgery in these animals. Interestingly, in birds that have had left hemisphere lesions early in life, subsequent lesions have the same effect as right-sided lesions in the intact birds (Nottebohm, 1984). These results suggest a certain amount of preprogramming of song control by the left hemisphere and, perhaps, that recovery is associated with a change in dominance to the right side when the left side is damaged.

Similarly, one of the mechanisms postulated to account for restitution of human language is the functional reorganization of the brain whereby homotopic structures in the intact nondominant hemisphere (usually the right hemisphere) are utilized to a greater or lesser extent, depending on particular circumstances, for language processing. The idea of shift of hemispheric dominance is attributed to Wernicke (1874) and was extended by Henschen (1922), Geschwind (1970), and Kinsbourne (1971). The possibility that the right hemisphere can, in fact, mediate language is supported by studies of commissurotomy (split-brain) patients, showing that the right hemisphere possesses some language-processing capabilities. However, direct evidence for right hemisphere involvement in recovery from aphasia derives mainly from the study of children with extensive left hemisphere damage and from clinical observations of adult aphasics. As early as the 1880s, Gowers observed that recovered aphasics who had sustained left hemisphere injuries relapsed following new lesions in the right hemisphere.

Kinsbourne (1971) has studied the effect of intracarotid injection of barbiturates in three aphasics with left hemisphere lesions. He found that injection into the left carotid artery did not affect residual speech in these patients, but injection into the right carotid resulted in arrest of speech of two of the three patients. More recently, Cummings, Benson, Walsh, and Levine (1979) reported recovery of language in a 54-year-old patient who was rendered globally aphasic due to extensive damage of his dominant left hemisphere after an embolic infarction. CT scans showed total destruction of the temporoparietal area of the dominant hemisphere. Therefore, the observed partial recovery of language in that patient was attributed to increased participation of his right hemisphere.

The role of the right hemisphere in restitution of language has also been inferred from the study of left hemidecortication, and hemispherectomy in infants and very young children who, despite total or nearly total incapacitation of their dominant hemisphere, develop apparently normal language.

The relative scarcity of unequivocal observations pertaining to shift of hemispheric dominance as one mechanism of language recovery after injury (e.g., trauma or infarct), as opposed to hemispherectomy, can be partly attributed to technical difficulties in directly establishing patterns of hemispheric asymmetries for language in the normal and injured brain. Recently, however, the establishment of patterns of hemispheric activity during a variety of linguistic and nonlinguistic cognitive tasks has become feasible through the use of cortical EPs and rCBF. The application of these procedures to the study of hemispheric reorganization in recovering aphasics will be detailed below.

PROBE EP STUDIES

Patterns of task-specific differential hemispheric activation have been obtained with the use of cortical EPs, especially in the context of the probe paradigm (Papanicolaou and Johnstone, 1985). This paradigm entails recording of EPs to an irrelevant probe stimulus (a tone or a flash of light) from left and right hemisphere sites during the performance of various cognitive tasks. When the task is purely linguistic, the amplitude of the probe EPs is attenuated significantly more over left hemisphere sites; whereas when the task involves nonlinguistic processing (e.g., visuospatial), the probe EPs show greater attentuation over the right hemisphere sites. It has been proposed that this task- and hemisphere-specific attentuation is due to competition for neuronal resources in the engaged hemisphere to process the probe stimulus and simultaneously perform the operations of the task (see, e.g., Papanicolaou, Levin, and Eisenberg, 1984).

Consistent patterns of regional brain activation indicating predominant left hemisphere involvement in language and predominant right hemisphere engagement in nonlinguistic tasks have been repeatedly obtained from normal dextral adult subjects. Significantly greater left hemisphere engagement has been observed during perception of speech, specifically, detection of phonetic and semantic targets embedded in the speech stream (Papanicolaou, 1980), performance of mental arithmetic tasks (Papanicolaou, Levin, Eisenberg, and Moore, 1983), production of covert speech (Papanicolaou, Eisenberg, and Levy, 1983), and writing (Galin and Ellis, 1975). Significantly greater right hemisphere activation has similarly been observed during perception of musical passages (Thomas and Shucard, 1983), perception of emotional content of speech conveyed by intonation (Papanicolaou, Levin, Eisenberg, and Moore, 1983), and performance of a block-design task (Galin and Ellis, 1975).

The reliability of the probe EP paradigm in revealing task-specific patterns of hemispheric asymmetries in normal subjects has encouraged its application to the study of development of hemispheric asymmetries in infants (Shucard, Shucard, and Thomas, 1977) and to the study of aberrant patterns of brain activation in children with developmental abilities. Moreover, the paradigm has been applied to the study of hemispheric activation in aphasic patients. Probe EP data (Selinger, Shucard, and Prescott, 1980) from five left-hemisphere-injured patients with varying degrees of linguistic impairment were collected during processing of verbal material. It was found that patients with mild language impairment displayed hemispheric activation patterns similar to those of normal subjects, but severely impaired patients displayed greater right hemispheric involvement. These preliminary data point to a shift of hemispheric control for language following injury to the language-dominant hemisphere.

Probe EP evidence of shift in hemispheric dominance for evidence has been obtained in our laboratory in a series of investigations involving closed focal head injury and stroke patients in the process of recovering from aphasia. In the first study of this series (Papanicolaou, Levin, and Eisenberg, 1984), six recovered aphasics (most with focal traumatic injuries in the left hemisphere), six nonaphasic diffuse injury patients, and eight normal volunteers were tested. EPs to probe click stimulus were recorded bilaterally from each subject and patient during a control condition of attending only to the click stimulus and during a verbal memory task involving encoding and silent rehearsal of a word list. During that task, EP amplitude attentuation occurred in the left hemisphere for the normal subjects (as expected) and for the nonaphasic patients but in the right hemisphere for the recovered aphasics. These contrasting asymmetries were interpreted as supporting the notion that the relatively intact right hemisphere is implicated in the spontaneous restitution of language.

To ascertain the reliability of these findings we repeated the experiment with four different groups of patients and control subjects (Papanicolaou, Moore, Levin, and Eisenberg, 1987). These consisted of a group of 11 recovering aphasics sustaining unilateral left hemisphere strokes, a group of 10 mild dysarthric patients sustaining mild strokes (primarily transient ischemic attacks), a group of 10 nonaphasic patients sustaining strokes in the right hemisphere, and a control group of 11 normal volunteers. In agreement with the previous study, the results of this investigation indicated greater right hemisphere activation in the recovering aphasics and, to a lesser degree, dysarthric patients and greater left hemisphere activation in both nonaphasic patients and normal control subjects.

Subsequently, we have applied the same probe EP method using a variety of language tasks including shadowing of word lists and phonological and semantic target detection in addition to the verbal memory task. We have collected EP data of cerebral activation during these tasks on 22 aphasics, 11 dysarthrics, 14 nonaphasic, right hemisphere stroke patients, and 20 normal control subjects. The results of this study (now nearing completion) are consistent with those previously reported. That is, the majority of the recovering aphasic patients show significantly greater right hemisphere activation in all language tasks whereas the nonaphasics, like the normal controls, demonstrate consistently the pattern of greater left hemisphere activation during the same tasks.

To further verify the phenomenon of increasing right hemisphere participation in language during recovery from aphasia and to cross-validate the EP procedure we have tested subgroups of the same patients using the rCBF procedure and a dichotic listening task. These procedures and the results of their application are presented in the next section.

rCBF AND DICHOTIC LISTENING STUDIES

rCBF, allowing assessment of local metabolic rates in the cortical convexity and, consequently, the degree of activation at the various brain regions during cognitive tasks, has become an important tool for investigating the issue of hemispheric reorganization of function, separately from or in conjunction with electrophysiological and behavioral procedures. The rCBF can be measured noninvasively by monitoring the buildup and washout of inhaled [133]Xenon gas in cerebral tissue with external scintillation detectors. Analysis of the xenon-desaturation curves yields values for gray matter flow in the cortical convexity, as well as several other indices of cerebral flow and tissue distribution (see, e.g., Obrist and Wilkinson, 1979). The interpretation of rCBF patterns as estimates of cortical activity levels is an accepted practice in normal subjects and most stabilized patients (Risberg, 1980) and is based on the fact that brain tissue regulates its blood supply in accordance with its metabolic demands (Sokoloff, 1977).

Studies of rCBF using the [133]Xenon inhalation technique have repeatedly shown differential hemispheric involvement in specific verbal and visuospatial tasks. The first major report of task-dependent asymmetries in hemispheric blood flow in a right-handed male subject was published by Risberg, Ali, Wilson, Wills, and Halsey (1975). These investigators showed greater increases of activity in the right hemisphere for a test of perceptual closure (visual task) and greater increase in the left hemisphere for a verbal reasoning test. Another study (Gur and Reivich, 1980) found similar results for the verbal test but reported greater right hemisphere increases during a perceptual-closure task only in the subjects who were most skilled on the test. These authors suggested that processing of verbal tasks may be more hard-wired to the left hemisphere, while spatial cognition is more affected by individual differences and situational variables.

Simple auditory stimulation has also been shown to result in hemispheric-flow asymmetries in normal subjects. One study (Knopman, Rubens, Klassen, Meyer, and Niccum, 1980) reported highly significant increases in rCBF in the posterior region of the left Sylvian fissuer during listening for word meaning. Another study reported left-right asymmetries in the rCBF in temporoparietal regions during listening to wood strings presented to one ear (Maximillian, 1982). Left or right ear stimulation resulted in higher flows in these regions of the left hemisphere.

Behavioral activation studies with stroke patients have shown an increase in rCBF, usually outside the lesion site, under several task condition (Ingvar and Risberg, 1967). Gur et al. have more recently reported that cognitive activation of patients with CT-scan-documented infarcts resulted in improved detection of these lesion sites by the rCBF technique—that is, the activation-accentuated abnormalities as recorded by rCBF (Gur et al., 1980). Also important is a study indicating there may be compensatory increases in right hemisphere flow in patients who recover from aphasia (Meyer, Sakai, Yamaguchi, and Shaw, 1980).

In our laboratory we have studied, up to this date, 11 recovering aphasics sustaining left hemisphere strokes and 5 nonaphasic patients sustaining strokes in the right hemisphere and who had shown a good recovery from initial hemiplegia or hemiparesis and visual-attentional problems including "neglect" and "denial" symptoms (Deutsch, Papanicolaou, and Eisenberg, 1987). rCBF was recorded during a baseline, resting condition, during a phonological target detection task, and during a visual rotation task that, in normal subjects, requires greater right hemisphere activation. The baseline rCBF results showed reduced hemispheric mean flow levels consistent with side of lesion. The stroke patients showed a striking activation pattern, significantly greater than that seen in our normal subjects, in both the impaired and spared hemisphere, suggesting a large demand on both the intact neural tissue and vasculature in the recovery process. The asymmetry in activation expected in the hemisphere-specific tasks was also altered in the stroke patients. The hemispheric (i.e., greater left hemisphere activation) asymmetry in flow increase expected during the phonologic task was diminished in the aphasics and exaggerated in the right hemisphere lesion patients. The asymmetry in flow increase expected during the rotation task (i.e., greater right hemisphere activation) was reversed in the right hemisphere lesion patients and exaggerated in the left hemisphere patients.

Six of the 11 left-stroke patients showed greater flow *increases* in the right rather than left hemisphere during the verbal task. This coupled with the magnitude of the increase, supports the idea of increasing participation of the nondominant hemisphere in the restitution of language in some aphasic patients. Correspondingly, 3 of the 5 right-stroke patients showed greater flow increases in the left rather than right hemisphere during the visuospatial task.

The hypothesis of increased participation of the spared hemisphere in the restitution of function normally subserved by a damaged hemisphere is supported by these findings—but with certain qualifications. It appears that intact tissue in *both* hemispheres is highly active during task performance, suggesting increased participation of both the intact hemisphere *and* spared areas of the damaged hemisphere.

Our data indicate that recovery of function following stroke depends on increased utilization of spared neural tissue and a consequent increased demand on the vasculature supplying that tissue. If this is confirmed it will provide more specific criteria for differential prognoses for different stroke victims, dependent on both type of stroke and condition of the remaining vasculature.

These preliminary rCBF data are in good agreement with the EP data obtained from the same patients in supporting the hemispheric reorganization hypothesis. Further support for this hypothesis is furnished by dichotic listening data obtained with subgroups of the same patients and normal subjects in our laboratory.

The dichotic listening technique (Broadbent, 1954; Kimura, 1961) has been repeatedly used with aphasic patients to address the question of whether language recovery following cerebral trauma to the left hemisphere involves increased contribution of the right hemisphere (Bavosi and Rup, 1984; Crosson and Warren, 1981; Johnson, Sommers, and Weidner, 1977; Niccum, Rubens, and Selnes, 1983; Petit and Noll, 1979; Schulhoff and Goodglass, 1969; Shanks and Ryan, 1976; Sparks, Goodglass, and Nickel, 1970). The basic finding in these studies has been that aphasics show a shift from the normal right ear advantage (REA) for verbal material to a left ear advantage (LEA). The interpretation of this shift has been the subject of much debate. Some investigators believe that left hemisphere aphasiogenic lesions trigger a shift in cerebral dominance for language resulting in LEA (Bavosi and Rupp, 1984; Johnson et al., 1977; Johnson, Sommers, and Weidner, 1978; Petit and Noll, 1979), while others believe the LEA occurs when lesions cause a degradation in auditory messages before they have a chance to be linguistically analyzed (Linebaugh, 1978; Niccum et al., 1983; Schulhoff and Goodglass, 1969).

We addressed these questions (Moore and Papanicolaou, 1988) in a study involving 31 stroke patients, with and without language disturbance, and 11 normal volunteers. The 31 patients were subdivided into three subgroups: (a) 11 patients showed CT-verified evidence of left hemisphere stroke and were initially aphasic but had regained much of their language abilities (Aphasia group); (b) 10 patients had suffered only mild strokes, typically transient ischemic attacks (TIAs), and had experienced only temporary dysarthria and mild symptoms of right-sided weakness or paresthesia (Dysarthric group); (c) 10 patients had suffered right hemisphere strokes which resulted in left hemiplegia but no symptoms of aphasia (Nonaphasic stroke group). In addition, 11 healthy adult volunteers served as the control group.

All patients and normal subjects were administered the dichotic listening test which consisted of dichotic presentation of 30 pairs of consonant-vowel nonsense syllables. During each presentation two of the syllables were presented simultaneously, one to each ear, and the subjects responded by saying what they heard.

Our results showed a clear REA in all but the recovering aphasics, the majority of whom (8 of the 11) showed an LEA.

Because there has been considerable debate over the possibility that sensory degradation of the verbal input rather than hemispheric dominance shift for language may be responsible for changes in ear preference of left-hemisphere-damaged patients, we addressed two additional questions. First, we asked if the dichotic detection performance differed in subjects with and without aphasiogenic lesions and, second, if there was a difference in the magnitude of the REA between the healthy control group and the group of nonaphasic patients. The rationale for these questions was as follows: Sensory degradation could conceivably occur because of lesions either to the primary auditory projection areas (Heschl's gyrus) or to the auditory association cortex. A lesion of Heschl's gyrus in the LH would degrade auditory information primarily from the right ear. This would result in a disadvantage for right ear input and, presumably, an LEA. It is not probable, however, that these aphasic patients had suffered lesions restricted to this area since they had initially displayed severe language deficits indicative of damage to LH speech areas. In addition, degradation of the right ear signal would negate the normal left ear/right ear competition for perception of dichotically presented material resulting not only in greater LEA but also better overall detection performance because of lessened inference. A lesion occurring in the speech areas of the left hemisphere, however, would degrade all sensory information from both ears resulting in *decreased* detection performance in these patients. Accordingly, we reasoned that a lesion to either the primary auditory projection area or the auditory association cortex would result in an increase or decrease, respectively, in the number of correct responses made by those subjects. Although there were small differences in the mean number of correct responses in the different groups (aphasics: 72%, dysarthrics: 75%, nonaphasic patients: 80%, controls: 79%) these were not statistically significant. Therefore, the presence of lesions does not appear to degrade the verbal messages as indicated by changes in level of detection performance.

To answer the second question, we compared the magnitude of the REA in the nonaphasic patients and in the healthy control subjects, both of which had never displayed symptoms of aphasia. We reasoned that a right hemisphere lesion would give an added advantage to right ear messages since left ear messages would be degraded before being transmitted transcallosally to the left hemisphere for linguistic analysis and would be less interfering with right ear messages. Therefore, if there is sensory degradation due to a right hemisphere lesion, the nonaphasic patients should show better detection performance and greater REA than the control subjects. Consequently, we submitted the number of correct responses of the control subjects and the nonaphasic patients in a two (group) by two (ears) repeated measures of analysis of variance. As expected, a significant main effect for ears was found indicating that both groups had more right than left ear responses (REA). However, the absence of a significant main effect for groups indicates that the control and nonaphasic patients did not differ in their levels of detection performance. In addition, the absence of a significant interaction indicates that these groups did not differ in the magnitude of their REA. Also, whereas 100% of the control subjects showed an REA, only 80% of the stroke patients did. Therefore, the hypothesis of sensory degradation was once again vitiated.

In summary, sensory degradation, whether conceived as operating at the level of transmission of verbal messages (primary auditory projection areas) or at the level of linguistic analysis (association cortex) does not suffice to explain the present results.

Although the aphasic patients had suffered left hemisphere stroke damage that initially produced aphasic symptomatology, the lesions appeared to have no effect on their ability to detect CV syllables at the time of testing. Detection performance was not different from that of either the control group, the dysarthric group with only mild transient expressive speech symptoms, or the nonaphasic patients who never displayed any language disturbance.

In addition, the magnitude of ear preference in the group of nonaphasic patients was not significantly different from the ear preference in the group of healthy control subjects. Their RH lesions apparently had little effect on their ability to process auditory stimuli coming through their left ear.

In conclusion, these data indicate that patients recovering from aphasia following left hemisphere trauma show a shift from the normal REA for dichotically presented verbal material. We believe that this is an indication of increased participation by the right hemisphere in the processing of verbal material, and we feel that an explanation based on a shift in language dominance is more viable than one based on signal degradation. This interpretation is corroborated by our rCBF and EP data reported above, which were obtained from the same patients.

CONCLUSIONS

The concurrence of rCBF, EP, and dichotic listening data in demonstrating task-specific differences in hemispheric activation in normal subjects is expected to allow assessment with greater precision of the nature and degree of long-term reorganization of brain function following injury to the dominant hemisphere. The hypothesis of functional reorganization of the brain involving shift of hemispheric dominance as one of the basic mechanisms of recovery of lateralized cognitive functions, particularly language, is also supported by our data. However, the conditions necessary for reorganization, such as extent of damage to the areas normally mediating language, the precise location of lesions, and the associated particular language deficits, have not been studied systematically. Moreover, the consequences of such reorganization, when, or if, it occurs, for the mediation of nonlinguistic functions normally lateralized in the intact nondominant hemisphere have also not been investigated.

Numerous important questions remain to be answered. For example: Does hemispheric dominance shift underlie recovery from all three basic types of aphasia, namely global, expressive (nonfluent), and receptive (fluent)? Is occurrence of dominance shift contingent on the size of lesion? Is the occurrence of dominance shift contingent on the initial severity of the aphasic deficit? Is the probability of dominance shift different for recovery from aphasia due to cortical and subcortical lesions? Is cerebral reorganization an incremental process covarying with the gradual process of language recovery? Is hemispheric dominance shift for language related to the integrity of nonlinguistic functions normally lateralized in the nondominant hemisphere? Is the frequency of occurrence of hemispheric dominance shift different for male and female patients? Does the age of the patient determine the occurrence of hemispheric dominance shift?

We believe that these questions can and will be eventually resolved. Moreover, their resolution is expected to facilitate the design of patient-specific strategies for rehabilitation that will enhance the efficiency of current language and cognitive retraining procedures used with head trauma and stroke victims.

Acknowledgment: This research was supported by Department of Education grant G008435031 and Dallas Rehabilitation Foundation Grant.

REFERENCES

Bavosi R, Rupp RR (1984): Dichotic abilities in children, normal adults and aphasic adults for open and closed context words. *The Journal of Auditory Research* 24:265–278.

Broadbent, D (1964): The role of auditory localization in attention and memory span. *Journal of Experimental Psychology* 47:191–196.

Crosson B, Warren RL (1981): Dichotic ear preference for C-V-C words in Wernicke's and Broca's aphasias. *Cortex* 17:249–258.

Cumming JL, Benson DF, Walsh MJ, Levine HL (1979): Left-to-right transfer of language dominance: A case study. *Neurology* 29:1547–1550.

Deutsch G, Papanicolaou AC, Eisenberg HM (1987): CBF during tasks intended to differentially activate the cerebral hemispheres: New normative data and preliminary application in recovering stroke patients. *Journal of Cerebral Blood Flow and Metabolism* 7:S306.

Galin D, Ellis R (1975): Asymmetry in evoked potentials as an index of lateralized cognitive processes: Relation to EEG alpha symmetry. *Neuropsychologia* 1:45–50.

Geschwind N (1970): The organization of language in the brain. *Science* 170:940–944.

Gur RG, Gur RE, Obrist WD, Hungerbuhler JP, Younkin D, Rosen AD, Skolnick BE, Reivich M (1980): Sex and handedness differences in cerebral blood flow during rest and cognitive activity. *Science* 217:659–661.

Gur RC, Reivich M (1980): Cognitive task effects on hemispheric blood flow in humans: Evidence of individual differences in hemispheric activation. *Brain and Language* 9:78–92.

Henschen SE (1922): *Klinische und anatomishe beitrage zur pathologie des gehirns*, vols. 5–7. Stockholm: Nordiska Bokhandelin.

Ingvar DG, Risberg J (1967): Increase of regional cerebral blood flow during mental effort in normals and in patients with focal brain disorders. *Experimental Brain Research* 3:195–211.

Johnson J, Sommers RK, Weidner WE (1977): Dichotic ear preference in aphasia. *Journal of Speech and Hearing Research* 20:116–129.

Johnson JP, Sommers RK, Weidner WE (1978): In response to dichotic ear preference in aphasia: Another view. *Journal of Speech and Hearing Research* 21:601–603.

Kimura D (1961): Cerebral dominance and the perception of verbal stimuli. *Canadian Journal of Psychology* 15:166–171.

Kinsbourne M (1971): The minor cerebral hemispheres as a source of aphasic speech. *Archives of Neurology* 25:302–306.

Knopman DS, Rubens AB, Klassen AC, Meyer MW, Niccum N (1980): Regional cerebral blood flow patterns during verbal and nonverbal auditory activation. *Brain and Language* 9:93–112.

Linebaugh CW (1978): Dichotic ear preference in aphasia: Another view. *Journal of Speech and Hearing Research* 21:598–600.

Maximilian VA (1982): Cortical blood flow asymmetries during monaural verbal stimulation. *Brain and Language* 15:1–11.

Meyer JS, Sakai F, Yamaguchi F, Yamamoto M, Shaw T (1980): Regional changes in cerebral blood flow during standard behavioral activation in patients with disorders of speech and mentation compared to normal volunteers. *Brain and Language* 9:61–77.

Moore BD, Papanicolaou AC (1988): Dichotic listening evidence of right hemisphere involvement in recovery from aphasia in left hemisphere stroke patients. *Journal of Clinical and Experimental Neuropsychology* 10:380–386.

Niccum N, Rubens AB, Selnes OA (1983): Dichotic listening performance, language impairment, and lesion location in aphasic listeners. *Journal of Speech and Hearing Research* 26:35–42.

Nottebohm F (1984): Learning, forgetting and brain repair. In: AM Galaburda & N Geschwind (eds.), *Cerebral dominance.* Cambridge, MA: Harvard University Press, pp. 93–113.

Nottebohm F, Nottebohm M (1976): Left hypoglossus dominance in the control of canary and white-crowned sparrow song. *Journal of Comparative and Physiological Psychology* 108:171–192.

Nottebohm F, Strokes T, Leonard C (1976): Central control of song in the canary. *Serinus canarius. Journal of Comparative Neurology* 165:457–486.

Obrist WD, Wilkinson WE (1979): The noninvasive xe-133 method: Evaluation of CBF indices. *Cerebral Circulation* 507:119–124.

Papanicolaou AC (1980): Cerebral profiles in language processing: The photic probe paradigm. *Brain and Language* 9:269–280.

Papanicolaou AC, Eisenberg HM, Levy R (1983): Evoked potential correlates of left hemisphere dominance in covert articulation. *International Journal of Neuroscience* 20:289–294.

Papanicolaou AC, Johnstone J (1985): Probe evoked potentials: Theory, method, and applications. *International Journal of Neuroscience* 24:107–131.

Papanicolaou AC, Levin HS, Eisenberg HM (1984): Evoked potential correlates of recovery from aphasia after focal left hemisphere injury in adults. *Neurosurgery* 14:412–415.

Papanicolaou AC, Levin HS, Eisenberg HM, Moore BD (1983). Evoked potential indices of selective hemispheric engagement in affective and phonetic tasks. *Neuropsychologia* 21:401–405.

Papanicolaou AC, Moore BD, Levin HS, Eisenberg HM (1987): Evoked potential correlates of right hemisphere involvement in language recovery following stroke. *Archives of Neurology* 44:521–524.

Petit JM, Noll JD (1979): Cerebral dominance in aphasia recovery. *Brain and Language* 7:191–200.

Risberg J (1980): Regional cerebral blood flow measurements by [133]xenon-inhalation: Methodology and applications in neuropsychology and psychiatry. *Brain and Language* 9:9–34.

Risberg J, Ali Z, Wilson E, Wills E, Halsey J (1975): Regional cerebral blood flow by [133]xenon inhalation: Preliminary evaluation of an initial slope index in patients with unstable flow compartments. *Stroke* 6:142–148.

Schulhoff C, Goodglass H (1969): Dichotic listening, side of brain injury and cerebral dominance. *Neuropsychologia* 7:149–160.

Selinger M, Shucard DW, Prescott TE (1980): Relationships between behavioral and electrophysiological measures of auditory comprehension. In RH Brookshire (ed.), *Clinical Aphasiology: Conference Proceedings*. Minneapolis: BRK Publishers.

Shanks J, Ryan WA (1976): A comparison of aphasic and non-brain-injured adults on a dichotic CV-syllable listening task. *Cortex* 12:100–112.

Shucard DW, Shucard JL, Thomas DG (1977): Auditory evoked potentials as probes of hemispheric differences in cognitive processing. *Science* 197:1295–1298.

Sokoloff L (1977): Local cerebral energy metabolism: Its relationship to local functional activity and blood flow. In *Cerebral vascular smooth muscle and its control* (Ciba Foundation Symposium, Vol. 56). Amsterdam: Elsevier.

Sparks R, Goodglass H, Nickel B (1970): Ipsilateral versus contralateral extinction in dichotic listening resulting from hemisphere lesions. *Cortex* 6:249–260.

Thomas DG, Shucard DW (1983): Changes in patterns of hemispheric electrophysiological activity as a function of instructional set. *International Journal of Neuroscience* 18:11–20.

Wernicke C. (1874): *Der aphasische symptomenkomplex*. Breslau: Cohn & Weigart.

11

Neurorehabilitation of Postacute Brain Injury: A Key to Optimizing Functional Motor Recovery

Richard Balliet, Ph.D.

Department of Rehabilitation Medicine, University of Wisconsin Medical School, and Neuromuscular Retraining Clinic, Madison, Wisconsin, U.S.A.

TREATMENT AND EXPECTED "TIME FUNCTION" OF RECOVERY

Approximately 30,000 to 50,000 people acquire serious disabilities annually as a result of traumatic brain injury. Most are young people with life expectancies between 35 and 50 years (Federal Register, 1987). This large and growing brain-injured population has, in part, resulted from advances in emergency and acute care. By reducing mortality, a tremendous need has been created for acute through postacute neurorehabilitation services. The term *neurorehabilitation* is defined as the process by which the central nervous system (CNS) is able to recover some amount of function. The term *postacute* is used to describe the later stage of the rehabilitation process, after the acute stage in which the patient is medically stable and has been discharged from initial hospitalization. Specifically, in current practice additional *early-postacute* treatment of a brain injury patient may be carried out for usually up to 1 or 2 years. Patients with residual dysfunction 2 years or more after their initial injury, and who are fortunate enough to have the resources for continued treatment, can be considered to be at the *late-postacute* stage (Bachy-Rita et al., 1988).

The neurorehabilitation of the individual brain-injured patient at some point includes deciding which of the numerous early-postacute rehabilitation services, available at various delivery costs, will be of most benefit to the patient. This is a particularly difficult question since brain-injured patients exhibit a wide range of recovery which may, or may not, be prognosticated by the evaluations that are available today. We can only be certain that the brain-injured person has individualized needs, both acutely and postacutely. Presently, the neurorehabilitation needs of early-postacute patients are mainly delivered by a system that utilizes a similar interdisciplinary, inpatient approach in the delivery of services to acute-care patients. If sufficient funds are available, this method of rehabilitation (usually $250 to $450 per day) is most effective if the patient needs many services and can rapidly benefit from a limited stay of 1 to 6 months. Patients not fitting this profile may receive more limited outpatient services, originating from the home or clinic as required over a similar period of time (e.g., physical therapy, occupational therapy, speech therapy, cognitive retraining, etc.). Unfortunately, these early postacute services are still relatively expensive; therefore many patients will only receive limited treatment or no treatment, depending upon their available funding.

The most problematic situation involves the late-postacute brain-injured patient who has been labeled "chronic." It is assumed that these patients have permanent cognitive or neuromuscular disabilities because their rate of recovery has apparently slowed or stopped, usually at a point 1 to 2 years after injury. This has been based on the traditional belief that spontaneous recovery (natural healing) effects have ended and therefore the patient would not be likely to recover significant function past this time. This belief has often led to the practice of "maintenance" of function rather than the application of long-term neurorehabilitation services to such postacute patients. The relatively small number of late-postacute neurorehabilitation services that are available are limited because of the time and cost required using the present inpatient or outpatient models, to treat these patients (Bach-y-Rita et al., 1988).

However, as times change, so do beliefs, and so do what we consider to be certain rigid cause and effect relationships. Recent research now indicates that neurorehabilitation may be possible at any time. It appears that *the expected "time function" of recovery depends upon the efficiency of the therapy methods more than upon how long after trauma therapy methods are applied.* In addition, it is becoming apparent that there is probably no particular "magic bullet" method of neurorehabilitation that can rapidly transform the brain-injured patient to "normal" on an acute or postacute basis. The common denominator to optimizing therapy effects of any type and at any stage of recovery seems to be as simple as maximizing informational processing and attentional factors. In general terms, this means the provision of high levels of sensory feedback information in low-noise environments over adequate periods of time (Bach-y-Rita and Balliet, 1987; Bach-y-Rita et al., 1988).

Remarkably, it was as early as 1915 that it was first reported that neurorehabilitation was not strictly time dependent and could occur with relatively simple techniques (Franz, Scheetz, and Wilson, 1915). This assertion came from three physicians who worked at the Government Hospital for the Insane, Washington DC, in 1915. In those days even relatively mild to moderately brain-injured patients were often treated and/or institutionalized alongside of insane individuals. They reported that with individualized training, brain-injured patients could obtain significant recovery of function as late as 20 years after injury. From their results and from other human and animal studies of the time they concluded:

> The possibility that conclusions regarding the permanency of paralysis from cerebral accidents were neither accurate nor scientifically grounded and that more attention should be paid to possible improvement in these cases. . . . Lesions of the motor cortex or the upper part of the pyramidal tract in man do not [necessarily] abolish function, but put the function in abeyance until such time as the appropriate condition is present for production of movement. . . . We should probably not [always] speak of permanent paralyses, but of uncared-for paralyses. This we say because many of the conditions which we have met appear to resemble . . . phenomena of disuse, rather than actual inabilities.

Franz et al. (1915) realized that the late-postacute recovery of function that they described was theoretically past the point of any apparent spontaneous recovery effects. They theorized that one explanation for their results may be "due to . . . another portion of the brain." Unfortunately, their results and hypotheses were far ahead of their time. It was not until the late 1960s and early 1970s that a significant number of animal studies and clinical demonstration studies were to appear, reporting the successful treatment of various types of late-postacute neurological disorders, including traumatic brain injury (reviewed by Bach-y-Rita and Balliet, 1987; Balliet, 1989; Balliet et al., 1987; Fields, 1987).

POSSIBILITY OF BRAIN REORGANIZATION: MORPHOLOGICAL AND FUNCTIONAL PERSPECTIVES

Over the past 20 years, the success of demonstration studies involving late-postacute recovery of function in the absence of spontaneous recovery effects has suggested that the brain may be capable of CNS reorganization or some form of "neuroplasticity." The hypothesized morphological mechanisms of late recovery developed primarily from animal research have included sprouting, denervation supersensitivity, unmasking, and diaschisis (as detailed by Bach-y-Rita, 1981a; Bach-y-Rita, 1981b; Bach-y-Rita et al., in press). Briefly stated, sprouting is defined as the growth of a cell body to another cell, such as in the case of collateral sprouting where new axonal processes bud off of an uninjured axon and grow into the tissue vacated by degenerated axons. Denervation supersensitivity involves a permanent increase in an axon's response from a relatively small input source. Similarly, unmasking involves the activation of secondary parallel pathways that would normally be inhibited. Diaschisis, as a mechanism of late recovery, assumes that remote structures connected to the site of an injury are depressed and that this suppression may be released through another mechanism, such as the addition of an agent that would selectively increase neurotransmission in the depressed area. All of these potential mechanisms of recovery have to some degree been demonstrated in experimental animal work. None, as yet, have been proven to be responsible for the recovery of function in man.

Because of the lack of conclusive proof, a more traditional perspective might conclude that the brain does not *need* to structurally reorganize itself but simply adopts relatively abnormal and inefficient "compensatory motor behaviors" to correct for the motor dysfunction associated with brain injury (Bach-y-Rita et al., 1988; Balliet et al., 1987; Harbst, Lazarus, and Balliet, in press). These types of "goal-directed behaviors" would develop as a substitute through simple associated usage. However, an issue of critical importance to this hypothesis is to consider what is meant by goal-directed behavior. What if the goal-directed behavior were not of a relatively general and unspecific directive but, instead, involved selective motor training of just the affected muscles? And, more importantly, what if such a noncompensatory training paradigm were successful with theoretically difficult patients, such as late-postacute brain injury patients?

The answer to these questions has often been ignored in the literature. There have in fact been many recent studies indicating that late-postacute patients can reacquire specific neuromuscular function if specific neuromuscular retraining is applied to the affected area (reviewed by Bach-y-Rita and Balliet, 1987; Balliet, 1989; Balliet et al., 1987; Fields, 1987). Therefore it can be argued that brain reorganization may have a higher probability of occurring when the brain has the opportunity to be presented with noncompensatory neuromuscular retraining strategies. In either case, both situations would seem to indicate that the CNS has some type of adaptive capacity and that it may have some ability to modify its own structural organization and function (Bach-y-Rita, 1980). *The only difference between compensatory and noncompensatory func-*

tional outcomes may often be one of nonspecific vs. specific training, respectively. The final proof will come from discovering factors that will lead to the optimization of positive adaptive effects and to the minimization of negatively adaptive responses. The answer to this question will depend primarily upon our ability to measure associated brain activity changes and secondarily upon applied clinical methodology.

Until such studies can be completed (see below) it is important to realize that at present the actual clinical retraining of the brain-injured patient at any point in time often may include inadequate and inappropriate information processing as mediated by various attentional factors. These factors are particularly important after the point at which spontaneous recovery has ceased, sometime during the late-postacute recovery stage. In general it must be stressed that *the brain-injured patient's potential for recovery depends not only upon the amount and location of brain injury but also upon the reestablishment of specific information inputs to the sensory-associational areas of the CNS that direct or redirect motor programming.* Having said this, it must be realized that there is a complexity of interactive variables that could either positively or negatively impact upon these information inputs (Bach-y-Rita and Balliet, 1987).

This notion is consistent with the observation that the brain's complexity of synaptic interactions must be incredibly dynamic in order to interpret and respond to the countless combinations of environmental circumstances impacting upon existing motor programs at any given moment. These existing motor programs have been established within certain normal or abnormal limits through past experiences, current conditions, and future outcomes as they are processed by some amount of genetically determined circuitry. The understanding of the brain's ability to modify motor control becomes more complex when these synaptic interactions are considered as "action systems" that translate into an infinite combination of interconnected or goal-directed behaviors. The structural abnormalities of a damaged nervous system effect a breakdown in the functional elements and relationships that comprise even simple actions. As a result, disorders or coordination are associated with underlying disorders involving tone and posture. Similarly, it is generally agreed that therapeutic interventions should involve not only the neuromuscular retraining of specific muscles but also should include functional and goal-directed actions as soon as possible. The use of this relatively hierarchial system allows the associational areas of the CNS to be more readily reestablished, thus facilitating lasting functional recovery (Lazarus and Balliet, in press).

In general terms, it appears from late-postacute recovery of function demonstration studies (i.e., in which spontaneous recovery is considered not to be a factor) that a very significant component of that *motor learn-*

ing depends upon the optimization of sensory feedback information (Bach-y-Rita and Balliet, 1987). This conclusion is derived from both work in motor learning and the therapeutic literature. To varying degrees both emphasize the use of immediate extrinsic sensory feedback information (e.g., proprioceptive and kinesthetic) to effect changes in intrinsic sensory feedback information (e.g., knowledge of results or performance) (Winstein, 1987). Since the term "optimization" is a relative term, this assertion is applicable regardless of the retraining methods or the motor tasks that are involved. It is the basis upon which future therapy methods for brain-injured patients will be developed. Similarly, sensory feedback information may also be a common denominator to the mechanisms of brain reorganization; i.e., a very significant component of *neural adaptation or plasticity of motor control reprogramming depends upon the optimization of sensory information* (Bach-y-Rita and Balliet, 1987). Once again, however, final proof will depend primarily upon our ability to measure potential brain activity changes that may be associated with motoric recovery.

THE APPLICATION OF LATE-POSTACUTE NEUROREHABILITATION AND NEW TECHNOLOGIES TO MEDICAL SCIENCE

Over the past three decades the field of rehabilitation has rapidly evolved in its approach to treating brain-injured patients. It has changed from basically an orthopedic physical therapy approach to a system that now involves an interdisciplinary team approach encompassing physicians (orthopedic, neurology, rehabilitation, etc.) psychologists (including neuropsychology), social workers, vocational counselors, as well as physical, occupational, speech, and recreational therapists. Most of these profesionals are to some degree also involved in community reentry, typically including the counseling of family members in approaches to adjustment, home therapy programs, independent living, vocational education, and the financing of care. Today many different professionals are required to deal with the specialized needs of the individual brain-injured patient.

However, this number is but a sample of the differing professionals that are actually required to solve the various problems in the neurorehabilitation of brain injury that remain today. Either directly or indirectly these professionals include specialists in various aspects of radiology, nuclear medicine, medical physics, computer sciences, digital electronics, applied mathematics, as well as the neurosciences including physiologists, neurophysiologists, anatomists, neuroanatomists, and kinesiologists. All of these people to some degree have been collectively responsible for the recent advancements in clinical diagnostics involving brain imaging techniques such as: computerized tomography (CT), magnetic resonance imaging (MRI), positron emission tomography (PET), electroencephalography (EEG), evoked potentials (EP), and electromyography (EMG). These rapidly evolving techniques and others currently under development either provide or have the theoretical potential to provide information concerning the neurophysiological mechanisms associated with the recovery of function.

It is clear that new technologies are essential to the research and development of more effective rehabilitation programs and the optimization of human potential after brain injury. In one possible application, such new technologies may be able to define the brain activity changes correlated with the return of function in patients with long-standing CNS damage. This type of baseline data is essential since, as previously mentioned, recovery of function that has been demonstrated in clinical studies has not been accompanied by solidly defined objective data. No method of therapy, either traditional or nontraditional, has been conclusively proven to be effective in stimulating brain reorganization or recovery of function that is beyond the limits of spontaneous recovery. It is still unknown exactly how, when, or where recovery of function takes place. Therefore, brain activity studies are required to determine if rehabilitation procedures have the capacity to actually effect recovery outside of the realm of treatments associated with spontaneous recovery effects. Issues regarding which therapy method and/or environmental condition is superior can be addressed only after this basic question is answered. Interdisciplinary cooperation is required to investigate the potential of these new technologies to better understand CNS recovery of function and to lead the way toward exacting clinical rehabilitation strategies not only for the brain-injured patient but also for other neurologically impaired individuals.

A key feature of a research design model for investigating such questions could initially include the late-postacute brain-injured (or stroke) patient with relatively focal damage, who is past the point of being influenced by confounding variables associated with spontaneous recovery effects. Once the patient is determined to be medically and neurologically stable, various methods of evaluating brain activity relative to different treatment effects could be assessed with the patients being used as their own control. Data from significant numbers of patients who were determined by evaluations to have certain similar or specified charcteristics could be compared or correlated. Since studies utilizing the late-postacute patient by definition (and evaluations) would not involve spontaneous recovery effects, it is more likely that such studies would be to some degree more applicable to the understanding of the acute-care patient than would studies designed the other way around.

In addition, it is also reasonable to assume that "moderately" involved patients would be ideal subjects of initial studies. Theoretically, the "mildly" involved patients might not demonstrate strong enough treatment or evaluation effects because they have relatively mild neuronal damage. Alternately, the "severe" patients have been to some degree classified as such because their likelihood and/or extent of recovery is relatively poor in comparison to other patients. For this reason, they might not demonstrate significant treatment effects, or because of extensive neural damage, they might not be within the useful range of certain evaluations (e.g., a coma patient taking a neuropsychology examination). The "moderately" involved late-postacute patients can be considered the best candidates for initial study because they have the greatest range for potential functional recovery.

SUGGESTED PROGRAMS TO CHARACTERIZE, CORRELATE, AND PROMOTE FUNCTIONAL MOTOR RECOVERY OF THE CNS

From the previous discussions, it can be seen that rehabilitation treatments that can be proven to promote actual functional recovery of the CNS after brain injury would have a significant interactive impact on long-term patient outcomes. New technology is required to measure these potential changes in neural activity leading to the assessments of various rehabilitation approaches and more accurate prognistication (Wilson et al., 1987). The suggested order of research priorities to accomplish this task could conceivably include the following seven successive research and development steps:

Step 1. Develop, test, and validate the reliability of objectively measured brain activity technology [e.g., computerized tomography (CT), magnetic resonance imaging (MRI), positron emission tomography (PET), electroencephalography (EEG), evoked potentials (EP), neuropsychology testing, etc.] and associated protocols specifically designed for late-postacute brain-injured (TBI) subjects with moderate (average) severity as well as in non-brain-injured normals. Patients would be at least 2.0 years post onset and would be determined to be functionally stable. Lack of change in brain activity measures as well as subjective and objective measures of physical performance for both TBI and normal subjects over a 6-month period involving no treatment would determine the success of this project. Intersubject comparisons between TBI and normal subjects without therapy over a 6-month period would result in objective information concerning the possible site of brain reorganization associated with the combination of previous acute-care therapy and spontaneous recovery effects.

Step 2. If Step 1 is successful, characterize and correlate objectively measured brain activity and therapy outcomes of the same stabilized late-postacute brain-injured patients (as previously determined in Step 1) over at least a one-year period. Therapy methods would consist of a combination of procedures that have been demonstrated to be effective in clinical trials. (Note: The question of which therapy method is the best is not being asked at this point.) Intersubject TBI comparisons before and after postacute therapy evaluations would result in objective information concerning the possible site and extent of brain reorganization as correlated to the degree of functional recovery not associated with spontaneous recovery. Assessments of brain activity measures and respective protocols utilized in future studies would be based on data collected in Steps 1 and 2 and/or by the availability of new technology. This assessment process would be continuous and included in all future steps.

Step 3. If Step 2 is successful in revealing differences, long-term therapy of more than one year (e.g., 2 or more years of therapy, as required to maximize function), evaluated by brain activity measures (as in Steps 1 and 2), would provide data regarding the potential "time function" of postacute neural recovery of function.

Step 4. Acute through late-postacute "longitudinal" intrasubject studies of brain activity changes associated with the combination of spontaneous recovery plus therapy through recovery of function associated primarily with therapeutic intervention, respectively. More acute changes in brain activity could then be compared to both early postacute and late postacute recovery stages.

Step 5. Steps 1 through 4 could be replicated with relatively mild or relatively more severe brain-injured patients.

Step 6. The data collected in Steps 1 through 4 (in which therapy involved a combination of therapy techniques) could then be used as baseline data for comparisons involving the reliability and validity of specific types of therapy used at various intervention times.

Step 7. At any point during Steps 1 through 6 differential brain activity effects associated with various pharmacological therapy interventions could be compared to "drug-free" controls.

BRAIN INJURY NEUROREHABILITATION AND THE ENHANCED FUNCTIONAL RECOVERY OF OTHER NEUROMUSCULAR DISABILITIES

Brain-injured patients (including those suffering from brain trauma and stroke) as well as other neurologically involved individuals such as those suffering from incomplete spinal cord injuries, peripheral nerve injures, progressive neuromuscular diseases, and various childhood traumas could all potentially benefit from research concentrated in the general area of CNS recovery of function. As an example, even lost function due to peripheral nerve injury or incomplete, lower motoneuron spinal cord injury conceivably may be recoverable because of the potential for CNS reorganization that could correctly rechannel the anatomically cross-wired neural efferent and afferent connections (Balliet, 1989).

In general, the neurophysiological components leading to the recovery of function in brain-injured patients must be shared to a large degree by other neuromuscular disabilities. This is not to say that we understand the interaction of common neuro-component tasks such as information processing, sensory-motor integration, memory, recognition, and learning, which allow even a "normal" person to accurately reach for a piece of food (i.e., produce a movement trajectory); but we are getting closer to understanding the complex normative and abnormal processes that must be shared by all central nervous systems regardless of disability.

A case in point involves recent discussions in *Science* that have compared motor problem solving in robotics to those problems faced by the central nervous system (Georgopoulos, Schwartz, and Kettner, 1987; Whitney, 1987). Even though it is not apparent that the CNS follows the same route to solutions that has been formulated in robotics, it is apparent that the relatively large number of muscles and joints in the human body produce a potentially more complicated situation for the CNS to solve. However, the implementation of a particular trajectory by the CNS involves "smart" solutions that might employ specialized neural networks that have been established by a long process of either actual or evolutionary "trial-and-error learning." This could involve programmable motor command centers of the brain, e.g., the cerebellum parietal cortex and basal ganglia, and even the spinal cord. Integral to spinal circuits are the convergent and divergent characteristics of interneurons. "For example, the propriospinal neurons involved in the implementation of reaching movements project to several motoneuronal pools that innervate muscles acting at several joints; these propriospinal neurons receive convergent inputs from several supraspinal structures [including corticospinal system of the motor cortex] and from limb afferents arising from many parts of the limb" (Georgopoulos et al., 1987). It can be concluded that "the essence of the interactive, multijoint, multimuscle nature of spinal and supraspinal motor control [and the learning] of reaching movements involving the whole limb still evades us. Its elucidation may provide the answer to the question of how the CNS actually implements a desired movement trajectory" (Georgopoulos et al., 1987). It is obvious that such basic data not only can help us better understand the essential components involved in neuromuscular control but can also help us understand the potential neurorehabilitation components involved in the reprogramming of the neurologically involved patient.

Similarly, a relatively more "generic" neuroscientific emphasis should be applied to the clinical delivery of what are currently identified as physical and occupational therapy services to brain-injured individuals. There is much to be learned from the field of neurorehabilitation and from programs that specialize in the neuromuscular retraining of a broad range of neurologically involved patients—not just the brain injured.

Such elementary changes in emphasis can lead to the enhancement of delivery systems and to the enhancement of functional recovery in neurologically involved patients. One such example is the concept of "neuromuscular retraining." These words connote the brain's active participation in the operation of the muscles. They also imply the patient's active participation in therapy. If it is assumed that there is a potential for a high level of patient participation (as well as that of a similarly trained family member or other person), the patient would only need to return to a central clinic or require a home visit for their individualized and intensive instruction on an occasional outpatient basis. Emphasis could then be placed primarily on retraining patients to train themselves in an extensive home program involving simple, but very slow, specific retraining procedures (e.g., therapeutic exercise) or other behavioral methods. Thus, the physical or occupational therapist would become an educator and guide and would need to be seen only infrequently. In this manner, patients could be followed for many months or years through the late-postacute stage of recovery. Certainly, this is but one of many possible solutions to maximize benefit while minimizing cost. That which is of most importance is the realization that the solving of such problems will be dramatically affected by our ability to modernize our mental constructs.

CONCLUDING COMMENTS: PRESENT KNOWLEDGE AND FUTURE DISCOVERY

It is well known that throughout history a society's consensus as to what it believes to be fact or to be of value has markedly influenced the direction of its scientific discovery. Accordingly, the basic terminology and methods that scientists choose to utilize, as influenced by society, will have specific impacts upon the immediate future of that society (Burke, 1985). To this extent scientists are not completely unbiased, neutral observers. They must constantly reevaluate what they consider to be basic and true as derived from their society's contemporary knowledge.

Consequently, present day brain injury researchers are making their future research plans in accordance with the most recent available data, methods, and technology as related to current gaps in patient treatment. Fortunately, these are exciting times, indeed. It is now apparent that recent successes in the neuromuscular retraining of late-postacute neurological patients (who are past the point of spontaneous recovery effects) will have a substantial influence on future research efforts. Most importantly, based on studies thus far completed, it now appears that *the CNS is not immutable and has the capacity for late brain reorganization, by some, as yet, unknown mechanisms.* The concept of brain reorganization as it relates to neuromuscular retraining gives new direction to the physical and occupational therapy potential of these patients. The term "neuromuscular" is a reminder that motor control involves the brain and that future clinical research efforts should be based on learning theory and neurophysiology, and not on tradition. This term is also pivotal to the concept that *a long-term goal of neurorehabilitation should be to assess whether it is the lesion or the strength of the therapy that is limiting the neurological patient's recovery of function, particularly at the late-postacute stage.* As a result, it is most probable that the optimization of (re)training paradigms will be able to facilitate significant amounts of functional recovery in great numbers of seemingly "chronic" postacute patients who previously appeared to be untreatable.

It is also clear that an increased knowledge of other neurological disorders involving specific aspects or areas of neurological damage will be of benefit in understanding the complexity of brain trauma and its neurorehabilitation. Areas of neurorehabilitation involving either basic or applied research, intrasubject or intersubject design, objective or subjective diagnostics, animal or human applications, brain injury or spinal cord patients (to mention but a few) will all be of great value in understanding the mechanisms of CNS reorganization and the clinical variables that will enhance its functional recovery. Finally, it seems apparent that the late-postacute brain-injured patient will be a principal player as well as a winner in the new interdisciplinary field of neuorehabilitation.

REFERENCES

Bach-y-Rita P (ed.) (1980): *Recovery of function: Theoretical considerations for brain injury rehabilitation* (pp. 225–263). Baltimore: University Park Press.

Bach-y-Rita P (1981a): Central nervous system lesions: Sprouting and unmasking in rehabilitation. *Arch Phys Med Rehab* 62:413–417.

Bach-y-Rita P (1981b): Brain plasticity as a basis for the development of rehabilitation procedures for hemiplegia. *Scand J Rehab Med* 13:73–83.

Bach-y-Rita P, Balliet R (1987): Recovery from stroke. In PW Duncan and MB Badke (eds.), *Motor deficits following stroke* (pp. 79–107). New York: Year Book Publishers.

Bach-y-Rita P, Lazarus JC, Boyeson MG, Balliet R, Myers T (1988): Neural aspects of motor function as a basis of early and post-acute rehabilitation. In JA Delisa, D Currie, B Gans, P Gatens, JA Leonard, Jr, M McPhee (eds.), *Prin-*

ciples and practices of rehabilitation medicine, pp. 175–195. Philadelphia: J.B. Lippincott.

Balliet R (1989): Facial paralysis and other neuromuscular dysfunctions of the peripheral nervous system. In OD Payton, RP DiFabio, SV Paris, E Protas, A Vansant (eds.). *Manual of physical therapy techniques* (pp. 175–213). New York: Churchill Livingston.

Balliet R, Harbst K, Kim D, Stewart B (1987): Chronic ataxia in traumatic CNS damage: the retraining of functional gait through the reduction of upper extremity weight bearing. *Int Rehab Med* 8(4):148–153.

Burke J (1985): *The day the universe changed.* Boston: Little, Brown & Company.

Federal Register (1987): RRTC in rehabilitation of moderate traumatic brain injury (TBI), 52, 108, June 5, 21348.

Fields RW (1987): Electromyographic triggered electric muscle simulation for chronic hemiplegia. *Arch Phys Med Rehab* 68:407–414.

Franz S, Scheetz M, Wilson A (1915): The possibility of recovery of motor function in long-standing hemiplegia. *JAMA* 65:2150–2154.

Georgopoulos AP, Schwartz AB, Kettner RE (1987): Neuronal coding and robotics: technical comments. *Science* 237:301.

Lazarus JC, Balliet R (in press): Brain reorganization and motor control theory: Recovery of function following brain injury. *J Motor Behavior,* 1–8.

Whitney, DE (1987): Neuronal coding and robotics: technical comments. *Science* 237:300–301.

Wilson MA, Perlman SB, Balliet R, Lazarus JC, Rowe B, Sacket SF, Sunderland J, Nickles RJ (1987): FDG cerebral studies during specific motor tasks in normal and traumatic brain injured patients. *73rd Scientific Assembly of the Radiological Society of North America,* November 29–December 4 (Abstract).

Winstein CJ (1987): Motor learning considerations in stroke rehabilitation. In PW Duncan, MB Badke (eds). *Motor deficits following stroke* (pp. 109–134). New York: Year Book.

IV

Rehabilitation Issues

12

Acute Care to Rehabilitation: Concepts in Transition

Nathaniel H. Mayer, M.D.

Drucker Brain Injury Center, Moss Rehabilitation Hospital, Philadelphia, Pennsylvania, U.S.A.

It is the thesis of this chapter that coordination of care and services between acute care and rehabilitation can only occur when each service delivery system understands the limits imposed by brain pathology on the possibilities for developing a social destination plan and a daily activity plan for the head-injured survivor.

Traumatic brain injury is best characterized as a diffuse injury to white matter of the brain along with predilection for damage to the frontal and temporal lobes. Diffuse brain damage, made worse by focal brain lesions and injuries to other parts of the body, impairs adequate behavioral problem solving in real life situations. Deficits in function are, therefore, apt to occur in wide ranging everyday skills which require differing degrees of mental alertness, processing of information, planning, execution, and mental monitoring of daily actions. Diffuse brain injury disrupts the performance of real life skills. Moreover, the inability of brain-injured patients to integrate skills, that is, to select and use a group of skills collectively and sequentially to solve real life problems, seems to be one of the most pernicious consequences of traumatic head injury. The patient is unable to generate integrative actions which are appropriate to context.

Two years after an automobile accident, a 20-year-old former college student was observed making purchases in a food store. She forgot to bring her well rehearsed shopping list as well as the monies given to her to make her purchases. She searched for items in trial and error fashion by going up and down all store aisles instead of taking a cue from clearly written categories at the head of each aisle. When selecting items, she displayed poor discrimination and judgment. She picked up the first vegetables in her line of sight without examining them. They turned out to be spoiled. She made no comment and offered no apology after accidentally bumping into another person with her shopping cart. She did not review the bill nor count her change when checking out at the checkout counter. She left the packages at the counter and had to be reminded to take them.

Classic rehabilitation aims at physical restoration through functional skills retraining with the expectation that the patient will use every restored skill as circumstances require. This approach assumes that the patient will integrate each restored skill within the context of the clusters of skills and routines needed for daily life. Head injury rehabilitation differs from this classic conception. The rehabilitation program must not only focus on training individual skills but must also concentrate on restoring the patient's ability to integrate these skills in problem-specific, context-specific ways. In the case above, staff had previously determined that the patient was capable of adequately performing individual skills needed for marketing. However, the trip to the community food store illustrated that this patient did not retrieve and integrate a variety of nested skills required of her in the context of the community setting. For this reason, "independence" in skill performance ("independent" in ambulation, "independent" in activities of daily living, "independent" in verbal communication) is not an acceptable standard of outcome when rehabilitating head-injured patients. Generally speaking, standards of independent skill performance assume that a patient can successfully integrate newly retrained skills within the context of the patient's activity patterns of daily life—an assumption that does not stand up well to clinical experience with head injury clients. Our idea of brain injury rehabilitation, our global goal so to speak, is to produce an individual who will be adaptive *(not independent)* in a stable social environment.

How are patients transitioned from acute care to rehabilitation? The Santa Clara Valley Medical Center Head Injury Rehabilitation Project reported in 1982 that patients were admitted to their rehabilitation unit when they met most of the following guidelines: (1) severe brain injury; (2) medical stability; (3) evidence of neurological improvement; and (4) require inpatient care. Exceptions are made when circumstances dictate. Investigators of that project state that all patients were admitted to rehabilitation with the explicit agreement of families that the initial 2 weeks were for evaluation to determine whether the patient (a) could benefit from rehabilitation care and (b) whether he or she was showing adequate responsiveness to treatment. If the patient improved, he or she was continued in the program. If not, the patient was discharged and received periodic follow-up.

At Santa Clara and elsewhere, admission and retention in an inpatient rehabilitation program tends to be an empirical procedure. Patients are admitted for evaluation and a trial of rehabilitation if they meet some very general admission criteria, and they are retained in the program until they stop improving or can be reasonably managed on an outpatient basis. Patients are not admitted on the basis of a predictive model for the interventions that are contemplated. Patients are not admitted with a particular prediction of social outcome but rather on the basis of estimated individual improvements. However, the need for predictive models is important clinically and economically. Questions of the same kind should be asked about rehabilitation as are routinely posed when drug treatment is under review. These include consideration of which patients to treat, when to treat, with what intensity, and when to stop. What are the predictable, desired effects; and are there adverse reactions?

In any discussion of goals and strategies of rehabilitation, it is important to clarify the associated terms and concepts:

1. *Impairment/disability/handicap.*
2. *Function/recovery of function/spontaneous recovery of function.*
3. *Restitution/remediation/restoration.*
4. *Alleviation/compensation/amelioration.*

The World Health Organization views *disability* as a restriction or inability to perform an activity resulting from an impairment or a pathology. (In principle, *impairment* reflects disturbances at the level of the organ.) Disability represents objectification of an impairment; it is the loss of function associated with an impairment reflecting disturbance at the level of the person. If Mike Schmidt, the baseball player, and I sustain amputations of a hand, we both lose function of the hand and are disabled with respect to functions of the hand. *Handicap,* as distinct from disability, is a disadvantage for a given individual, resulting from an impairment or a disability, that limits or prevents the fulfillment of a role that is normal (depending on age, sex, social, and cultural factors) for that individual. Because of the hand amputation, Mike Schmidt can no longer perform his job and is handicapped. I, as a physician, can still practice medicine without one hand and, therefore, am not handicapped though I have a disability. Handicap, thus, represents socialization of an impairment or disability; and as such, it reflects the consequences for the individual—cultural, social, economic, and environmental—that stem from the presence of impairment and disability.

Rehabilitation concerns itself with the *alleviation* of handicap, typically by using strategies that allow the patient to *compensate* for lost function. Pathology is not reversed. Specific disability is not undone.

Yet, handicap is lessened or even totally obviated by appropriate interventions. For example, Mike Schmidt could be taught to be a baseball manager—a job he could do with one hand. In the aftermath of brain injury, Miller believes that *amelioration* is a much more sensible and potentially attainable goal than *restitution*. In Miller's opinion, functional adaptation is the major mechanism for recovery of function following brain injury. The general idea behind functional adaptation is that the injured individual might be able to regain the ability to achieve a certain goal affected by brain damage by means other than those originally employed. The classic rehabilitation approach is to do just that: train an individual to achieve similar goals by means different from those used premorbidly in order to eliminate handicap despite the presence of disability.

According to Miller, neither of the terms contained in the phrase "recovery of function" is simple or straightforward. Luria states that the term *function* can be understood in two completely different ways. Function can refer to the activities of a small unit such as a particular tissue. The function of the pancreas is to secrete insulin. The function of muscle tissue is to contract. Such functions are specific and are strongly localized in the particular tissues. Function can also be understood as a complex adaptive activity aimed at the performance of some vitally important task. For example, locomotion, speech, and mathematical calculation can be understood as activities of complex systems whose components have been put together from more elementary central nervous system processes. These adaptive activities are performed by complex functional systems that pursue constant goals through complex, interchangeable means. Luria gives the following example:

> The function of respiration is to supply air to the alveoli of the lungs. However, the fulfillment of this task requires expansion of the chest; and this act in turn requires the participation of a system of muscles, particularly the muscles of the diaphragm. However, if the muscles of the diaphragm are paralyzed the person does not die from asphyxia. The intercostal muscles are brought into action, and to a large extent, they take over the function of the muscles of the diaphragm. If for some reason the intercostal muscles are also out of action, the person can swallow air by utilizing the apparatus of the pharynx and larynx not previously concerned with the act of respiration.

Luria thus regarded respiration not as a function of a fixed tissue but rather as the product of a complex functional system. Constraints imposed upon task performance resulted in the utilization of other means to achieve the desired outcome (air supplied to the lungs). From Luria's perspective, patients with brain injury have disturbances in "higher psychological processes" and these processes are not "functions" in the first meaning of the word but rather complex and variable functional systems capable of carrying out specific ends through a variety of different means.

The term function can also be used to refer to some kind of overt performance. For example, the ability to walk in the community for a specified distance may be used as the defining characteristic of a functional community ambulator. On the other hand, the function involved could be assumed to be some sort of hypothesized ability, such as motor control or voluntary function, considered to be necessary for adequate performance in tasks requiring cyclical movements. Thus function can refer to goals (e.g., walking to a mailbox in the community) or to means (the underlying voluntary movement process).

In regard to goals and means, *recovery* is ambiguous in the same way as function. Recovery in a hemiplegic patient may be considered solely in terms of meeting certain ends. The goal might be recovery of everyday walking without falling or fatigue. This goal may be achieved by using a brace and cane. Alternatively, recovery may refer to an improvement in the means (i.e., voluntary motor control processes) by which a person is enabled to walk. Walking without a cane in the home is a sign of recovering "similar" premorbid means of motor control. In general terms, recovery of means implies recovery of the ability to achieve end goals. However, the reverse is not necessarily true since the person may learn to achieve the same goals, such as going to the store, by different means, such as using a wheelchair to compensate for poor leg control. The term *recovery of function,* unless clearly specified in the context in which it is used, can lead to ambiguities both from the perspective of conceptualizing function and conceptualizing recovery.

Matters may muddle a bit more when the term *spontaneous* is merged with recovery of function to produce the superficially clear phrase: "spontaneous recovery of function." Some think spontaneous refers to recovery that takes place in tissue that is temporarily but not permanently damaged. A favorite example is the resolution of edema following a central nervous system lesion. The recovered function was never permanently lost but rather temporarily blocked. Loss of facilitation or increased inhibition (according to von Monakow's theory of diaschisis) as a result of a lesion may be another mechanism that, when reversed, can result in the clinical appearance of spontaneous recovery. Another view of the concept of spontaneous functional recovery centers on the *absence of intervention,* which could account for the recovery. Improvement is considered to be spontaneous because no direct intervention is "causal." An example comes from Geschwind, who describes the following patient recovering from aphasia:

> One patient whom I followed closely had shown no change between 3 months and 1 year and I advised him that I doubted that he would ever get back to

his old job. A year later, 2 years from onset, he turned up in my office. Over the intervening year with *no specific treatment* he had improved to the point of being able to return to work as a salesman. I know of other cases in which significant recovery has gone on over as many as 6 years.

Later Geschwind summarizes: "Although spontaneous useful recovery in aphasia, therefore, occurs in many cases, we should not forget that poor recovery is still the fate of probably the majority of aphasics." Geschwind appears to equate spontaneous recovery with changes occurring without specific treatment.

The need for rehabilitation is not necessarily obviated by spontaneous recovery. First, our ability to predict that spontaneous recovery will take place is limited. Second, resolution of edema or diaschisis occurs over weeks, and patients easily develop deconditioning or a variety of bedrest complications. Though the neurological signs and symptoms recover spontaneously the patient may lose overall functional capacity which can be restored through formal rehabilitation programs. More typically, the commonest type of problem seen in the rehabilitation clinic is the case in which neurological recovery is incomplete and rehabilitation techniques are needed to deal with impaired function associated with the neurological residual. For example, a case of Guillain-Barre syndrome can show neurological recovery for many months. Complete recovery doesn't necessarily occur, and residual neurological weakness and the attendant reduction in functional capacity can be dealt with by a variety of rehabilitation techniques.

Rehabilitation does not make claim to reversing pathology or causing recovery. Rehabilitation techniques take advantage of recovery when it does occur to assist the individual in achieving practical end goals through a variety of means that generally were not employed before the injury. Treatment strategies can be broadly categorized into three classes: remediation/restitution/restoration, compensation/amelioration/alleviation, and environmental modification. Remediation/restitution/restoration are terms that are most referable to the concept of anatomical or functional reorganization. In a sense, a rehabilitation training program that aims at remediation/restitution/restoration attacks the pathology directly and, in some way, hopes to capitalize on reorganization, assist reorganization, and promote functional recovery by improving means processes that approach or attain premorbid levels of operation. If the rehabilitation aim is to compensate/ameliorate/alleviate the functional consequences of neurological impairment, then functional adaptation as an explanation for recovery provides a more appropriate fit to this intervention strategy. Modification of the environment, such as providing a wheelchair ramp into a building, also falls under the general category of compensation/alleviation/amelioration from a strategic point of view.

Miller strongly feels that functional adaptation is the primary mode of recovery of function in brain-injured survivors and should be considered the basis for current rehabilitation programs in this population. Luria's training method, which emphasizes alternative means to accomplish specific functional goals, is a good approach to follow. In the area of memory impairment, Schacter and Glisky come down strongly in favor of alleviation of memory problems in specific situations as opposed to restoration of memory processes in a general way. Similarly, Mayer, Keating, and Rapp have advocated a skills-specific, context-specific approach based on the functional adaptation model of recovery.

How does the clinic integrate theory with practice? Every clinician who is an advocate for his patient hopes for reestablishment of function. He shares hope with the family that function is not really lost but merely blocked by a treatable pathology or by one that will remit on its own. When matters are known and interventions can be tried, the clinician will attempt to intervene. He will try steroids for edema, burr holes for a subdural hematoma, and a shunt for normal pressure hydrocephalus. However, complete reestablishment of premorbid function is uncommonly seen in the rehabilitation clinic where partial recovery is the general rule. Therefore, techniques of compensation and environmental modification are most commonly used by the rehabilitationist to augment the partial recovery that has taken place. A direct attack on the pathology might also be considered, depending on the degree of functional recovery, i.e., how much it approaches the premorbid level of operation. For example, as a patient with Guillain-Barre syndrome reestablishes strength in his or her lower extremities, restorative gait training, which supplants wheelchair ambulation, is usually appropriate. But while training for restitution of gait function goes on, the rehabilitationist will utilize compensatory strategies to achieve functional end goals even while working on strengthening process means. He may, for example, prescribe a brace to be used by the patient who is recovering from Guillain-Barre syndrome in order to help the patient achieve stability in locomotion. Without compensatory bracing, it might not be possible for the patient to ambulate at all. The priorities of the clinic are, for the most part, to achieve function as ends rather than means.

Since most patients who enter the rehabilitation system do so directly from acute care, rehabilitation practitioners seem most familiar with early recovery issues. The problems faced by patients and families during early recovery, particularly after catastrophic central nervous system insults, are usually more dramatic and globally significant to the patient and his or her social support system. Late recovery issues tend to be more focal and are better circumscribed. They are usually raised in regard to patients who are highly motivated and who can participate actively in a concentrated way on a specific retraining paradigm. Much remains to be developed in the area of late recovery, particularly mechanisms that can be identified through clinical techniques that would enable the practitioner to target specific patients for late recovery training.

Jennett has pointed out that the temporary crises of the first few days after a head injury fade into insignificance beside the life-long handicap that many survivors of severe injury are destined to suffer. What do we know about that handicap? Livingston, Brooks, and Bond (1985) reported that social maladjustment of relatives of head-injured persons increased over the course of the first year after head injury. Thomsen (1974) found that the main problem identified by patients 1 to 6 years after severe head injury was lack of social contact. Most of the patients she described had lost contact with old friends and had little opportunity to make new friends because they spent nearly all their time at home. In an in-depth interview with 142 families of traumatic head-injury survivors in the metropolitan Los Angeles area, Jacobs (personal communication) indicated that families constituted the major sources of support, socialization, and assistance to the head-injured survivors across all life skill areas that were surveyed. The hidden costs to the family that were associated with caring for a head-injured survivor were most telling. In approximately 37% of the families surveyed, a family member had to continuously supervise the head-injured survivor, and in half of these cases, this family member had given up a job or full-time schooling to meet this need. Thus, the family suffered the loss of one person's income to meet this need. In agreement with others, Jacobs also found that behavioral, emotional, and cognitive problems were more difficult to cope with than physical problems and that long-term financial issues were always a source of concern for everybody.

As Bond and others had previously reported, Jacobs found that head injury was a significant cause of stress in most areas of family living including marital, parental, and sibling relations; family activities; and the long-term goals of most family members. Families reported playing highly significant roles in both the daily lives and futures of head injury survivors. Not only were most families highly involved during initial rehabilitation programming but many families reported providing perpetual care and treatment to meet the needs of their disabled members. Most of the deficits identified in the Jacobs survey precluded the independent functioning and self-sufficiency of the head-injured survivor. With a poor prognosis for employment, impaired community functioning, and a life expectancy similar to the noninjured population, this expanding group of individuals could be dependent upon others for 50 years or more. "Ultimately at some point the care and rehabilitation of the survivor becomes a social issue." Jacobs charitably concludes:

Although it is not clear how effectively newly developing rehabilitation programs will be able to help the survivor return to independent status, and how much perpetual support each survivor will require over their lives, it is clear that a wide range of services and programs are required to meet these needs.

Clinical experience along with a review of the available literature on social outcome strongly suggests that current rehabilitation programs are not able to help the severely head-injured patient return to independent status. Perpetual support for the survivors will be required over their lifetimes. Predictive models of the degree of that support are clearly needed. These models will likely be based on theoretical underpinnings for social system dynamics. For example, systems analysis research may help to clarify the kinds of supports that should be provided to families and members of social networks who are managers and caregivers for head-injured survivors. Rehabilitation potential should not be defined strictly in terms of the individual with a head injury but rather should be viewed from the perspective of rehabilitating the entire social system of which the head-injured individual is a part. Prediction of outcome, therefore, would not simply relate to the outcome status of the individual but rather to the outcome status of the nuclear social system that includes the patient.

Because the author views the problem of head injury as social in nature, it is his belief that fundamental issues for every patient with a head injury center on the stability of (a) destination and (b) activity pattern. By destination, we mean: (a) Where will the patient live; (b) who will be the managers; (c) who will be the caregivers; (d) what will be the costs; (e) what social rearrangements will be necessary (i.e., what will be the social burden?); and (f) most importantly, what prediction of stability can be made with regard to the destination plan and what supports are necessary to preserve that stability? By activity pattern, we mean: (a) What does the patient do with his time; (b) how can the individual contribute to the stability of the caregiving system that has been developed around him; (c) how much management is required to implement an activity pattern; (d) what are the economic and social costs of maintaining an activity pattern; and (e) how does the activity pattern relate to the quality of life of the individual? An effective outcome would be one in which social burden is minimized, destination stability maximized, and activity patterns established to the satisfaction of the head injury survivor and his or her caregivers and managers. Of course, rehabilitating the individual to an independent status that is restoring his or her ability to make responsible decisions and to take control of his or her life would be most desirable but is certainly unrealistic at the present time.

Oddy reiterates the wide-ranging effects that closed head injury has on the survivor's life as well as on the lives of those around the survivor. Social isolation was a strong theme that he identified in the group of patients he studied, and this was particularly true for patients who had received treatments in rehabilitation centers and were acknowledged to be the most severely injured population. Oddy concluded that here was a clear need to broaden the aims of rehabilitation. He felt that there was a strong argument for the reallocation of resources to cover mental as well as physical rehabilitation. His work, as does the work of others cited above, points to the significant social consequences of head injury, which need reassessment by rehabilitation professionals in terms of the goals that they pursue.

The classical definition of rehabilitation is from the National Council on Rehabilitation (1942): ". . . restoration of the handicapped to the fullest physical, mental, social, vocational and economic usefulness of which they are capable." The World Health Organization (1969) definition is similar. "Rehabilitation is combined and coordinated use of medical, social, educational and vocational measures for training or retraining the disabled individual to the highest level of functional ability."

As emphasized in the classical definition, the practice of rehabilitation today is very much oriented to *rehabilitation of the individual* but the functional consequences of brain injury affect not only the injured people but also their immediate families, their extended social networks, their immediate communities, and society at large. It is the author's view that emphasis should be shifted to *rehabilitation of the nuclear social system* that includes and supports the disabled individual. Head injury is a social disorder of which the chief handicap is characterized by the shift of responsible decision making from the brain-injured individual to targeted managers and caregivers. The focus of rehabilitating the individual to his or her maximum ability or maximum potential is out of sync with the clinical pathology that dictates a shift of responsible decision making by the patient to responsible decision making for the patient by caregivers and managers. Though degree of management and caregiving may be altered by rehabilitation, the permanent loss of complete executive control sets a limit on the possibilities of rehabilitation and requires clinicians to reflect on the fundamental questions that emerge after acute care stabilization, namely: How do clinicians predict the rehabilitation potential of *this* patient in terms of social outcome? (Translate *outcome* as demands made on the nuclear social system.) Rehabilitation of whom? The patient? No. The nuclear social system that includes the patient. What predictions of destination and activity pattern can clinicians make for this patient? Where will clinicians find effective rehabilitation and reeducation programming consistent with the social predictions of long-term burden? When viewed from the perspective of social disorder, brain injury produces a variety of handicaps for the nuclear social system, and it is these handicaps which need our rehabilitative efforts. To date, the efforts of rehabilitation have been focused largely on the injured person and away from the caregivers and managers. This is a mistake for two reasons: (a) The considerable population of patients with severe and moderate head injury requires managers and caregivers despite clinicians' best efforts to rehabilitate the individual "out" of this requirement, and (b) the consequences of the head injury epidemic to society will continue to generate pressures for relief of the societal burdens of this population. The danger of such pressures lies in enacting solutions that may benefit society at large but may, nevertheless, be detrimental to the brain-injured population we are seeking to serve. Our future research agenda should include themes relevant to theories of recovery of function for the individual and their implications for clinical practice. However, the agenda should also include a new emphasis on theories of *recovery of social function,* namely, functional adaptation within the nuclear social system of which the brain-injured person is a part.

REFERENCES

Bach-y-Rita P (1980): *Recovery of function: theoretical considerations for brain injury rehabilitation.* Baltimore: University Park Press.

Bond MR (1975): Assessment of the psychosocial outcome after severe head injury. Outcome of the severe damage to the CNS. *CIBA Foundation Symposium* 34:141–153.

Brooks N (1984): *Closed head injury: psychological, social and family consequences.* New York: Oxford University Press.

Gouvier WD, et al. (1987): Reliability and validity of the disability rating scale and the levels of cognitive functioning scale in monitoring recovery from severe head injury. *Archives Physical Medicine & Rehabilitation* 68:94–97.

Jennett B, Teasdale G (1981): *Management of head injuries.* Philadelphia: F.A. Davis Company.

Livingston MG, Brooks DN, Bond MR (1985): Patient outcome in the year following severe head injury and relative psychiatric and social fuctioning. *Journal of Neurology, Neurosurgery and Psychiatry* 48:876–881.

Luria AR (1975): Neuropsychology: its sources, principles, and prospects. In: *The neurosciences: paths of discovery.* Cambridge, MA: The MIT Press.

Mayer NH, Keating DJ, Rapp D (1986): Skills, routines, and activity patterns of daily living: a functional nested approach. In: BP Uzell, Y Gross: *Clinical neuropsychology of intervention.* Boston: Martinus Nijhoff Publishing.

Miller E (1984): *Recovery and management of neuropsychological impairments.* New York: John Wiley & Sons.

Oddy M, Humphrey M (1980): Social recovery during the year following severe head injury. *Journal of Neurology, Neurosurgery, and Psychiatry* 43:798–802.

Schacter DL, Glisky EL (1986): Memory remediation: restoration, alleviation, and the acquisition of domain-specific knowledge. In: BP Uzell, Y Gross: *Clinical neuropsychology of intervention*. Boston: Martinus Nijhoff Publishing.

Stein D, Rosen J, Butters N (1974): *Plasticity and recovery of function in the central nervous system*. Orlando, FL: Academic Press.

Thomsen IV (1974): The patient with severe head injury and his family—a follow-up study of 50 patients. *Scandinavian Journal of Rehabilitation Medicine* 6:180–183.

World Health Organization (1969): WHO Expert Committee on Medical Rehabilitation Second Report. WHO Technical Report, Series 419.

13

Improvement in the Context of Rehabilitation

Brigitta Rees, M.D.

Rehabilitation Research and Training Center, Emory University, Atlanta, Georgia, U.S.A.

Rehabilitation of the traumatically brain-injured individual was initiated to meet a tremendous need that had only become identified within the last 10 to 15 years. A considerable effort has been made throughout the world to affect the overall outcome of this complex population through specific programmatic designs and systems of care. Outcome, outcome predictors, and outcome measures have been intensely studied, but relatively little is known about the impact of rehabilitation interventions on overall outcome.

We are involved in research as well as the clinical care of individuals with traumatic brain injury. The proper use of the terms *outcome, improvement,* and *recovery* is a constantly recurring issue, and it appears that the terms need some clarification. In this chapter, I will attempt to define the terms, present an algorithm to relate the terms to one another, and relate them to the current knowledge about the terms in the context of traumatic brain injury.

Outcome is the overall status of an individual with traumatic brain injury at any point relative to the status immediately postinjury.

Improvement is the difference in status between two assessments in time and can be assessed between any chosen points.

Recovery is the process in time occurring because of actual neural, spontaneous recovery over time without the impact of rehabilitation interventions.

Therefore, improvement could be viewed as the functional gains resulting from both neural recovery and therapeutic interventions (Corthell and Tooman, 1985). Outcome could be viewed as the functional status due to improvment at any chosen point in relation to the status immediately after the occurrence of the traumatic brain injury. Outcome, therefore, would require an assessment at a chosen point compared to the baseline assessment done at the immediate acute stage following traumatic brain injury. Improvement would be the difference between at least two assessments in time as compared to one another. The two individual components determining both outcome and improvement would be the result of spontaneous recovery as well as improvement secondary to rehabilitation interventions.

OVERVIEW

In an attempt to conceptualize the above defined terms, outcome, improvement, and recovery, we propose the following algorithmic model (see Figure 13-1).

In the proposed model, outcomes and improvements are subdivided into relative contributory units in major life areas. PH represents the physical motor component, C the cognitive behavioral component, CM the communicative component, and PS the pscyhosocial component. The relative value of any component is shown by the height of the column in which it is represented, and time is shown for each component in 3-month bins. Outcome could be viewed as the sum of PH at the last mea-

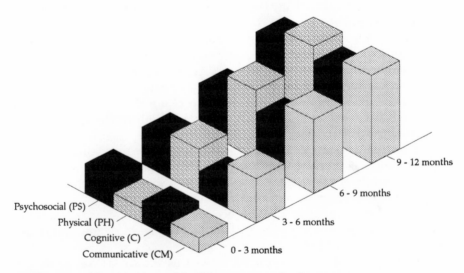

FIG. 13-1. Algorithmic model of the components of recovery.

sured point in time minus PH at the time zero, plus C at the last measured point minus C at point zero, plus CM at the last measured point in time minus CM at zero, plus PS at the last measured point in time minus PS at the onset.

Improvement, unlike outcome, can be referenced to any two points in time. Overall improvement at any moment could be viewed as the sum of the differences between two points in time for all components. For example, PH_n is a moment for variable PH representing, let us say, a 6 to 9 month value. PH_{n-1} is some moment before PH_n, say a 3 to 6 month value. Improvement in the physical component would be PH_n minus PH_{n-1} for the time interval between 6 to 9 months and 3 to 6 months.

The diversity of the traumatic brain-injured population and the attempts at classifying and identifying subgroups pose the next biggest problem. There seems to be a current consensus to classify acute traumatic brain injury into mild, moderate, and severe according to scores on the Glasgow Coma Scale. Severe head injury would be a score on the scale from 3 to 8; moderate, a score of 9 to 12; and minor, a score of 13 to 15 (Rimel et al., 1982; Heiden et al., 1979). There appears to be some controversy as to when an assessment on the Glasgow Coma Scale is a reliable predictor of outcome. Some studies are based on assessments within 2 to 4 hours of admission (Rimel et al., 1982) and some within the first 24 hours of admission (Heiden et al., 1979). We have some evidence that assessments done too early may lead to an unduly pessimistic prognosis (Jennett et al., 1979).

It is well known that scores on the Glasgow Coma Scale can change rapidly within the first hours or first days. Depending on the intracranial lesion, scores are also apt to change in both directions. For example, a patient originally admitted with a Glasgow Coma Scale of 13 to 15 may develop a hematoma hours to days later, with the Glasgow score changing to 3 to 5. Obviously, this change makes the prognosis much bleaker (Gennarelli et al., 1982). On the other hand, a patient admitted with a Glasgow Coma Scale below 7 but making a rapid recovery to a Glasgow Coma Scale above 8 may have a significantly better outlook than predicted at the time of emergency room admission.

Outcome predictions based on the Glasgow Coma Scale, especially when combined with the presence or absence of midline shifts on the CAT scan (Young et al., 1981), have been found to be useful predictors of overall outcome. We know that at 3 months postinjury, 38% of the moderate head injury category and 75% of the minor head injury category present with a good outcome (Rimel et al., 1982), whereas only 12% of those falling in the severe category within the first week have a favorable outcome (Young et al., 1981). When the Glasgow Coma Scale is compared to the Glasgow Outcome Scale (Jennett and Bond, 1975) at one year postinjury in the severe category, 35% of patients show moderate disability or good recovery, 13% remain severely disabled or vegetative, and 52% die (Heiden et al., 1983). In longitudinal follow-up, there may be a need for a somewhat more refined tool than the Glasgow Outcome Scale to identify more subtle progress during the course of rehabilitation (Hall et al., 1985).

The data mentioned in the two preceding paragraphs were gathered without specific attention to the presence of rehabilitation intervention strategies, and it remains the case that there is a significant lack of data demonstrating the impact of rehabilitation on the overall outcome in traumatic brain injury. Indeed, we know quite a bit about general recovery rate tendencies but very little about the actual impact of influencing factors such as rehabilitation.

There is, however, one recent publication (Aronow, 1987) on a study using a quasi-experimental method in studying the effect of rehabilitation in severe traumatic brain injury. This particular study concludes: (1) There seems to be better long-term outcome with rehabilitation. (2) There is a difference in the reported persisting problems and symptomatology between the two populations: (a) the subjects who had undergone rehabilitation reported more cognitive and emotional symptoms, and (b) the population without rehabilitation reported more physical symptoms. (3) There seems to be a significant impact on overall cost with the use of rehabilitation. As in many studies, the population that was referred to rehabilitation was the more severely affected traumatically brain-injured population. Once this factor was considered, there seemed to be a decrease in overall cost on a long-term basis in the traumatically brain-injured population that had undergone rehabilitation.

There is evidence that the greatest part of recovery occurs within the first 3 to 6 months after the injury (Heiden et al., 1983; Bond and Brooks, 1976; Diller and Ben-Yishay, 1983). Only 10% of patients who were in the severely or moderately disabled category at 6 months were in the next better category at 1 year (Jennett et al., 1981). After 1 year, only 5% of patients followed beyond the 12-month period to more than 18 months showed sufficient improvement to move on to a better category.

It has been postulated (Bond and Brooks, 1976) that the improvement within the first 6 months reflects actual physical reparation of the brain, whereas improvement beyond that point is primarily concerned with adaptation to fixed mental and physical deficits. When we follow patients over a 2-year period (Hall et al., 1985), there appears to be continued improvement in all areas. It is quite evident that rehabilitation strategies would make a significant difference in overall outcome, especially if implemented after 6 months when the presumed physical reparation of the brain is mostly completed.

Three stages of recovery have been proposed (Bond, 1979). The first stage is the period of unconsciousness. During the second stage, the patient regains full consciousness as signified by the end of posttraumatic amnesia and accompanied by rapid improvements in basic physical and mental functioning. The third stage is that of permanent residual disabilities. Each stage will require very specific and carefully tailored physical, psychological, and social intervention techniques. Also, there is evidence that individual impairments may be of varying importance depending on the particular stage of recovery and may have to be specifically addressed relative to the stage of recovery.

Again, there is a paucity of evidence that outside factors significantly change the overall outcome, and this is again identified as an area of great need for further study. More fascinating, though, would be to see whether specific interventional strategies in psychophysical retraining could significantly alter the seemingly natural recovery curve. Conceivably, if we could alter recovery in its early stage, we might, to some extent, change the overall outcome as well as the duration of the rehabilitation progress. This may have significant fiscal implications in terms of which rehabilitation strategy is introduced at what time.

Recovery curves and their potential alteration with interventions constitute one of the more fascinating, unstudied areas in traumatic brain injury. We know that recovery tends to occur at different rates within individual components of recovery as outlined above (Bond and Brooks, 1976). It is interesting, therefore, to speculate whether this is a natural course of events or whether our current approach in therapeutic measures addresses one aspect of recovery more efficiently than another. For example, does the relatively rapid recovery of verbal functioning (Mandleberg and Brooks, 1975) as compared to other functioning reflect our specific approach in the domain of communication, or does it reflect the natural healing tendencies of the brain? Obviously, many questions in this area remain to be answered, and this seems to be a fertile field for future research.

Across the numerous studies, various predictors of outcome have been identified. If it would be possible to change the predictive factors within themselves, overall outcome could conceivably be affected. The obvious, most important predictive factor at onset appears to be the premorbid state of the brain and the overall functioning within important life areas (Hagel, 1982). This is a given entity, amenable only to change in one direction. Age at the time of injury is another identified crucial factor that is not subject to change. Length and depth of coma are factors that are possibly subject to change through intervention. It would be of interest, however, whether use of psychotropic medications, specifically stimulants, could enhance recovery by their effect on arousal. Restlessness and agitation and their occurrence during the recovery seem to predict final outcome somewhat (Rao et al., 1985); but whether proper management of restlessness and agitation may indeed influence severity, duration, and/or final outcome merits investigation. It is conceivable that the overall state of health, infections, associated injuries, and general nutritional state may alter, to some extent, recovery curves (see "Nutritional Assessment of Closed Head Injured Patients" performed under Grant G008300041 from the National Institute on Disability and Rehabilitation Research, U.S. Department of Education).

In looking at overall outcome and improvement, one important aspect of health care delivery that has not been addressed so far is fiscal feasibility, even though major insurance carriers for a long time have studied cost factors of individual rehabilitation programs and of specific therapeutic interventions. Some of the following seems fairly common knowledge: Rehabilitation outcome statistics look much more favorable when patients are treated in larger, identified rehabilitation centers. Also, there seems to be an overall cost benefit of specifically identified programs, such as spinal cord injury programs and head injury programs, with a certain number of dedicated beds. There is at least some evidence that the more money initially spent in restoration and rehabilitation, the better the long-term fiscal outcome. A combination of the above factors seems to translate into decreased recurrent morbidity and hospitalizations and, therefore, saves a significant amount of money. Patients who benefit from a combination of the above factors seem to be more functional and are more likely to be able to live in less expensive living arrangements on a long-term basis. Also, a combination of the above factors may lead to increased employment or vocational reentry.

Unanswered questions include: (a) When is the best time for intervention? (b) What is the best type of intervention? (c) What should be the frequency and duration of the intervention for the best, and quickest, results? and (d) What is the cost benefit of individually identified programs? Also, it seems important fiscally to provide an adequate system of care, carrying a patient from the acute stage through the rehabilitation stage into the long-term care living arrangement and vocational stage. At least one study (Dekaban and Robinson, 1984) showed that after rehabilitation of severe closed head injury, 23.1% could be expected to return to full-time employment; 38.5% were able to perform part-time, lesser work; 13.8% were able to perform nonremunerative chores at home; 25.6% were not able to return to any work; and one third of the latter permanently required a long-term care facility. Another study showed that 30% of severe TBI patients returned to work 1 year after injury (Dekaban and Robinson, 1984). These studies, however, look at the cases after comprehensive rehabilitation only and do not necessarily reflect overall outcomes without rehabilitative intervention.

This section was an attempt to outline current knowledge about the effect and value of rehabilitative techniques in the context of our current knowledge of overall outcomes. It is evident that there are many unanswered questions and much need for future research in many of these areas. In the next section, the individual components of improvement and outcome as outlined in the proposed algorithms will be more specifically addressed.

PHYSICAL COMPONENT

Neurological dysfunction and secondary physical impairment are common consequences of traumatic brain injury. The variability of the type of involvement as well as the severity of involvement is one of the hallmarks setting traumatic brain injury and its consequences apart from other conditions causing central nervous system dysfunction. To some extent, the type and severity of involvement have been linked to the areas of the brain affected. But, in general, correlation with CAT scan findings and with resulting physical involvement is rather poor (Cohadon and Richer, 1983).

The following physical dysfunctions have been identified as occurring after traumatic brain injury: hemiplegia/diplegia, spasticity, rigidity, ataxia, sensory dysfunction including proprioceptive loss, apraxia, and multiple cranial nerve dysfunction secondary to brain stem lesions (Roberts, 1979). One series has found hemiparetic involvement in 40% of the severe traumatic brain-injured population; brain stem cerebellar involvement was the next most common, with 20% of that population affected; and only 5% showed athetoid and pseudobulbar type involvement.

Some stages of physical recovery have been recognized (Cohadon and Richer, 1983). The first stage is nonarousal, Glasgow Coma Score 3 to 8. This is frequently accompanied by severe neurovegetative disorders and decerebrate rigidity. In this stage, patients often require ventilatory assistance. The second stage is decorticate rigidity, in which the patient usually shows signs of receding neurovegetative disorders and ventilatory assistance can be discontinued. This may happen after a few days or weeks. In the third stage, awakening begins and the patient is starting to either localize response or follow a command. At this point, the actual physical deficits will become more obvious and symptoms of ataxia, paresis, and so forth may emerge more clearly. In general, this stage is still marked by significant hypertonicity. The recovery of motor activity at this stage will often closely parallel the ontogenesis of motor activity in early life (Cohadon and Richer, 1983). Characteristically, after traumatic brain injury the physical disability will steadily decrease with the passage of time; and in one study (Roberts, 1979), 71% of victims of severe traumatic brain injury were left with no or only insignificant motor disability.

As we look at physical disability, we can isolate the impairment of individual functions such as ataxia, hemiplegia, and sensory disturbances, or we can look at the overall functional state of a patient given certain physical limitations. A number of studies (Goodwin, 1982) have shown that in terms of overall outcome, physical impairments are relatively minor contributors to overall functioning in major life areas. In overall functioning in major life areas, the total functional outcome seems to be of a greater clinical importance than individual physical impairments. An excellent suggestion in the correlation of the two issues is given in a proposed rating scale (Dekaban and Robinson, 1984). It has been found (Cohadon and Richer, 1983) that even in cases of extremely severe traumatic brain injury, motor recovery or learning compensation tends to be striking and leads to a normal level of function in 50% of the cases.

It is self-evident that associated injuries as well as complications such as contractures (Najenson et al., 1974), heterotopic ossification, and decubitus ulcers will have a significant impact on improvement as well as on overall outcome. It has been shown, for instance, that fracture stabilization within the first 24 hours after traumatic brain injury has a significant impact on duration of ventilatory assistance as well as on death rate (Hanscom, 1987). Complications will naturally significantly retard improvement and possibly affect overall functional outcome.

We have little information about the validity of rehabilitation as a whole and about individual strategies affecting physical improvement and, possibly, recovery. For instance, we have some information about the superiority of certain gait training approaches (Nelson, 1983). Forced use has shown improvement of motor performance in a chronic head-injured population (see "Forced Use in Improving Function of Upper Extremity in Traumatic Head Injured Patients" performed under Grant G008300041 from the National Institute on Disability and Rehabilitation Research, U.S. Department of Education).

In summary, the natural history of recovery, improvement, and outcome of physical impairments incline toward a favorable result. There is, however, little information about either the necessity or the validity of rehabilitation interventions versus spontaneous recovery only.

COGNITIVE AND BEHAVIORAL COMPONENT

In this section, and in the limited context of this particular chapter, only a very cursory attempt can be made to illustrate the area of cognition and behavior in overall outcome, recovery, improvement, and therapeutic interventions. Cognition is used in this chapter as defined by Prigatano (1986). It is the basic ability of the brain to process, store, retrieve, and manipulate information to solve problems. The common cognitive dysfunctions are the following: (a) disorders of attention and concentration, (b) disorders of initiation and planning, (c) disorders of judgment and perception, (d) disorders of learning and memory, and (e) disorders of speed of information processing.

The last group, disorders of communication, will be dealt with in the next section. It has been known for quite some time and studies repeatedly reaffirm the fact that disturbances in cognition and behavior are the major determinant of overall outcome and of an individual's long-term functioning within himself or herself, the family, and society as a whole (Jennett et al., 1981; Bond, 1975). The overall intellectual functioning in the context of formalized testing, both in recovery as well as outcome, is probably the best studied area in cognition over time. Studies have shown that WAIS IQ scores reached an average plateau for adults at 6 months for verbal IQ and 13 months for performance IQ (Levin et al., 1982; Brooks, 1984). Apparently, recovery of intelligence to within the average range is common after traumatic brain injury, not necessarily meaning that return to premorbid functioning in terms of intellectual functioning is common after traumatic brain injury. Remediation strategies are many, and a number of programs have shown a significant impact of therapeutic interventions on intellectual and cognitive functioning using certain strategies (Diller and Ben-Yishay, 1983; Goldstein and Levin, 1987). We do have some evidence that neuropsychological rehabilitation results in a greater improvement in neuropsychological functioning on selected variables than outcomes unaffected by rehabilitation intervention (Prigatano et al., 1983; Prigatano et al., 1986).

The next area of cognition that has been studied to some extent is memory functioning. Apparently memory impairment, time and time again, has been shown to be a significant factor in the functional outcome of traumatically brain-injured patients (Wood, 1987). Rates of recovery seem to parallel those of general cognitive recovery. In memory retraining, the following facts seem to emerge: (a) Rehabilitation strategies have been quite effective in a patient population with a capability of learning memory compensation strategies and translating them into daily life, and (b) actual memory retraining, however, has shown rather disappointing results and usually shows improvement only in the laboratory with no carryover into functioning in major life areas.

Behavior is the next major determinant of overall functional outcomes. Behavior appears to be determined by certain stimulus events such as physical, social, or internal; organismic variables due to biological condition of the person involved; responses, either motor, cognitive, or physiological; and the consequences that follow from responses, such as self-generated anxiety or depression—physical or social (Wilson, 1987). Again, behavior seems to respond to behavioral remediation employing different conditioning procedures and principles. Behavioral techniques can be successfully applied to many areas of brain injury rehabilitation (Grafman, 1984).

In the area of cognition and behavior, we certainly do have some evidence of significant effectiveness of rehabilitation strategies. However, there still are many unanswered questions; questions such as timeliness and necessary intensity of involvement, as well as necessary duration, need to be studied further.

LANGUAGE AND COMMUNICATIVE COMPONENT

This component of overall impairment has been identified as another major determinant of overall functional outcome. It is quite often dealt with in the context of impairments of cognition. Because recovery tends to be somewhat different, as illustrated before, and impairments in this area can exist in isolation, it is dealt with as a separate entity in the context of this chapter. Impairment in language and communication can be divided into the following subgroups: (a) The mute or nonverbal vocal individual presenting with global language impairment (this may occur in up to 3% of the severe traumatically brain-injured population [Levin et al., 1983]; when associated with diffuse brain injury, this condition is often a predictor of long-term significant linguistic deficits); (b) the non-vocal patient with intact understanding; (c) the patient with fluent expression but dysphasic involvement or language disorganization; and (d) the nonaphasic dysarthric patient (Sarno and Hook, 1980; Sarno and Levita, 1986).

Significant improvement in language functioning will occur within the first month and be noticeable at a monthly rate up to 6 months (Groher, 1977). In our own population (see "The Relationship Between Cognitive Status, Objective Language Skills and Functional Language During Recovery From Severe Closed Head Injury" performed under Grant G008300041 from the National Institute on Disability and Rehabilitation Research, U.S. Department of Education), evidence shows that 18 months to 5 years posttraumatic brain injury, 20% of involved individuals still demonstrate some degree of aphasic impairment.

So far, little has been done to validate the effects of individual intervention strategies in improved communication. The fact that linguistic functions tend to recover either parallel or faster than any other function possibly points toward our most efficient approach currently in this particular area. Still further studies need to be done in timeliness, efficiency, and feasibility of intervention.

PSYCHOSOCIAL COMPONENT

Changes in psychosocial functioning after traumatic brain injury are the major determinants for patient and family distress. Traumatically brain-injured patients present themselves with increased levels of depression and decreased self-esteem, translating into impaired social and interactional skills of an increasing severity with increasing temporal distance from head injury (Tyerman and Humphrey, 1984). This will translate, socially, into loss of relationships, decreased leisure activity, and vocational losses. Factors working within the family unit are role changes and conflicts arising from this issue; loss of revenue; coping of relatives with the traumatic incidents; coping of family members, specifically spouses, with the behaviorally altered individual; and parent/child relationship problems. Interestingly enough, psychosocial problems tend to increase in severity (Brooks et al., 1986) with family-reported distress levels being much more severe at 5 years after the injury than at 1 year. There is one study, however, that demonstrates improvement over the second year. It is interesting to note that in this particular study, all patients were in a therapeutic program (Weddell et al., 1980). At least one study of late outcome 10 to 15 years posttrauma showed psychosocial problems presenting the most serious problems at that time after injury (Thomsen, 1984).

This particular area is interesting. With the exception of a few studies reporting on patients mostly in rehabilitation settings, reported stress levels, social dysfunctions, and depression appear to worsen over time. All other areas of posttraumatic brain injury dysfunction show a natural gradual tendency toward improvement with the exception of this one (Lezak, in press; Fordyce et al., 1983; Novack et al., 1984).

There is only suggestive evidence that effective therapeutic intervention in psychosocial aspects could lead to dramatic results in psychosocial functioning and distress on the part of patients and their families or others close to them.

Acknowledgment: The author would like to acknowledge the valuable assistance and cooperation of Drs. Gonnella, Banja, Wolf, Auerbach, Stringer, Daniel, DeBacher, and Cording, and Ms. Sullivan.

REFERENCES

Corthell DW, Tooman M (1985): *Rehabilitation of TBI (traumatic brain injury).* Louisville: Twelfth Institute on Rehabilitation Issues.

Rimel RW, et al (1982): Moderate head injury: completing the clinical spectrum of brain trauma. *Neurosurgery* 11:344–351.

Heiden JS, et al (1979): Severe head injury and outcome: a prospective study. In: Popp R (ed.), *Neural trauma.* New York: Raven Press, pp. 181–193.

Jennett B, et al (1979): Prognosis of patients with severe head injury. *Neurosurgery* 4:283–289.

Gennarelli TA, et al (1982): Influence of the type of intracranial lesion on outcome from severe head injury. *Journal of Neurosurgery* 56:26–32.

Young B, et al (1981): Early prediction of outcome in head-injured patients. *Journal of Neurosurgery* 54:300–303.

Jennett B, Bond M (1975): Assessment of outcome after severe brain damage: a practical scale. *The Lancet* 1:480–484.

Heiden JS, et al (1983): Severe head injury: clinical assessment and outcome. *Physical Therapy* 63:1946–1951.

Hall K, et al (1985): Glasgow outcome scale and disability rating scale: comparative usefulness in following recovery in traumatic head injury. *Archives of Physical Medicine and Rehabilitation* 66:35–37.

Bond MR, Brooks DN (1976): Understanding the process of recovery as a basis for the investigation of rehabilitation for the brain injured. *Scandinavian Journal of Rehabilitation Medicine* 8:127–133.

Aronow HU (1987): Rehabilitation effectiveness with severe brain injury: Translating research into policy. *Journal of Head Trauma Rehabilitation* 2(3):24–36.

Diller L, Ben-Yishay Y (1983): *Severe head trauma: a comprehensive medical approach to rehabilitation.* New York: New York University Medical Center, Institute of Rehabilitation Medicine.

Jennett B, et al (1981): Disability after severe head injury: observations on the use of the Glasgow Outcome Scale. *Journal of Neurology, Neurosurgery, and Psychiatry* 44:285–293.

Bond MR (1979): The stages of recovery from severe head injury with special reference to late outcome. *International Rehabilitation Medicine* 1:155–159.

Mandleberg I, Brooks DN (1975): Cognitive recovery after severe head injury. I. Serial testing on the Wechsler Adult Intelligence Scale. *Journal of Neurology, Neurosurgery, and Psychiatry* 38:1121–1126.

Hagel KH (1982): Prognose und rehabilitationsaufgaben nach schweren Schaedel-hirn-verletzungen [Prognosis and rehabilitation after severe cranio-cerebral trauma]. *Unfallheilkunde* 85:192–200.

Reyes RL, Bhattacharyya AK, Heller D (January 1981): Traumatic head injury: restlessness and agitation as prognosticators of physical and psychologic improvement in patients. *Archives of Physical Medicine and Rehabilitation* 62(1).

Bhoomkar A, Barbour P (1986): Nutritional assessment of closed head injured patients. Annual Progress Report to the National Institute of Disability and Rehabilitation Research, Grant G008300041, pp. 127–131.

Dekaban AS, Robinson CE (1984): Application of a new rating scale of brain dysfunction to monitoring rehabilitation in 65 patients with severe head injury. *Bulletin of Clinical Neuroscience* 49:89–92.

Cohadon F, Richer E (1983): Recovery of motor function after severe traumatic coma: a clinical description and discussion of mechanisms involved. *Birth Defects: Original Article Series* 19:375–387.

Roberts AH (1979): *Severe accidental head injury.* London: Macmillan Press, Ltd.

Goodwin DM (1982): Cognitive and physical recovery trends in severe closed-head injury (doctoral dissertation, Pacific Graduate School of Psychology, 1982). *Dissertation Abstracts International* 43:3066B.

Najenson T, et al (1974): Rehabilitation after severe head injury. *Scand J Rehab Med* 46:5–14.

Hanscom DA (1987): Acute management of the multiply injured head trauma patient. *Journal of Head Trauma Rehabilitation* 2:1–12.

Nelson AR (1983): Strategies for improving motor control. In: Rosenthal M, et al (eds.). *Rehabilitation of the head injured adult.* Philadelphia: FA Davis Company.

Wolf SL (1986): Forced use in improving function of upper extremity in traumatic head injured patients. Annual Progress Report to National Institute of Disability and Rehabilitation Research (grant G008300041), pp. 67–85.

Prigatano GP, Fordyce DJ (1986): Cognitive dysfunction and psychosocial adjustment after brain injury. In: Prigatano GP, et al (eds.). *Neuropsychological rehabilitation after brain injury.* Baltimore: The Johns Hopkins University Press.

Bond MR (1975): Assessment of the psychosocial outcome after severe head injury. In: *Outcome of severe damage to the central nervous system (CIBA Foundation Symposium #34).* New York: American Elsevier, pp. 141–157.

Levin HS, et al (1982): *Neurobehavioral consequences of closed head injury.* New York: Oxford University Press.

Brooks N (1984): Cognitive deficits after head injury. In: Brooks N (ed.). *Closed head injury: psychological, social, and family consequences.* Oxford: Oxford University Press, pp. 44–73.

Goldstein FC, Levin HS (1987): Disorders of reasoning and problem-solving ability. In: Meier M et al (eds.) *Neuropsychological rehabilitation.* New York: The Guilford Press, pp. 327–354.

Prigatano GP, et al (1984): Neuropsychological rehabilitation after closed head injury in young adults. *Journal of Neurology, Neurosurgery, and Psychiatry* 47:505–513.

Prigatano GP, et al (1986): The outcome of neuropsychological rehabilitation efforts, In: Prigatano GP, et al (eds.). *Neuropsychological rehabilitation after brain injury.* Baltimore: The Johns Hopkins University Press, pp. 119–133.

Wood RL (1987): *Brain injury rehabilitation: a neurobehavioral approach.* Rockville, MD: Aspen Publishers, Inc.

Wilson BA (1987): *Rehabilitation of memory.* New York: The Guilford Press.

Grafman J (1984): Memory assessment and remediation in brain-injured patients: from theory to practice. In: Edelstein BA, Couture ET (eds.). *Behavioral assessment and rehabilitation of the traumatically brain damaged.* New York: Plenum.

Levin HS, et al (1983): Mutism after closed head injury. *Archives of Neurology* 40:601–606.

Thomsen IV (1980): Evaluation, outcome and treatment of aphasia in patients with severe head injuries. In: Sarno MT, Hook O (eds.). *Aphasia: assessment and treatment.* Stockholm: Almqvist & Wiksell International, pp. 181–185.

Sarno MT, Levita E (1986): Characteristics of verbal impairment in closed head injured patients. *Archives of Physical Medicine and Rehabilitation* 67:400–405.

Groher M (1977): Language and memory disorders following closed head trauma. *Journal of Speech and Hearing Research* 20:212–223.

Peach R (1986): The relationship between cognitive status, objective language skills and functional language during recovery from severe closed head injury. Annual Progress Report to the National Institute for Disability and Rehabilitation Research (grant G008300041), pp. 108–121.

Tyerman A, Humphrey M (1984): Changes in self-concept following severe head injury. *International Journal of Rehabilitation Research* 7:11–23.

Brooks N, et al (1986): The five year outcome of severe blunt head injury: a relative's view. *Journal of Neurology, Neurosurgery, and Psychiatry* 49:764–770.

Weddell R, et al (1980): Social adjustment after rehabilitation: a two year follow-up of patients with severe head injury. *Psychological Medicine* 10:257–263.

Thomsen IV (1984): Late outcome of very severe blunt head trauma: a 10–15 year second follow-up. *Journal of Neurology, Neurosurgery, and Psychiatry* 47:260–268.

Lezak MD (in press): Relationships between personality disorders, social disturbances, and physical disability following traumatic brain injury. *Head Trauma Rehabilitation* 2(3):57–70.

Fordyce DJ, et al (1983): Enhanced emotional reactions in chronic head trauma patients. *Journal of Neurology, Neurosurgery, and Psychiatry,* 46:620–624.

Novack TA, et al (1984): Factors related to emotional adjustment following head injury. *The International Journal of Clinical Neuropsychology* 6:139–142.

14

Assessment in Traumatic Brain Injury

Leonard Diller, Ph.D., and Yehuda Ben-Yishay, Ph.D.

Rusk Institute of Rehabilitation Medicine, New York University Medical Center, New York, New York, U.S.A.

The purpose of this chapter is to review the knowledge base in assessment in the rehabilitation of individuals with traumatic brain injury (TBI). The review takes into account, first, issues concerning the development of valid and reliable knowledge, dealing primarily with methodologic considerations, and, second, the knowledge that has actually been established with instruments that have been used. Both methodology and content will then be examined to formulate suggestions for future directions. Furthermore, since the field is so large and bewildering, it might be helpful to consider the literature from the two major perspectives that have served as an impetus for the studies. These are from the vantage point of recovery and from the vantage point of rehabilitation. While both vantage points overlap, they also differ. The communalities and differences are important in considering further knowledge needs in this field.

Before examining accomplishments we note that the assessment instrument developer, who is generally a researcher, and the instrument user, who is generally a clinician, usually operate in different contexts with different constraints. A useful way of looking at this may be from a historical perspective.

Future generations of students of assessment of TBI rehabilitation may look back on our current activities much as we look back at the efforts of earlier generations of mapmakers and of navigators. Mapmakers had to struggle with balancing existing domains of knowledge with different degrees of credibility to establish new reliable points of knowledge. These points were determined by considerations of how gross/refined a map should be, how boundaries will be established and confirmed, and who would be using the map. A navigator was concerned with fashioning a path by using markers that were as trustworthy as possible to arrive at a destination. As students of cognitive theory have pointed out, navigators had to make decisions by taking into account knowledge of geography, elements of weather, oceanography, astronomy, and the means at their disposal including their ships, crews, and finances to estimate what was doable. The scientists among us are much like the early map-makers who wanted to establish reliable information. The clinicians among us are like the early navigators who needed knowledge to make decisions in terms of which paths of opportunity should be pursued. Both researchers and clinicians may be interested in recovery and rehabilitation.

The perspectives of recovery and rehabilitation share overlapping concerns in wishing to describe behavior, to formulate predictions, and to conduct research. They differ in relative emphases. For example, studies of recovery, which have by far the largest number of papers, have typically been concerned with brain behavior relationships. Most of the explications of behavior have been in the domain of impairments because the work emerged from neurosurgical settings with a strong emphasis on neurological, neuropathological, and neuropsychological measurements. Measures of disability and handicap were defined in rather gross terms as seen in the Glasgow Outcome Scale (Jennett, 1983). The impairment measures that were used (Brooks, 1984), for the most part, were derived from conventional neuropsychological tests which had to be adapted to the special considerations of TBI populations. By way of contrast, measures derived from rehabilitation settings that emphasize interventions and are more concerned with disabilities and handicaps tend to emphasize observations of behavior in naturalistic and seminaturalistic settings. These contrasting emphases tend to lead to somewhat different perspectives on assessment and measurement of behavior.

RECOVERY

What Have We Learned about Methodology?

Population Issues

1. The heterogeneity of TBI from neurological and neuropathological standpoints has been well described (Levin, Benton, and Grossman, 1982; Uzzel, 1986). A major way of categorizing subtypes of TBI is in terms of duration and depth of coma, for example, Glasgow Coma Scale (Teasdale and Jennett, 1974). Numerous studies suggest the usefulness of this ap-

proach. However useful this approach for describing groups, many investigators believe other measures must be added for individual prognosis (Eisenberg and Weiner, 1987). Furthermore, it has been shown that classification of individuals in terms of neurobehavioral syndromes leads to useful information. Thus Alexander (1987) has shown that TBIs divided on the basis of diffuse axonal injury, focal cortical contusions, and hypoxic-ischemic injury and combinations of these may show important clinical consequences and outcome. Similarly, distinctions between closed and penetrating TBI may have important clinical implications (Grafman and Salazar, 1987). Many of the studies of cognitive impairments have not examined the variations associated with etiology and other salient parameters of TBI.

2. Demographic considerations have also entered in terms of age, which may account for some of the variance in predicting recovery and social background and history. The latter are particularly important since it has been shown that traumatically brain-injured individuals may have a higher incidence of sociopathological background, which may influence outcome. Social factors in patient selection may affect who enters a study (Diller and Ben-Yishay, 1983) as well as attrition in follow-up. For example, patients without family support systems (Diller and Ben-Yishay, 1983) tend to drop out of follow-up as do patients with mild disabilities or those who deny disabilities (Brooks, 1984). Growing sophistication in retaining subjects may be seen when considering Conkey's (1938) study conducted 50 years ago when only 4 of 38 subjects returned one year later for follow-up. Dikmen and Temkin (1987) have drawn attention to problems created in recovery studies when patients are selected on the basis of convenience rather than on the basis of theoretical considerations. They found that a mild/moderate group of traumatically brain-injured patients performed relatively well when matched against norms used to standardize a test but showed a marked decline when compared with the test results of a group of friends who volunteered to serve as a comparison group.

Testing Issues

1. Neuropsychological tests have grown out of a blend of tasks used in clinical psychology, experimental psychology, and refinements and extensions of clinical neurological examinations. The same test items can be passed/failed for different reasons so that while a test score can be interpreted against some type of normative data base, the clinical significance of the score may not be obvious and its meaning may be ambiguous. Furthermore, major constructs such as attention or memory can be defined in many ways and measured by multiple indicators. It is,

therefore, important to use families of tests which may reflect the same underlying construct.

2. When tests are used on two or more occasions in recovery studies, it is unclear as to whether changes in performance may be attributed to genuine improvement, practice effects, or intratest variability. This critical question cannot be ignored. Various solutions have been offered, but each in turn has its own problems. Suggestions include using alternate forms of a test or using variations of sequential and cross-sectional designs (Brooks, 1987). It also may be necessary to titrate for the effects of severity. Severity of brain damage may be important with regard to practice effects because it is possible that an impaired group will improve with practice while an intact group will not or vice versa (Dikmen and Temkin, 1987). Finally, the issue of what happens between testing is generally ignored in reporting of results of recovery studies, yet it is clinically apparent that people go through major life experiences which might influence test results.

3. Ceiling-floor effects also enter because it is difficult to have a single test that is equally sensitive to performance differences at the lower range of functioning and at the upper range of functioning. Strauss and Allred (1987) have discussed many of the statistical issues concerning the discrimination power of test items and attempt to deal with problems in this area by statistical adjustments and the use of suitable control groups.

4. Changes in test scores or lack of changes in test scores have also surfaced as a methodologic issue in two additional ways. First, earlier studies, which had noted plateaus in recovery on intelligence test scores (Mandleberg and Brooks, 1975), were based on the use of group means. A look at recovery curves for individual patients suggests wide variation in recovery rates and plateaus so that individual prediction is more hazardous than the literature suggests (Brooks, 1984; Kay, Ezrachi, and Cavallo, 1986). Indeed, some of the variation may be due to the heterogeneity of traumatically brain-injured patients which are cited above. Second, statistical change or lack of statistical change on a test repeated on two or more occasions may or may not be associated with clinically significant change. In fact, it is not uncommon to find a statistically significant change although the amount of absolute change may be trivial. One solution to both of these problems has been offered by Kay, Ezrachi and Cavallo (1986), who plotted individual recovery curves that showed vast differences among traumatically brain-injured patients although group differences on tests administered on two occasions were not significant. They used as a measure of change on an individual test score one standard deviation (plus or minus) as a significant marker and were able to show different subtypes.

5. What types of norms are to be used? In theory, norms may be de-

rived from the standardization data, from other groups of traumatically brain-injured individuals who are recovering, and from pretraumatic data, where the individual serves as his or her own reference point for comparison. All of these approaches have practical and/or conceptual problems associated with them. If a comparison group is to be used, should the cohort group consist of individuals who haven't suffered brain damage but come from the same social background, a group that has suffered trauma without brain damage, or a group with an equivalent pattern of functional disability? Since it is difficult to control for all of these factors, investigators must often choose from among them. The unknowing reader or user of an instrument must be made aware of the limitations with regard to interpretation. With an increasing number of longitudinal studies, which are beginning to generate data (McClean et al., 1984; Acker, 1986; Meier, Strauman, and Thompson, 1987), there is increasing information about recovery for sizeable numbers of people. However, these studies were, for the most part, not designed for the purpose of serving as references for normative data with descriptions of procedures that would be found in test manuals.

6. Temporal issues also pose a methodologic problem. Different investigators have used time since onset as opposed to time since recovery from coma or posttraumatic amnesia as zero points to measure recovery. It is recognized that the starting point and point of initial testing will depend on factors such as severity of TBI because severe patients are untestable. Also, most of the published data on recovery in TBI has been confined to the first year post onset. This is largely due to matters of convenience and logistics. However, as there is a growing concern with management issues after rehabilitation has been completed, there will be increasing interest in tracking people over long periods of time.

7. While tracking studies conducted a decade ago were able to deal with significant population groups who received a minimum amount of care after the acute medical phase, this is less likely because TBI programs have grown so rapidly. Currently, interventions or the lack of interventions may be influenced by considerations of ability to pay so that social biases may partially determine who get treated.

8. Other issues emerge in different ways. It is increasingly recognized that problems in arousal, executive functions, self-regulatory behaviors, memory, and personality surface when the individual with TBI returns to the community. While there is effort being made to develop frontal lobe tests (Stuss, 1987; Goldberg and Bilder, 1987), these measures have seldom been included in studies of recovery. Many of the phenomena observed have, therefore, been at a gross descriptive level, using ratings or checklists rather than controlled samples of behavior which can be calibrated, scored, and matched against norms.

The major conclusions are that (a) experience with recovery studies shows increasing precision in subject and test selection and strategies for maintaining patients in a follow-up group, and (b) that better-designed studies should permit us to state a richer array of results with more confidence.

What Facts Have We Learned about Recovery?

1. In recovery basic skills return before complex skills.
2. WAIS verbal I.Q. scores recover before performance I.Q. scores.
3. Visual acuity for fine print is slow to recover and is sensitive to length of coma.
4. Memory variables improve later than most other variables.
5. While most recovery takes place during the first 6 months, there is evidence that language functions and other cognitive functions continue to improve at least during the first 24 months.
Linguistic disorders outside of dysphasia and dyspraxia occur in approximately one third of the patients referred to medical rehabilitation programs.
6. Clusters of cognitive disorders—attention, concept formation, executive functions, self-regulation of affect and memory—have all been identified. However, their coincidence and independence from each other have not been defined.
7. Personality disturbances have been noted but their assessment remains less precise than is the case in cognitive disturbances.
8. Various combinations of neurologic, neuropsychologic, and demographic variables can predict various outcomes. However, even though there are more than 40 studies published (Acker, 1986; Meier, Strauman, and Thompson, 1987), there is an absence of replications wherein investigators have used the same assessment instruments and criteria in different settings.
9. There is greater intraindividual variability in recovery than initial studies presumed.

REHABILITATION IN TBI

A rehabilitation perspective is, of course, concerned with issues of recovery. It emphasizes, however, a functional approach to assessment in terms of assistance needed to carry out the demands of daily living. It draws on a wide array of professional skills and combinations of resources for interventions and, finally, it attempts to reduce the dependency and enhance the satisfaction of the patient and family in order to pursue paths to normalization as much as possible. An important by-product of functional assessment is that it must be understood by a wide range of people including patients, families, service providers, administrators, resource providers, and researchers. Although the language of functional assessment is nontechnical, to be useful clinically and scientifically the vocabulary of functional assessment must be defined precisely.

Before proceeding, we can raise several caveats that should be considered. The field of rehabilitation appears to be evolving toward developing a taxonomy of distinctions in the domains of impairment, disability, and handicap (Fuhrer, 1987). While a discussion of these categories is beyond the scope of this chapter, it should be noted that this taxonomy evolved from experiences with people whose disabilities were primarily motoric. When the motoric problems are embedded in a complex of cognitive/behavioral/emotional dysfunctions or when this complex of dysfunctions is the problem, the distinctions and the usefulness of the taxonomy of the instruments used for categorizations may not be adequate. Thus, traditionally, levels of assistance for activities of daily living in spinal cord patients are predictable from degrees of motor impairment. But this need not be the case for individuals recovering from TBI, where cognitive factors must be considered. There appear to be phases/stages in recovery in which the management issues require systematic observations and interventions that are outside of the traditional domains of rehabilitation. This appears to be the case in individuals emerging from coma (Grimm and Bleiberg, 1985). To take a further example, what if the individual does not dress himself or herself, not because he or she is paralyzed but because the individual sits on the bed without initiating any movement?

What Have We Learned about Methodologic Issues?

1. In testing for outcomes of intervention, one must provide for a way of distinguishing between those subjects who have responded to the specific treatment and those who have not. It is possible that those who do not improve were never involved in the treatment (Freyer and Haffey, 1987; Prigatano, 1987).

2. Currently there are more than 18 systems for functional assessment that have been developed for the field of rehabilitation that are applicable to tracking TBIs (Forer, 1985). Only one of these, the Disability Rating Scale, has been developed specifically for TBI (Hall et al., 1985) and only one, the Functional Assessment Inventory Crew, has been used to assess program effects. Which of the functional assessment instruments should be used? At the present time, it is difficult to judge the merits of the individual instruments. Some of the issues concerning instrument selection have been discussed in general (Brown, Gordon, and Diller, 1984) and in specific reference to TBI (Diller and Ben-Yishay, 1987). Among the issues are relevance (Does the instrument reflect

disturbances in TBI? Does it capture the goals or content of the program? Does it measure change sensitive to case management or programs outcome?), feasibility (cost, duration of administration, ease), and validity and reliability.

3. Some of the considerations in designing methods for assessing effects of interventions must include specification of what is being treated, as measured by what stimuli and responses; how it is being treated, by whom, and for what length of time and frequency; and how outcomes are described (Diller and Gordon, 1981).

4. A major problem in assessing treatment effects is to demonstrate transfer of gains to situations outside of the treatment and to situations that are not task specific. One solution to this problem is to build in tests for generalization of skills that are taught in the program. For this reason pre and post measures of disabilities as well as of impairments should be included in test procedures. Examples of such an approach may be found in case studies of cognitive retraining (Cicerone, 1986) as well as in programs using a more holistic approach (Ben-Yishay et al., 1985).

What Have We Learned about Assessment Based on Observations in Rehabilitation?

1. In rehabilitation, performance in naturalistic situations is sampled and targeted for treatment. This is seen in the case of activities of daily living in medical rehabilitation, in work samples in vocational rehabilitation, and in learning academic samples in special education. In the case of cognitive deficits, a task analysis from the perspective of cognitive disturbances might be one strategy for assessment as well as for treatment. This approach has been used in the analysis of tooth brushing behavior in TBI (Nagele et al., 1986), driving behavior (Van Zomeren et al., 1987), patterns during occupational trials (Ben-Yishay, Silver, Ezrachi, in prep.), and—from a neighboring population—stroke patients learning to transfer to and from wheelchairs (Diller, Buxbaum, and Chiotelis, 1972).

Another approach has been to develop naturalistic tasks to sample cognitive disabilities. This may be seen in a test of memory in which individuals with TBI are required to remember different aspects of performing "natural" tasks such as following instructions (Baddeley et al., 1987) on the Rivermead Behavioral Memory Test.

A third approach has utilized observations of deviant behavior which can be monitored during rehabilitation. These observations can be used as criteria for interventions as seen in the work of Corrigan et al. (1985), who developed a measure of reality orientation that could be used as a criterion for a reality orientation group. Examples of this approach can be seen in methods of monitoring recovery from amnesia (Levin et al., 1979) and agitation (Corrigan et al., in press).

This approach to assessment is in keeping with "a process approach" in neuropsychology (Kaplan, 1987) wherein response style is said to reflect the manifestations of disturbances. However, instead of looking at performance on neuropsychological tests as the key, one looks at behavior manifested in the rehabilitation setting outside of the structured test.

2. Assessments of patterns of behavior exhibited by individuals with TBI have been shown to be reliable and sensitive to change while the individuals participated in medical rehabilitation programs. In the case of the Levels of Cognitive Functioning Scale, the so-called Ranchos Los Amigos Scale (Hagen et al., 1979), the Stover-Zeiger Scale (Stover and Zeiger, 1976), and the Disability Rating Scale (Hall et al., 1985) can be used in an interdisciplinary team setting.

3. More conventional approaches have also been shown to be sensitive to changes in activities of daily living skills (Panikoff, 1983), and variations of conventional scales have also been shown to be sensitive to change (Sehgal and Heinemann, 1986; Jellinek et al., 1982).

4. Rating scales can be used to assess a wide range of behaviors for individuals with TBI attending outpatient programs with holistic approaches (Ben-Yishay et al., 1987) and to track different dimensions of behavior for follow-up on a long-term basis (Lezak, 1986).

5. Scales for employment have been utilized in many studies (Ben-Yishay et al., 1986). Ben-Yishay et al. (1987) have developed a 10-point scale of employability to track vocational outcomes at periodic intervals. The refinement in methodology also is important because the question of job stability is a vital one in the case of TBI.

6. Can the self-reports of individuals with TBI be used in assessment? Self-reports of symptoms have been used in follow-up studies (Barth et al., 1983; Dikmen et al., 1983) and as ways of specifying complaints and needs in TBI cases. External validity of self-report is, of course, difficult to establish. However, it should be noted that individuals with TBI tend to minimize cognitive disabilities and that performance on psychological tests is related to family reports of dysfunctional behaviors but not to patient self-reports (Sunderland et al., 1984).

While most measures in rehabilitation utilize changes in skilled performance, attitudinal factors are important. In the case of TBI a vital factor appears to be that of denial/acceptance. Acceptance of disability is a critical factor in treatment compliance. Fordyce and Roueche (1986) have measured denial/acceptance by examining discrepancies of ratings among patients, families, and staff and found them to be related to treatment. Ben-Yishay et al. (in prep.) found that acceptance is the most powerful predictor of vocational outcome. The finding is striking because conventional prediction studies of outcomes have generally used neurologic, demographic, and neuropsychologic test performance as predictors. It might be argued that such studies fail to sample what is being treated whereas acceptance of disability is a major variable being treated in a holistic outpatient treatment program.

Finally, there is a suggestion that patients' perceptions of memory problems differ from the problems being assessed by conventional tests of memory. This raises the possibility that patients' primary concerns with prospective memory are not evaluated or treated. Since tests are derived from laboratory and psychometric considerations, and memory remediation has been difficult to demonstrate in TBI, perhaps the failure may be due to the fact that the wrong dimension of memory is being treated. Mateer et al. (1987) argue that this type of assessment, which is basically consumer driven, may indicate a need for a paradigm shift in assessment as well as treatment in TBI.

7. In addition to attempts at quantifying observations relevant to inpatient rehabilitation for TBI noted above, some attempts to quantify relevant observations for outpatients may also be noted. One such approach (Ben-Yishay et al., 1982) integrates neuropsychologic data, samples of daily life functioning, assessment of personal (self-awareness understanding, and acceptance) and interpersonal (intimacy and small group interactions) behaviors. A profile based on all of these measures is established. The neuropsychologic domains-psychomotor, integrative memory, and verbal-ideational skills use multiple tests to sample each of these domains. Redundancy of tests is used to test for the effects of generalization of skill training within a domain. The areas of competence in daily life involve dimensions of behavior that are sensitive to disturbances common in TBI, such as orientation to familiar and unfamiliar environments, memory for daily life routines, and appropriateness of interpersonal behavior. In addition to these measures, which are administered at the beginning and end of the program, two other sets of measures are used including (a) process measures such as a cognitive learning index, a small group assimilation index (or interpersonal inputs), and a malleability index (i.e., willingness and capacity to modify pathologic behaviors that interfere with normal functioning/acceptance in everyday life); and (b) outcome measures (e.g., competence in daily life functions, measures of employability and work skills, and measures of personal and social adjustment).

While pre and post studies have been conducted to test for the effects of interventions (Ben-Yishay et al., 1987), it is apparent that the process measures are related to both initial competence and vocational outcome measures. While initial competence measures predict vocational outcomes, when the process measures are partialed out of the correlation the prediction drops. Hence while initial competence is related to vocational outcome, the relation is mediated by the person's ability to learn and assimilate interpersonal inputs. Finally, when a process measure labeled acceptance index was used to predict outcome, it added considerably to the prediction.

Many of the critical behaviors observed in the course of the program become part of the treatment. While not assessed on formal tests, they are capable of reliable observation and become major components of the treatment and appear to relate highly to outcomes.

ISSUES/NEEDS FOR FUTURE STUDY

1. Conventional neuropsychologic tests and functional assessments derived from other populations and applied to TBI, versus measures derived from observations of individuals with TBI and program content, or combinations of both—what is the best mix?

2. Psychometric tests to measure frontal lobe functions, for example, executive functions, process functions, and acceptance/awareness, need to be developed.

3. Appropriate taxonomies of TBI for rehabilitation purposes, that is, methods of integrating indexes of pathology, impairment disability, and outcome measures, need to be developed.

4. There is a need for measures that sample what is being treated.

5. With the multiplication of a variety of outpatient treatment programs, for example, vocational, day treatment, cognitive rehabilitation, with overlapping program content, there is a need for an assessment of instruments to help decide who needs what program.

6. There is further need for ecologically relevant measures in all phases of rehabilitation.

7. There are specific assessment tools that are needed to monitor behavior at both ends of the TBI continuum, the very severe and the very mild.

REFERENCES

Jennett B (1983). Scale and scope of the problem. In: M Rosenthal, ER Griffith, MR Bond, JR Miller (eds.). *Rehabilitation of the head injured adult*. Philadelphia: FA Davis.

Brooks N (ed.) (1984). *Closed head injury: Psychological, social and family consequences*. New York: Oxford University Press.

Levin H, Benton AL, Grossman R (1982). *Neurobehavioral consequences of closed head injuries*. New York: Oxford University Press.

Uzzel BP (1986). Pathophysiology and behavioral recovery. In: BP Uzzel, Y Gross (eds.). *Clinical neuropsychology of intervention*. Boston: Martinus Nijhoff Publishing.

Teasdale G, Jennett B (1976). Assessment and prognosis of coma after head injury. *Acta Neuro (Wien)* 34:45.

Eisenberg HM, Weiner R (1987). Input variables: how information from the acute injury can be used to characterize groups of patients for studies of outcome. In: HS Levin, J Grafman, HM Eisenberg (eds.). *Neurobehavioral recovery from head injury*. New York: Oxford University Press.

Alexander MJ (1987): The role of neurobehavioral syndromes in the rehabilitation and outcome of closed head injury. In: HS Levin, J Grafman, HM Eisenberg (eds.). *Neurobehavioral recovery from head injury*. New York: Oxford University Press.

Grafman J, Salaza A (1987): Methodological considerations relevant to the comparison of recovery from penetrating and closed head injuries. In: HS Levin, J Grafman, HM Eisenberg (eds.). *Neurobehavioral recovery from head injury*. New York: Oxford University Press.

Diller L, Ben-Yishay Y (1983): *Final report on severe head trauma. A comprehensive medical approach to rehabilitation* (National Institutes of Handicapped Research). New York: New York University (grant No. GT13-P-59082).

Conkey RC (1938): Psychological changes associated with head injuries. *Archives of Psychology* 232:1–62.

Dikmen S, Temkin N (1987): Determination of the effects of head injury and recovery in behavioral research. In: HS Levin, J Grafman, HM Eisenberg (eds.). *Neurobehavioral recovery from head injury*. New York: Oxford University Press.

Brooks N (1987): Measuring neuropsychological and functional recovery. In: HS Levin, J Grafman, HM Eisenberg (eds.). *Neurobehavioral recovery from head injury*. New York: Oxford University Press.

Strauss ME, Allied LJ (1987): Measurement of differential cognitive deficits after head injury. In: HS Levin, J Grafman, HM Eisenberg (eds.). *Neurobehavioral recovery from head injury*. New York: Oxford University Press.

Mandelberg J, Brooks AN (1975): Cognitive recovery after severe head injury. I. Serial testing on the Wechsler Adult Intelligence Scale. *J Neurol Neurosurg Psychiatry* 38:1121–1132.

Kay T, Ezrachi O, Cavallo M (1986): Plateaus and consistencies: Long term neuropsychological changes following head trauma. In: Proceedings 94th Annual Convention of The American Psychological Association, p. 175.

McClean E, Tembib N, Dikmen S, Wyler AR (1984): The behavioral sequelae of head injury. *J Clin Neuropsychol* 5:361–375.

Acker MB (1986): Relationships between test scores and everyday life functioning. In: BP Uzzel, Y Gross (eds.). *Clinical neuropsychology of interventions*. Boston: Martinus Nijhoff Publishing.

Meier MJ, Straumann S, Thompson GW (1987): Individual differences in neuropsychological recovery: an overview. In: MJ Meier, AL Benton, L Diller (eds.). *Neuropsychological rehabilitation*. New York: Guilford Press.

Stuss D (1987): Contribution of frontal lobe injury to cognitive impairment after closed head injury. Methods of assessment and recent findings. In: HS Levin, J Grafman, HM Eisenberg (eds.). *Neurobehavioral recovery from head injury*. New York: Oxford University Press.

Goldberg E, Bilder R Jr (1987): The frontal lobes and hierarchical organization of control. In: E Perceman (ed.). *The frontal lobes revisited*. New York: RBN Press.

Fuhrer M (ed.) (1987): *Rehabilitation outcomes analysis and measurement.* Baltimore: Paul H Brookes.

Fryer J, Haffey WJ (1987): Cognitive rehabilitation and community readaptation: outcomes from two program models. *J Head Trauma Rehabil* 2(3):51–63.

Prigatano G (1987): Neuropsychological rehabilitation after brain injury: some further reflections. In: JM Williams, CJ Long (eds.). *The rehabilitation of cognitive disabilities.* New York: Plenum Press.

Forer S (1985): Rehabilitation outcome and evaluation systems for traumatic brain injury. *J Organiz Rehabil Evaluation* 5:52–74.

Grumm BH, Bleiberg J (1985). Psychological rehabilitation in traumatic brain injury. In: SB Filskov and TJ Boll (eds.). *Handbook of clinical neuropsychology,* vol II. New York: John Wiley & Sons.

Hall K, Cope N, Rappaport M (1985): Glasgow outcome scale and disability rating scale: comparative usefulness in following recovery in traumatic head injury. *Arch Phys Med Rehabil* 66:135–137.

Brown M, Gordon WA, Diller L (1984): Rehabilitation indicators. In: AS Halpern, MJ Fuhrer (eds.). *Functional assessment in rehabilitation.* Baltimore: Paul H Brookes.

Diller L, Ben-Yishay Y (1987): Analyzing rehabilitation outcomes of persons with head injury. In: M Fuhrer (ed.). *Rehabilitation outcomes: analysis and measurement.* Baltimore: Paul H Brookes.

Diller L, Gordon WA (1981): Interventions for cognitive deficits in brain injured adults. *J Consult Clin Psychol* 49:822–834.

Cicerone KD (1984): *Strategy training and generalization in the cognitive remediation process.* Paper presented at the 5th Annual Traumatic Head Injury Conference, Braintree, MA.

Ben-Yishay Y, Rattok J, Lakin P, et al. (1985): Neuropsychologic rehabilitation: quest for a holistic approach. *Semin Neurol* 5:525–529.

Nagele DA (1985): Neuropsychological inferences from a tooth brushing task: A model for understanding deficits and making interventions. *Arch Phys Med Rehabil* 66:58.

Van Zomeren AH, Brouwer WH, Minderhoud JM (1987): Acquired brain damage and driving; a review. *Arch Phys Med Rehabil* 68:697–705.

Ben-Yishay Y, Silver S, Ezrachi O (1987): A manual for occupational trials. In: Progress Report: RTC stroke and head trauma. NYU Medical Center. Submitted NIDRR, Washington, D.C.

Diller L, Buxbaum J, Chiotelis S (1972): Relearning motor skills in hemiplegia; error analysis. *Genet Psychol Monog* 85:249–286.

Baddley AM, Harus J, Sunderland A, Watts KP, Wilson B (1987): Closed head injury and memory. In: HS Levin, J Grafman, HM Eisenberg (eds.). *Neurobehavioral recovery from head injury.* New York: Oxford University Press.

Corrigan JD, Arnett JA, Houches LJ, Jackson RD (1985): Reality orientation for brain injured patients: group treatment and monitoring of recovery. *Arch Phys Med Rehabil* 66:626–632.

Levin HS, O'Donnell VM, Grossman RG (1979): The Galveston orientation and amnesia test: a practical scale to assess cognition after head injury. *J Nerv Ment Dis* 167, 675–684.

Hagen C, Malhmus D, Durham P (1979): Levels of cognitive functioning in rehabilitation of the head injured adult. Downey, CA: Rancho Los Amigos Hospital.

Stover S, Zeiger HE (1976): Head injury in children and teenagers: functional recovery correlated with duration of coma. *Arch Phys Med Rehabil* 57:201–205.

Panikoff L (1983): Recovery trends of functional skills in the head injured adult. *Am J Occupat Ther* 37:735–743.

Jellinek HM, Torkelson R, Harvey R (1982): Functional abilities and distress levels in brain injured patients at long term followup. *Arch Phys Med Rehabil* 63:160–162.

Lezak MD (1987): Relationships between personality disorders, social disturbances and physical durability following traumatic brain injury. *J Head Trauma* 2(5).

Ben-Yishay Y, Silver SL, Piasetsky E, Rattok J (1987): Relationship between employability and vocational outcome after intensive holistic cognitive rehabilitation. *J Head Trauma Rehabil* 2(1):35–40.

Barth JT, Macciocchi SN, Giordani B, Rimel R, Jone JS, Boll TJ (1983): Neuropsychological sequelae of minor head injury. *Neurosurgery* 13:529–537.

Dikmen S, Recton R, Temkin N (1983). Neuropsychological recovery in head injury. *Arch Neurol* 40:333–338.

Sunderland A, Harris J, Gleave J (1984): Memory failures in everyday life following severe head injury. *J Clin Neuropsychol* 6(2):127–142.

Fordyce DJ, Roueche JR (1986): Changes in perspectives of a disability among patients, staff and relatives during rehabilitation of brain injury. *Rehabil Psychol* 31:231–241.

Mateer CA, Sohlberg MM, Crinean J (1987): Focus on clinical research: perceptions of memory function in individuals with closed head injury. *J Head Trauma Rehabil* 2(3):74–84.

15

Rehabilitation Interventions After Traumatic Brain Injury*

George P. Prigatano, Ph.D.

Section of Neuropsychology and Division of Neurological Rehabilitation, Barrow Neurological Institute and St. Joseph's Hospital and Medical Center, Phoenix, Arizona, U.S.A.

Rehabilitation interventions after traumatic brain injury (TBI) can be defined as those actions or events that theoretically and practically facilitate the recovery process. The term *intervention* is used to imply that without such actions or events, not only will the recovery process be less likely to proceed to its maximum potential but complications may well occur that interfere with recovery and adaptation. These ideas have come mainly from stroke rehabilitation (Stern et al., 1971). They are based on the observation that a patient's neurological deficits may remain "static," while functional or day-to-day self-care activities can improve with rehabilitative help (see Prigatano, 1986).

This chapter addresses current knowledge of *how* rehabilitation services contribute to improve "functional outcome" in TBI patients. It also emphasizes *issues* related to the case management process, recognizing team concepts as well as the role of specific rehabilitation professionals. Finally, new approaches such as supported employment and microcomputer use are reviewed and their implications for research and training are identified.

HOW DO REHABILITATION SERVICES CONTRIBUTE TO IMPROVE FUNCTIONAL OUTCOME?

Ten practical services that rehabilitation specialists provide that seem to improve functional outcome in TBI patients are listed below.

---

*This chapter appeared in the *BNI Quarterly* 4(2):30–37, 1988.

1. Restraining patients' activities when they are easily confused and behave in an impulsive and harmful manner to themselves and others.

2. Teaching them to cooperate with others and appropriately respond to environmental demands.

3. Providing guided practice and self-care activities despite neurologic deficits.

4. Providing guided practice at improving control or mastery over partially damaged functional systems (i.e., the ability to ambulate, the ability to manipulate objects with one's hands, the ability to communicate with others, etc.).

5. Providing compensatory techniques and equipment to minimize the effects of neurologic mediated disabilities on daily activities.

6. Listening to the frustrations, anger, and depression of patients (and family and rehabilitation staff) and providing strategies for coping with these and other emotional/motivational disturbances.

7. Teaching the patient (and family and rehabilitation staff) about the nature of neurologic deficits, presumed recovery courses, and useful rehabilitation interventions to attempt.

8. Providing altered or adjusted home and/or work environments that allow a person to function as independently and productively as possible.

9. Providing realistic hope, comfort, and when possible a forum for understanding the "meaning" of this tragedy in their lives.

10. Coordinating financial resources of the patient and family to achieve as many of the activities listed above as possible.

These activities cut across different time frames of patient care (i.e., acute, intermediate, and long-term or chronic stages of care). They emphasize the need for a wide variety of allied health services. Certainly the varied neuropathological insults associated with TBI produce many types of motor, linguistic, cognitive, and personality disorders (see Hagan, 1981; Levin, Benton, and Grossman, 1983; Prigatano et al., 1986). Also, premorbid characteristics of patients are equally variable and further contribute to many different types of symptoms and syndrome pictures.

Scientific investigation on the effectiveness and efficiency of various rehabilitation services after TBI unfortunately has been rather sparse. Jennett and Teasdale (1984) have pointed out that there is a "lack of good evidence as to the effectiveness of specific rehabilitation procedures on disability caused by brain damage" (p. 267).

Some of the major research questions regarding how rehabilitation services contribute to improve functional outcome follow.

1. Can various rehabilitation services (e.g., occupational therapy (OT),

physical therapy (PT), nursing, speech and language services (SP), psychological services, etc.) reduce the period of posttraumatic amnesia (PTA) and facilitate the rate at which patients accomplish self-care activities?

2. Can various rehabilitation services influence functional motor outcome given hemiparesis or hemiplegia?

3. Can various rehabilitation services influence the functional communication outcome given aphasia, dysarthria, and subclinical language disorders?

4. Can various rehabilitation services influence the functional outcome of problem-solving skills (memory included) at home and/or at work?

5. Can various rehabilitation services improve functional outcome of interpersonal competency (i.e., getting along with others) at home or at work?

6. Given the individual efforts of specific rehabilitation therapists, integrated rehabilitation teams, or various rehabilitation programs (supported employment programs included), is there evidence that (a) a greater proportion of patients receiving such services function more independently in the home than patients not receiving such treatments (see Prigatano, Klonoff, and Bailey, 1987); (b) a greater proportion of patients receiving rehabilitation services are functioning in gainful employment (even nongainfully employed volunteer jobs) than nontreated or minimally treated patients (see Prigatano et al., 1986); and (c) a greater proportion of patients receiving rehabilitation interventions need less acute medical care and less intermediate and long-term medical and psychiatric care for their disabilities than those not receiving interventions? Within the confines of this chapter, a few examples of how these questions could be approached will be suggested.

Roberts (1976) reports that 40% of a large number of TBI patients studied 10 to 25 years postinjury showed residual hemiparesis. He suggests, as does the stroke literature, that the first few months postinjury predict motor outcome. Yet, precise data on recovery of various motor functions and functional outcome are lacking. Partridge, Johnston, and Edwards (1987) have recently reported on the functional motor recovery of 368 stroke patients using a simple "does perform" or "does not perform" judgment of 13 simple motor behaviors. Figure 15-1 illustrates the recovery curves of these patients. Such data would be useful for various types of TBI patients. Against this type of baseline data, specific rehabilitation interventions could be better assessed.

A second example concerns verbal impairment associated with traumatic brain injury. Sarno, Buonaguro, and Levita (1986) report that in a sample of 125 closed head injury (CHI) patients with a history of coma, three types of verbal impairment are noted approximately 6 months postinjury. One third showed clear aphasic symptomatology. Another third showed dysarthric difficulties associated with what is termed sub-

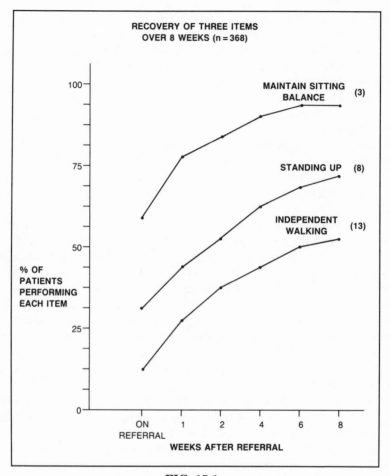

FIG. 15-1.

clinical aphasia. The remaining third showed no evidence of aphasia or dysarthria but on formal language testing have impairment involving naming, sentence repetition, and word fluency (i.e., show subclinical aphasia). These authors suggest that at least two thirds of all CHI patients with a history of coma appear more linguistically intact than they actually are (p.404). Research on the natural recovery course of these types of verbal impairments is also lacking. Until baseline data are presented, the efficacy of various forms of speech and language therapy, as well as certain forms of cognitive retraining, cannot be adequately assessed.

A third example involves efforts at improving higher order cerebral functions after TBI. A recent paper by Ben-Yishay, Piasetsky, and Rattok (1987) addressed the question of whether or not disorders of attention can be "ameliorated." They report that some patients improved their ability to maintain focused attention and thereby process information more efficiently. However, these authors interpret their data as reflecting greater use of "residual cognitive skills, rather than an increase in the capacity levels of their underlying cognitive abilities" (p.258). These patients were several months postinjury. Research is needed to evaluate the efficacy of various forms of cognitive retraining at different stages following traumatic brain injury.

As early as 1947, Zangwill raised issues that remain unanswered concerning the efficacy of various forms of training programs following brain injuries (see Prigatano et al., 1986; Prigatano, 1987).

A fourth example comes from the use of speciality programs aimed at helping patients specifically return back to work. Two studies (Ben-Yishay et al., 1985; Prigatano et al., 1986) suggest that a greater portion of TBI patients can be returned to work given specialty programs after traditional rehabilitation activities have failed. Further research is needed to document this claim.

A final research example centers on the assumption that TBI produces relatively "static" lesions, with relatively permanent neuropsychological deficits several months postinjury. On the positive side, some patients seem to show continued behavioral recovery several months postinjury (see Prigatano, 1987). On the negative side, some patients may actually show decline in their neuropsychological status with the passage of time. Lezak (1979) has reported this in a group of TBI patients studied over time on various memory measures. Individual case studies have also appeared that show the same pattern (see Prigatano, 1987). Further research is needed to evaluate whether some traumatic brain lesions may actually be progressive in nature. Basic and clinical neuropathological and neuroradiographic studies should help improve our understanding of this question, and the implications for rehabilitation intervention should be explored.

TYPOLOGIES IN TBI REHABILITATION SERVICES

The types of rehabilitation interventions TBI patients receive are undergoing some interesting changes compared to traditional approaches to brain dysfunctional patients. These changes reflect not only the complexity and variability of their neurological deficits but also reflect the response of family members, insurance carriers (or third party payers), and the rehabilitation staff to these patients and their problems.

Traditionally, the focus of neurorehabilitation was inpatient care. During the acute phase of recovery, patients were provided with 24-hour supervision and rehabilitation therapies aimed primarily at orientation, ambulation, self-care, and communication skills. Physical therapists, occupational therapists, and speech and language pathologists with nursing services *were* the rehabilitation team. Social workers helped counsel families and arranged for financial services and coordinated transfers from one medical facility to the next. Physicians oversaw the treatment and provided medical advice/intervention to avoid mainly physical complications. In fact, inpatient neurological rehabilitation still emphasizes the importance of avoiding physical complications and teaching patients and families to live with neurological impairments and resultant behavioral disabilities.

Given the relatively young age of TBI patients (vs. stroke patients) and the fact that they tend to survive their injuries, a shift in emphasis on the types of rehabilitation services these patients receive has occurred.

Outpatient programs historically were there to provide continued physical therapy, occupational therapy, and speech services. However, as the higher cerebral deficits of these patients became more obvious and began to negatively impact home life and influence occupational choices (see Bond, 1975), psychologists and vocational rehabilitation specialists progressively became involved. Cognitive retraining by a number of specialists became an integral part of both inpatient and outpatient rehabilitation (see Rosenthal, Griffith, and Bond, 1983). A definite shift has occurred from providing therapies aimed at avoidance of physical and medical complications to attempting to help reintegrate patients into complicated social systems despite physical and cognitive disabilities.

Part of the problem in doing this, however, has been our continued difficulty conceptualizing the higher order disturbances of these patients. While one can give these patients a wide variety of tests to document their performance on neurological and neuropsychological dimensions, there has still been relatively little advance in our ability to conceptualize the nature of these problems and thereby develop adequate interventions (see Prigatano, 1986; Prigatano et al., 1986).

This is not a criticism of rehabilitation specialists but simply a reemphasis of the fact that as long as we are not able to adequately define what the higher cerebral functions are, it is impossible to adequately measure and treat these disturbances (see Prigatano, 1986). In order to develop relevant typologies of rehabilitative services for TBI patients, three major advances need to occur in the field.

1. An integration of basic science and applied clinical observation on the nature of brain dysfunction and its impact on higher and lower brain functions is needed. For example, there is a growing appreciation that patients may be organically less aware (vs. denying) of cognitive and personality deficits than was previously thought. This has led to inter-

vention approaches that traditionally have not been applied and may yield a greater portion of patients reentering the work force (see Prigatano et al., 1986).

2. Intervention strategies based on these conceptualizations need to utilize appropriate reeducational materials that have motivational appeal for the patients. One major problem in this field is that rehabilitation tasks given to patients may appear to have little direct relevance to the patients' day-to-day activities. Tasks that are seen as typical of "school work" or not reflecting occupational interests and histories of TBI patients are less likely to involve the patients. Consequently, patients may prematurely terminate rehabilitation services because of the inappropriateness of the teaching materials from the patients' perspectives.

3. Individual therapists must understand how impairments outside of their range of expertise actually impact on their treatment activities with a given patient. For example, physical therapists need to understand the nature of cognitive and personality disorders as they attempt to help brain-injured patients ambulate (see Prigatano, 1988). Disorders of memory, impulsive control, etc. may directly interfere with a patient's ability to maintain an appropriate posture or to attempt to coordinate motor activities as he or she walks.

The concept of the interdisciplinary team vs. the multiple disciplinary team has emerged to theoretically handle this latter problem (see Fordyce, 1981). Yet, in day-to-day clinical practice it is difficult to develop truly interdisciplinary neurological rehabilitation teams (see Prigatano, 1987). This common failure to establish such teams, despite the fact that many rehabilitation programs describe themselves as interdisciplinary in nature, seems to have led to the development of the case management model.

While the physician is theoretically and legally in charge of a given patient's care, the physician's attention is often split across patients and he or she may have difficulty tracking a given patient's progress and needs. Also, the physician frequently is concerned with avoidance of medical complications and treating physical disabilities. Yet most, if not all, TBI patients have cognitive and personality disorders that overshadow their various therapies and medical management. These disorders have the greatest negative impact on the patient's ability to return to a productive life and be integrated back into the family (see Oddy et al., 1985). Consequently, the concept of the case manager has emerged to oversee the myriad of problems these patients experience and to arrange for various services for a given patient. It certainly seems appropriate that someone should oversee the entire range of a given patient's needs, problems, and financial resources. Time will tell whether or not the case management model is a substantial improvement over present approaches to patient care. At this point, however, it is interesting that the case management model has emerged and different case management profiles are seen in the TBI population.

SPECIFIC CASE MANAGEMENT PROFILES

Despite the great deal of variability in the symptoms and syndromes seen in TBI patients, four major types or profiles are encountered by rehabilitation specialists. Before describing these four types, however, I will explicitly exclude those cases which are in a semicomatose or vegetative state. They provide a host of medical problems that go above and beyond the realm of rehabilitation interventions that are aimed at returning people back to work or becoming more independent in the home.

Table 15-1 lists four types or profiles of TBI patients that frequently require case management.

The first type of patient presents major physical disabilities. In Roberts' (1976) series of 291 patients, 5% demonstrated "severe bilateral pyramidal damage with postural dystonia and often striking bradykinesia and fragmentary athetosis." An additional 20% showed evidence

Table 15-1.   *Types of TBI Patients Requiring Case Management Services*

Types	Major characteristics	Estimated percentages[a]
Type I	Major physical disabilities with associated higher cerebral deficits.	25% of severe TBI patients
Type II	Hemiparesis with or without aphasia and associated higher cerebral deficits.	40% of severe TBI patients
Type III	No major motor or language disorder present, but significant higher cerebral deficits.	35% of severe TBI patients
Type IV	No major motor, linguistic, higher cerebral dysfunction present, but major psychiatric disability.	Typically seen in patients with a history of mild to moderate TBI. % unknown.

[a]Percentages estimated from data reported by Roberts, 1976; Gilchrist and Wilkinson, 1979; Sarno et al., 1986; and Prigatano et al., 1987.

of cerebellar and pyramidal lesions demonstrating significant ataxia, spasticity, and hemiplegia. Perhaps, then, 25% of severe TBI patients have a complicated and bilateral neuromuscular disorder.

While they frequently have associated speech, language, and cognitive deficits, the limits posed by their motor disorders require that first consideration be paid to this dimension. These patients need a tremendous amount of input from nursing, physical therapy, and occupational therapy. Speech pathology services may also be important when dysarthria and swallowing difficulties are present.

The second type of patient seen has a definite hemiparesis or hemiplegia with or without language disorder. Again, according to Roberts' (1976) data this may include as many as 40% of the patients. These patients most resemble the stroke victims and often are treated as such. Many of these patients, however, have diverse higher cerebral dysfunction, including alterations in personality secondary to bilateral and fronto-temporal lesions. Many of these patients receive traditional PT, OT, and speech and language therapies for their obvious deficits. They may or may not receive neuropsychological or clinical psychological services for subtle higher cerebral disturbances. Many of them are able to eventually function in the home, but a good portion of them have very limited job success without special rehabilitation programs (see Gilchrist and Wilkinson, 1979).

A third type of patient has no obvious physical or linguistic difficulties but demonstrates significant disorders of higher cerebral functioning. These are the patients who literally "walk and talk and look good from a galloping horse." They frequently fail to return to gainful employment given traditional methods of rehabilitation. Perhaps this group constitutes as much as 30% to 40% of the patient population. Prigatano et al. (1986) have recently summarized many of the cognitive and personality difficulties of members of this group and have proposed a milieu or holistic approach to their rehabilitation.

While the above three categories typify the most common types of cases seen following *severe* traumatic brain injury (i.e., 25% with severe physical disability and associated cognitive deficits; 40% with hemiparesis with or without aphasia but with associated cognitive disorders; 35% with primarily higher cerebral disturbance but no obvious motor or linguistic deficits), there is perhaps even a larger number of patients with a history of mild or moderate TBI who can pose significant challenges to the case manager. The actual number or percentage of these patients is undetermined. These patients, who neurologically seem to have "mild" or "moderate" brain injuries with no obvious neuromuscular or linguistic impairment, show a great many emotional/motivational disturbances. They frequently are involved in litigation or have a pre-trauma history of marginal psychosocial adjustment or significant psychiatric disturbance. Patients who fall within this category often have a myriad set of psychiatric disturbances which can include depression, anxiety, phobias, and paranoid thinking. These patients frequently have a preoccupation with bodily discomforts and disabilities (e.g., low back pain, headache). They also can become quite explosive when frustrated. At times, some of these patients can be dangerous, particularly if they are paranoid. As a group, they are extremely difficult to return to work. Traditional rehabilitation services have not worked with them. Even when they are placed in special programs and are seen by experienced psychiatrists and psychologists, they often are not adequately helped. No clear cut rehabilitation approach to this group of patients has yet emerged.

In addition to the problems presented by these four "case" profiles, there are at least two other major influences on the case management process after TBI that should be recognized. One influence centers around the family's reaction to the TBI patient, the rehabilitation process, and litigation. At times, direct intervention with families is necessary if rehabilitation interventions are going to proceed at all. Family members can and do experience a great deal of anxiety, anger, and depression; and their behavior is felt by the rehabilitation team, including the case manager (see Prigatano et al., 1986; Klonoff and Prigatano, 1987).

The second external influence centers around economic realities associated with a patient's care. What is done for a patient will clearly be influenced by the services that can be afforded. Also, the pressures from insurance carriers to expedite putting a patient back to work can influence the case management process. There are instances in which patients are put back to work prematurely. By the nature of their higher cerebral deficits, some patients may be unaware of their limitations. They perceive themselves as being able to return to work before they are ready. If rehabilitation teams encourage this, patients can return to work only to experience needless frustration and failure. The end result can be that the patient quits or is fired and thereby loses insurance benefits. This is a true disservice to patients and something that should be carefully monitored. Eventually the early return to work could have massive legal repercussions.

A second economic influence is that produced by litigation. Attorneys can directly or indirectly influence a patient's attitudes toward rehabilitation. Some patients may simply go "to rehabilitation" because their attorney has requested it so their case may look more favorable. In some instances, patients may actively or passively resist rehabilitation for disabilities because they may view this as jeopardizing their future claims. The social-economic influences produced by litigation and the insurance carrier have a profound impact on case management and, indirectly, on the practice of medicine and the allied health professions.

PROBLEMS WITH INTERDISCIPLINARY TEAMS AND MANAGING DIFFERENT SOURCES OF INFORMATION

While the concept of the interdisciplinary team approach to traumatic brain-injured patients is difficult to argue with, there are clear problems with this approach. As a team, the rehabilitation therapists experience predictable group dynamics and conflicts. These group influences can have either a positive or negative effect on patient care. On the positive side, therapists can feel a "sharing of the burden" involved in patient care. They can exchange information concerning patients' needs and treatment approaches and learn from other therapists. This can frequently lead to patients receiving a more holistic or comprehensive approach to their treatment.

However, within the context of an interdisciplinary team approach certain negatives can and do emerge. For example, if there are differences of opinion between therapists, who will eventually have the last say on how to approach a given patient about a particular problem?

If the therapists disagree, who will ultimately make the final decision and resolve the disagreement? Since there are different therapists and different types of therapies the same problem that a patient experiences (such as a memory difficulty) may be approached quite differently by the different therapists. Problems of "professional turf" and "authority" among disciplines quickly emerge and can be destructive to the team process. These and other inherent problems have been described elsewhere (Prigatano, 1987). They have led, in my opinion, to the emergence of the case manager model. But how does the case manager manage different sources of information from various rehabilitation team members?

The answer is: With caution! Therapists may be technically well trained but lack common sense about how a patient is actually functioning in the real world. Therapists may be overly protective or even hostile (see Gans, 1981) toward certain patients. They may agree with other therapists' opinions concerning a patient's care out of friendship rather than out of solid clinical decision making. Likewise, they may disagree with other therapists simply because of interstaff conflict.

In evaluating information from different specialties, the case manager has to determine how reliable a given therapist's observations are, how practical his or her suggestions are concerning interventions, and how effective the interventions actually are once they have been attempted. The case manager has to keep clearly in mind the goals of a given patient in order to effectively determine how to use the input from various rehabilitation specialists. There are, in my opinion, three major goals that should be kept in mind in order to adequately interpret and utilize different sources of information concerning patient care. The first goal is to help the patient become independent or semi-independent in the home. The second goal is to return the patient to gainful employment (or some level of productivity). The third goal is preventive: Help the patient and family require less future psychiatric and/or medical care.

The actual combining and sequencing of rehabilitation services to accomplish these goals is indeed a complicated matter. There are different types of patients with varying symptoms and syndrome pictures. There are the external financial and internal family influences. There is a great variability in the sophistication of various therapists and the role of group dynamics in influencing their judgments and practices. Truly, the effective case manager must have considerable managerial and clinical skill and at the same time, a command of scientific knowledge to facilitate the recovery course for a given patient.

NEW APPROACHES

The use of the microcomputer in neurological rehabilitation has begun. TBI patients use microcomputers to practice visual spatial scanning, speech and language function, learning, and memory. Basic arithmetic, reading, and spelling skills can also be taught via the computer. In some instances the computer programs are sold as so-called "memory training" or "cognitive retraining" devices. While the computer is undoubtedly an extremely important adjunct to the armamentarium used in educating brain-injured patients, it is highly doubtful that the software developed to date has substantially improved *cognitive deficit*. Schacter and Gliskey (1987) have reviewed the literature on memory remediation and particularly the role of the computer in this regard. They point out the lack of systematic research findings demonstrating that these activities substantially improve underlying memory. More recent authors (Wilson, 1987) have emphasized the role of helping patients learn compensatory methods to get around these deficits. The computer may fall within this category as Schacter and Glisky (1987) point out. They suggest that some brain-injured patients may actually be taught to program microcomputers to organize their days and compensate for deficits that interfere with day-to-day functioning.

A second new approach to TBI rehabilitation is the development of models for helping patients return to work. Ben-Yishay et al. (1985) and Prigatano et al. (1986) emphasize the importance of working with patients in individual and group settings to prepare them for the interpersonal stresses involved in work.

In our present model at the Barrow Neurological Institute, for example, patients are seen for formal therapies in the morning and, in the afternoon, placed in voluntary work settings. Rehabilitation staff frequently visit job settings and obtain information from both patients and supervisors about how patients are doing. The therapists then work with patients on specific difficulties they are having on the job in order to make sure they can maintain their job responsibilities. Many of these patients are progressively weaned off this type of help and are able then to maintain full-time employment.

The supportive employment model used with developmental disability patients is also being applied to TBI patients (Wehman et al., in press; Kiernan and Stark, 1986). The supportive employment model emphasizes placing TBI patients in competitive jobs and training them to function at those jobs. Job coordinators do a lot of on-site problem solving to help patients adequately compensate for cognitive and physical disabilities in performing the job tasks.

The problem we have experienced, however, is that many TBI patients have unrealistic appraisals of their skills and abilities and often behave inappropriately in job settings. Behavioral methods, such as an extinction technique, in and of themselves frequently do not eliminate the behavior. This is because the behavior is the end result of complicated brain-behavior disturbances as well as of premorbid personality characteristics. TBI patients have some cognitive and personality skills that are "normal" and others that are not. They can also remember what they "used to be like" (something not true of developmental disability patients).

They require, in my opinion, a combination of individual and group rehabilitation activities aimed at dealing with cognitive and personality deficits *while* they are also placed in the job setting. We accomplish this by having individuals work with us in neuropsychologically oriented rehabilitation in the morning and putting them in job trials in the afternoon as indicated above.

Very chronic TBI patients who have experienced a lot of failure prior to coming to rehabilitation may be able to utilize a direct supportive employment model, because they have experienced enough failure that they are willing to be more realistic in their aspirations. However, frequently this occurs when patients are anywhere from 2 to 4 years post-injury, and this is a long time for them to remain unemployed. I believe, therefore, that the concept of supported employment should be incorporated in ongoing neuropsychologically oriented rehabilitation to return more patients to work at a faster rate and to keep them there.

IMPLICATIONS FOR RESEARCH AND TRAINING

Some of the implications of these observations for research and training are as follows:

1. Rehabilitation interventions seem to improve the functional out-

come of TBI patients, but there are several unanswered research questions. These questions focus on the efficacy of helping patients emerge from the period of posttraumatic amnesia; improve motor, linguistic, and cognitive function; and ultimately achieve a greater degree of independence at home and at work.

2. The concept of an interdisciplinary team approach is useful but is fraught with a number of difficulties. Group dynamics and conflicts of rehabilitation teams need to be adequately researched and managed.

3. The training materials and activities that are involved in rehabilitation intervention have to have greater motivational appeal for TBI patients.

4. Professional graduate and undergraduate training of rehabilitation therapists must be interdisciplinary in nature. It cannot be put off until the therapists are a part of a rehabilitation team.

5. Revision of our conceptualization of underlying brain disorders and of the syndromes they produce is needed. As this is done, the development of special programs for different types of TBI patients will be more effective.

6. The use of microcomputers as a sophisticated adjunct to teaching patients to compensate for higher cerebral deficits should be clearly explored and, as technology emerges, applied to the home as well as the work setting.

7. The external influences of families, third-party payers, litigation, and other sources on how a patient's case is managed needs systematic investigation.

8. The impact of family perceptions of rehabilitation and the rehabilitation staff's reactions to both family and patient must be thoroughly understood to adequately manage a patient.

CONCLUSIONS

The conclusion of this section on rehabilitation intervention can best be summed up in a quote taken from Jennett and Teasdale's (1984) book, *Management of Head Injuries.*

> Questions of the same kind should be asked about rehabilitation as are routinely posed when drug treatment is under review. These include consideration of which patients to treat, when to treat, with what intensity (e.g., dosage), and when to stop. What are the desired effects, and are there adverse reactions? Is there evidence of a placebo effect, and can patients become dependent on therapy (if not actually addicted)?" (p.268)

When these types of questions are asked and answered, rehabilitation interventions after TBI will make substantial gains and the care of these patients and their families will be greatly improved.

REFERENCES

Ben-Yishay Y, Rattok J, Lakin P, Piasetsky EB, Ross B, Silver S, Zide E, Ezrachi O (1985): Neuropsychologic rehabilitation: quest for a holistic approach. *Semin Neurol* 5(3):252–258.

Bond MR (1975): Assessment of the psychosocial outcome after severe head injury. In: Ciba Foundation Symposium, R Porter, DW Fitzsimons (eds.). *Outcome of severe damage to the central nervous system* (pp. 141–157). New York: American Elsevier/Excerpta Medica/North-Holland.

Fordyce W (1981): On interdisciplinary peers. *Archives of Physical Medicine & Rehabilitation* 61:51–81.

Gans JS (1983): Hate in the rehabilitation setting. *Archives of Physical Medicine and Rehabilitation* 64:176–179.

Gilchrist E, Wilkinson M (1979): Some factors determining prognosis in young people with severe head injuries. *Archives of Neurology* 36:355–358.

Hagen C (1982): Language-Cognitive disorganization following closed head injury: A conceptualization. In: LE Trexler (ed.). *Cognitive rehabilitation: conceptualization and intervention*, pp. 131–172. New York: Plenum Press.

Jennett B, Teasdale G (1984): *Management of head injuries*. Philadelphia: FA Davis Company.

Kiernan W, Stark JA (1986): Employment options for adults with developmental disabilities: A conceptual model. *RASE* 7:7–11.

Klonoff P, Prigatano GP (1987): Family and staff's reactions in the rehabilitation of brain injured patients: clinical and research findings. *Adult head injury rehabilitation: community re-entry*. San Diego: College Hill Press.

Levin HS, Benton AL, Grossman RG (1983): *Neurobehavioral consequences of closed head injury*. New York: Oxford University Press.

Lezak MD (1979): Recovery of memory and learning functions following traumatic brain injury. *Cortex* 15:63–72.

Oddy M, Coughlan T, Tyerman A, Jenkins D (1985): Social adjustment after closed head injury: A further follow-up seven years after injury. *J Neurol Neurosurg Psychiatry* 48:564–568.

Partridge CJ, Johnston M, Edwards S (1987): Recovery from physical disability after stroke: normal patterns as a basis for evaluation. *Lancet* 1 February 14, 373–375.

Prigatano GP (1986): Higher cerebral deficits: the history of methods of assessment and approaches to rehabilitation: Part II. *BNI Quarterly* 2(3):15–26.

Prigatano GP (1987): Problems encountered in establishing "truly" interdisciplinary neurological treatment teams. Paper presented at 2nd Annual Symposium on Advances in Head Injury Rehabilitation, Dallas, Texas, March 5–7.

Prigatano GP (1987): Recovery and cognitive retraining after craniocerebral trauma. *Journal of Learning Disabilities* 30:603–663.

Prigatano GP (1988): Emotion and motivation in recovery and adaptation to brain damage. *Brain and recovery: Theoretical and controversial issues*. Finger S, et al. (eds.), New York: Plenum Press, pp. 335–350.

Prigatano GP, Klonoff PS, Bailey I (1987): Psychosocial adjustment associated with traumatic brain injury: Statistics BNI neurorehabilitation must beat. *BNI Quarterly* 3(1):10–17.

Prigatano GP, et al. (1986): *Neuropsychological rehabilitation after brain injury,* The Johns Hopkins University Press, Baltimore and London.

Roberts AH (1976): Long-term prognosis of severe accidental head injury. *Proceedings of Royal Society of Medicine,* 69, 137–140.

Rosenthal M, Griffith ER, Bond MR, Miller JD (1983): *Rehabilitation of the head injured adult* Philadelphia: FA Davis Company.

Sarno MT, Buonaguro A, Levita E (1986): Characteristics of verbal impairment in closed head injured patients. *Archives of Physical Medicine & Rehabilitation,* 67:404.

Schacter DL, Glisky EL (1986): Memory remediation: restoration, alleviation and the acquisition of domain-specific knowledge. In: BP Uzzel, Y Gross (eds.). *Clinical neuropsychology of intervention.* Boston: Martinus Nijhoff, pp. 257–282.

Stern PH, McDowell F, Miller JM, Robinson M (1971): Factors influencing stroke rehabilitation. *Stroke* 2:213–218.

Wehman P, Kreutzer J, Wood W, Morton MV, Sherman P (in press): Supported work model of competitive employment for persons with traumatic brain injury: Toward job placement and retention. *Rehabilitation Counseling Bulletin*

Wilson BA (1987): *Rehabilitation of memory.* New York: Guilford Press.

Zangwill OL (1947): Psychological aspects of rehabilitation in cases of brain injury. *British Journal of Psychology* 37:60–69.

16

Understanding and Optimizing Family Adaptation to Traumatic Brain Injury

Mitchell Rosenthal, Ph.D.

Department of Psychological Medicine, Marianjoy Rehabilitation Center, Wheaton, Illinois, U.S.A.

The significance of the family in the process of brain injury rehabilitation can be traced to several major sources: (1) research studies that have documented how families are impacted by traumatic brain injury (Brooks and McKinlay, 1983; Brooks, Campsie, Symington, Beattie, and McKinlay, 1987; Lezak, 1978; Livingston, 1987; Oddy, Humphrey, and Uttley, 1984; Romano, 1974; Panting and Merry, 1972); (2) emergence of consumer organizations, such as the National Head Injury Foundation in the United States and Headway in Britain; and (3) the widespread incorporation of families into the rehabilitation process within comprehensive brain injury rehabilitation programs.

The pervasive neurobehavioral deficits that result from injury to the brain are now commonly recognized as those which primarily comprise the brain-injured person's capacity to think, reason, make adequate judgments, remember, perceive, plan and execute actions, manifest emotion, behave in a socially appropriate fashion, and exist as a productive member of society (Levin, 1982). In cases of severe brain injury, the victim of head injury, though often physically intact and superficially recognizable to the family, thinks and acts in a manner that is unlike his or her preinjury behavior and quite socially maladaptive. The "burden" of care and management of this "changed" person, after acute neurosurgical and medical management ends, are often squarely on the shoulders of the relatives.

In this chapter, I will examine (1) the specific types of deficits that most directly impact the family; (2) the emotional adjustments often seen on the part of family members; (3) the changes in roles and responsibilities so often necessary for family members; (4) the methods used by health care professionals to facilitate the family adaptation process; and (5) research questions that should be addressed in future studies.

In understanding the nature of the impact of brain injury on the family, a few principles derived from research should be stated. As Bond (1975, 1984) and others have noted, after the first year postinjury, the family is more troubled by the behavioral or personality disturbances exhibited by their relative than by any other sphere of difficulty—e.g., cognitive, physical. Though families learn to understand the nature of brain injury and develop coping strategies, the degree of felt burden does not significantly decline after the first year. In fact, Brooks (1987) has recently reported on a series of 134 patients up to 7 years postinjury and noted that the level of burden remains significant. There is some correlation between severity of injury (as measured by duration of post-traumatic amnesia) and degree of burden, but it is not a 1:1 relationship. It should be kept in mind that survivors of *minor* head injury (i.e., those who sustain a brief loss of consciousness) can experience significant psychosocial disability for months and years after the injury and create great stress for families (Gronwall, 1986).

The burden upon the relatives after head injury is complicated even further by the loss of social support from significant others, such as close friends and other members of the community. Kozloff (1987), in a recent study of the social networks of 37 severely head-injured patients and 39 of their significant others, concluded:

> The results of the present study show that after the initial phases of recovery, the patient is dependent on his primary kin for financial, emotional and task-oriented support. This pattern of dependency causes problems within the structure of the family (p. 20).

Thus, the understanding of long-term family adaptation to brain injury is partly dependent on the analysis of the social support system, which is likely greatly diminished after severe traumatic brain injury.

SPECIFIC DEFICITS THAT IMPACT THE FAMILY

One of the most frustrating problems for head-injured patients and their families is *impairments in attention and memory*. Even after the initial period of posttraumatic amnesia resolves, the brain-injured person often has significant difficulty in maintaining attention on a task, storing information in short-term memory, and retrieving the information at a later time (Whyte, 1986). These deficits are often easily demonstrated on standardized neuropsychological tests but may be more apparent to families in everyday situations. Forgetting a telephone message or an appointment, inability to remember several items on a shopping list, inability to focus in on a conversation when other persons are talking or when there is background noise (such as radio or TV noise) are examples. These difficulties are even more troublesome in a school situation or on the job where ongoing focused attention or memory is critical to success.

Damage to the frontal lobes often is responsible for the manifestation of so-called *executive deficits* (Lezak, 1982). This category of deficits encompasses the abilities to initiate, plan, organize, monitor, and sustain behavior. Even a casual observer of brain injury will often note that the brain-injured patient tends to be more directed by external than by internal stimuli. That is, without structure, verbal and physical guidance, frequent coaxing and positive reinforcement, and close supervision, many brain-injured patients will fail to spontaneously generate any goal-directed behavior or, if a behavior is started, will fail to monitor the correctness of their actions or fail to complete the intended task. In a severe case of executive deficits, the patient will be asked to brush his or her teeth, start to put the toothpaste on the brush, and lose his or her attention while in the midst of performing the activity. Or in a work situation, the patient may be addressing envelopes for mailing from a pretyped list but not doublecheck the list to see if the finished label is correct. In the home environment, this inability to monitor activities often necessitates full-time supervision by family members, who fear for their relative's safety.

Inappropriate social behavior is a broad category of dysfunction, which includes altered affect and emotions, childlike dependency, disinhibition, excessive talkativeness, and lack of awareness or frank denial of deficits (sometimes referred to as anosognosia). This sphere of disability is often the one that imposes the greatest amount of stress upon the family. The brain-injured patient is often childlike and excessively dependent upon family members. Often, the social network of the patient dissipates within weeks of return to the community. Therefore, the patient is left without external social supports and must rely on family members exclusively. A childlike brain-injured spouse will often display jealousy when the partner leaves the home for even short periods of time and may display temper tantrums in response. Excessive talkativeness may be clearly manifested when the family visits a restaurant and the head-injured relative talks loudly and inappropriately to strangers and causes great embarrassment. The frank denial of deficits may lead a head-injured patient to reject or fail to cooperate with postacute treatment programs and thus block any further progress in recovery. In sum, the inappropriate social behavior leaves the relative the unenviable task of managing a person who is chronologically an adult but more of a young child, from a psychosocial standpoint.

This is a very brief overview of several key deficit areas that impact the family. There are many other important neurobehavioral problems that occur, such as depression and suicidal behavior, communication deficits, apathy and lethargy, and decreased sexual drive. It is important to recognize that each brain injury produces a unique constellation of deficits and resultant family problems, owing to the specific location of brain damage, severity of injury and associated injuries, and preinjury strengths and weaknesses of the patient and family system. In each case, a careful assessment of these factors is necessary to successfully intervene with the family of the brain-injured person.

EMOTIONAL ADJUSTMENTS AND COPING STRATEGIES

A common early reaction to traumatic brain injury is denial (Romano, 1974) in which the "fact" of having sustained a catastrophic life-threatening injury is blocked from objective reality. Family members who observe their loved ones in a coma, tied to tubes and medical apparatus, may feel that this is a terrible nightmare and is unreal. After the patient emerges from coma, there is a gradual recognition and acknowledgment of the injury but an inability to fully comprehend the immediate and long-term effects. In the period of emergence, the patient starts to exhibit agitated, confused, sometimes bizarre behavior, which is completely unlike his or her former personality. Upon entry into the acute rehabilitation phase, families are often provided with extensive information about the effects of brain injury and the likelihood of some permanent alterations in cognitive and behavioral function. This information is difficult to accept and often evokes a secondary denial, in which the family refuses to accept the notion that long-term or permanent changes will remain. This is understandable, in view of the fact that families often observe rapid improvement in all areas of physical and neurobehavioral function in the rehabilitation hospital and naturally are reinforced in their belief that the observed deficits will be transient.

Following discharge from the acute hospital to home (usually within 3 to 6 months of injury), the initial reaction is one of great joy and happiness. The family and patient are so relieved to be within the "safe" home environment that there is little immediate attention directed toward the changes in everyday life that are necessitated by the limitations in function.

After the initial "honeymoon" period at home, there are feelings of discouragement and a sense that perhaps the changes in their relative may last for a very long time. The brain-injured person may be attending outpatient therapy or day treatment, but the rate of improvement has slowed in many areas and problems in day-to-day management of behavior at home become more prominent and frustrating. Financial hardships may be present, as residual hospital bills pile up, lost wages are missed, alternate sources of disability support have not yet been approved, a pending legal case starts to drag on, and future prospects of returning to normalcy in the family are dashed if not destroyed.

At this point, many families start to experience feelings of depression or despair (Lezak, 1986). Conflicts between family members begin to surface, as the tension of living with a brain-injured relative creates friction and disrupts healthy communication patterns. During this period, family members may first gain a fuller appreciation and acknowledgment of the permanence of certain deficits and the realization that their loved one may never resemble the person that they formerly knew and lived with. A process of disengagement may begin where the relative and patient spend more time apart. A process of mourning for the "partial death" of their loved one is frequently observed (Rosenthal and Muir, 1983). Family members may now actively seek professional intervention or peer support through local chapters of the National Head Injury Foundation. It is not uncommon for families of head-injured patients to seek out medication (Panting and Merry, 1972) to deal with their own anxiety.

Finally, the family often reaches a stage of reorganization (Lezak, 1986), usually after 18 to 24 months, by which time the family has experienced a great deal of inner turmoil and pain, understood more fully the meaning of brain injury, accepted the reality that permanent limitations in function are likely, and is engaged in the process of seeking out community-based social and vocational programs that can help upgrade their relative's capacity to function more independently.

EFFECTS ON ROLE RELATIONSHIPS AND FAMILY RESPONSIBILITIES

A variety of changes within role relationships is often necessitated by traumatic brain injury. At least 50% of survivors of brain injury are unable to return to work within the first few years postinjury, if ever. Those who do return to work often are employed at a lower capacity than their premorbid employment. The net result is often a diminished amount of earnings and need for other family members to become employed or to be a primary source of income for the family. Thus, the brain-injured person who previously was employed and independent may need to assume the role of a financially dependent person.

Though not often recognized, the presence of a head-injured relative within the family system can dramatically impact the siblings within the family. Siblings may experience guilt feelings about their brain-injured relative due to the circumstances of the accident. They may also feel resentment toward the overwhelming amounts of attention their sibling is receiving. When the sibling of the brain-injured person is an adolescent, these feelings are rarely directly expressed. Instead, it may be manifested in school failure, acting out behavior, or failure to accept the brain-injured sibling in his or her new condition. Because families tend to handle their newly injured relative in a protective manner, many previously held jobs within the family may be redirected toward the healthy sibling(s), which causes additional resentment. The chronologically younger sister may now be functionally the "big sister," a change which may be very difficult for both the head-injured person and sibling to accept.

One of the most common problems in role relationships after traumatic brain injury is the marital relationship. Though there are no available statistics that cite increased divorce rates, clinicians who work with brain-injured people are fully aware of the changes in marital relationships that occur. Due to the emotional and physical dependency, it is difficult for the healthy spouse to view his or her loved one as a sexual partner. In a study of the wives of brain-injured Israeli soldiers, Rosenbaum and Najenson (1978) found that ". . . wives of brain-injured men go through a crisis period one year following their husbands' injury. At that time, hopes for a complete recovery vanish and they are faced with living with a person whose needs are great while he can give little in return" (p. 881).

Though it is commonly believed that mothers can adapt better to assuming the role of primary caregiver after brain injury, the recent study by Brooks and co-workers (1987) has indicated that there is no significant difference between levels of burden as reported by wives and mothers several years after brain injury. For the head-injured adult who may have lived independently for many years moving back to the parental home can be traumatizing in and of itself. Indeed, the need to live with parents again may reinforce an emotional regression that had been initially produced by brain damage. To be sure, some gratification is obtained through the reestablishment of a close parent-child bond, but eventually the bond may become symbiotic and may negatively impact on future growth and change in the head-injured person.

METHODS OF FAMILY INTERVENTION

The unique and complex nature of traumatic brain injury causes great confusion and anxiety for family members. They are often bewildered by the many changes in both physical and neurobehavioral function in their relatives. For this reason, a variety of family intervention strategies may be considered.

First, it is now commonplace for most rehabilitation programs to include a *family education* component in their protocol. This part of the rehabilitation program is designed to give families a good understanding of the nature of brain injury, what types of specific deficits can be related to sites of brain damage, how the rehabilitation process aids in recovery and promotes readaptation, and what methods can be used by families to facilitate growth and improvement. A variety of methods may be used to accomplish family education, including individual sessions with a physician, social worker, or neuropsychologist; group sessions with members of families of brain-injured patients and rehabilitation specialists; "family education days" in which family members spend the entire day in the rehabilitation hospital, accompanying their relatives to therapies and being instructed in methods of care by the health care professionals; and educational brochures, instructional videotapes, and books that can be obtained through the National Head Injury Foundation or at a local rehabilitation facility.

Another common type of intervention is termed *family counseling*. The purpose of family counseling is to assist the family in dealing with the overwhelming feelings of loss and helplessness. It is also designed to help the family understand and accept the disability and its potential consequences (e.g., increased dependence, impaired cognitive and behavioral functioning, decreased physical abilities). Family members are given the opportunity to express their feelings of guilt, anguish, anger, sadness, and loss. As discharge approaches, families can become apprehensive since they have been given an implicit or explicit message that a plateau has been reached. During the transition from hospital to community, the family counselor can play a key role in helping the family anticipate future problems and be more psychologically and physically prepared to assume the burden of care. Frequently, the patient and family maintain unrealistic expectations that restoration of function will "magically" occur when the patient can return home. The counselor can gently prepare the family for the realities of life with a brain-injured relative and maintain close communication to provide the support so often needed but rarely requested.

For a select number of families, a more intensive type of intervention may be needed—*family therapy*. Family therapy may be defined "as a professionally organized attempt to produce behavioral changes in a disturbed marital or family unit by essentially interacting non-physical methods" (Glick and Kessler, 1974, p. 1). In the case of brain injury, family therapy can be useful for families with a premorbid history of dysfunction or for those in which the presence of a head-injured relative has created catastrophic reactions on the part of certain family members, which produces maladaptive communication and interaction within the family.

The goals of family therapy are (1) to provide a supportive environment in which all family members can freely verbalize feelings about the trauma and its effects upon the family; (2) to educate the family about the nature of the deficit in communication and develop methods for resolving conflicts within the relationship patterns of the family system; and (3) to examine, clarify, and restructure roles and responsibilities within the family system. Some techniques often used include (1) emphasizing the mutuality of responsibility for the family problems and shifting the burden of guilt from the identified patient to the family system; (2) analyzing, focusing on, and strengthening the positive aspects of the family system; (3) exploring dysfunctional patterns of interaction by reenacting family conflicts and assisting family members to problem-solve to alleviate these conflicts; and (4) prescribing "homework assignments" for the family to practice outside the sessions to foster generalization of behavior change. The aforementioned framework for family therapy is also easily applied to a marital counseling situation, as well.

Another major form of family intervention would be the use of *family support* groups. As family-initiated organizations have grown within the past decade, there has been a proliferation of local family support groups that are conducted by the families of brain-injured people, *without* professional leadership or participation. For many families, this type of intervention is better accepted than professional help. Those who have personally experienced the trauma of head injury have much to offer those who are in the process of trying to make sense of their experience. Besides receiving emotional support from the sessions, families often form inter-family friendships and support systems that assist them on an ongoing basis. Also, concrete information about the merits and deficiencies of certain treatment facilities and about the availability of certain types of financial or social agency support is provided.

RESEARCH QUESTIONS

Concept of Burden and Long-term Adaptation

A means of assessing the impact of head injury on family members has been to ask the relatives to rate their distress on a seven-point scale, with a low score representing little distress and a high score signifying the highest level of felt distress (Brooks et al., 1987). By categorizing relatives' response into low-, medium-, and high-burden categories, Brooks and co-workers have attempted to correlate the relationship among posttraumatic amnesia, changes in residual deficits, and parent vs. spouse relationships, and the degree of felt burden. In following up patients to 7 years postinjury, results suggested that the level of burden did *not* diminish, that severity of injury (specifically length of posttraumatic amnesia greater than 14 days) often resulted in high relative burden, and that there were no differential ratings of reported burden by wives as compared to mothers. This study, as well as others utilizing the concept of burden as a means of quantifying the relatives' levels of distress, was performed in the United Kingdom, in which formal, extended late rehabilitation programs do not exist. It would be of great value for researchers in the United States to attempt to replicate this study to determine whether the findings reported to date have universal generalizability or may be partly a function of the extent to which patients and their relatives have received extended rehabilitation services. It would also be useful to prospectively analyze how burden and family distress change over time and stage of recovery.

Effectiveness of Family Intervention Techniques

Though families have become a focus for educational and therapeutic intervention in the rehabilitation process, there are no data that clearly document the manner and degree to which family involvement in the rehabilitation process affects outcome. Specifically, controlled studies are needed to document whether structured family education programs produce changes in knowledge, attitudes, and behavior in family members. Are occasional family conferences during inpatient rehabilitation helpful? Do family members benefit more from weekly counseling sessions with a psychologist or social worker? Are therapeutic weekend passes beneficial? Should families become involved with support groups prior to patient discharge from acute rehabilitation? Can family therapy significantly impact a family with dysfunctional interaction predating the brain injury?

Effects of Head Injury on the Family System

Though a number of studies (Brooks et al., 1987; Livingston, 1987) have documented the presence of burden on the part of relatives, there exists a need to examine the impact of head injury on the entire family system. In what manner are family conflict, communication, cohesion, organization, role-relationships, and the like affected by traumatic brain injury? An instrument such as the McMaster Family Assessment Device (FAD), recently used to examine the relatives of stroke patients by Evans and co-workers (1987), or the Family Environment Scale (Moos, 1972), might be used to prospectively analyze family system functioning. Within an analysis of family system function, some attention should be directed toward assessing sibling relationships. Anecdotally, clinicians have noted that the siblings of the head-injured person have difficulty accepting the changes in their head-injured brother or sister, may experience school problems, or may display attention-seeking behaviors.

Specific Effects on the Family

Though it has been documented that a head injury negatively affects the family, few large-scale studies have addressed and documented the frequency and nature of social dysfunction after head injury. There need to be large-scale, multicenter studies that document the frequency of divorce, marital separation, remarriage, financial hardship, job change, emotional disorder, etc. and make comparisons to a comparable "normal" population. This may be accomplished through state or national head injury registries, a national data collection system, or through studies similar to the one recently performed by Jacobs (1987) in Southern California, in which 142 families responded to a 750-question survey about daily living activity patterns. In addition, the question of whether and to what extent family members experience psychological disorders after injury and seek and receive psychotherapy or psychotropic medication has only been occasionally and incompletely addressed in previous research. Furthermore, there is a need to differentiate between the effects of pediatric head injury on the family and adult head injury and to determine what the resulting needs might be.

Need for Specialized Services

There are a variety of services that families often need but may not have access to after traumatic brain injury. Some of these services include respite care, legal advice regarding conservatorship or guardianship, professional case management, financial assistance, ongoing social support, transportation, and in-home therapy services. Though the availability of these services has increased greatly over the past 5 years, there are likely many rural or undeserved geographic areas where families have limited access to these services. The development of a coordinated national data base and state brain injury registries may be a mechanism for identifying the magnitude of this problem—i.e., the number of families who are in need but unable to access these important family services.

Training Family Members as "Therapists"

Though family members have been accorded a central role in the rehabilitation process and routinely receive education and supportive counseling, it may be that they could be more effective if they received formal, structured training in cognitive and behavior management skills. This notion derives from the behavior therapy literature in which parents have been effectively trained as "therapists" to manage noncompliance, temper tantrums, and other behavior problems exhibited by their own children. With the application of cognitive rehabilitation and behavioral management to brain injury patients, families have been eager to learn how they can apply these "new" techniques at home. Currently, Jacobs (1986) and co-workers at UCLA are attempting to test the efficacy of a family training model. This technique holds great promise for providing families with an increased feeling of confidence in being able to better care for their relatives and perhaps create more optimal family adjustment.

REFERENCES

Bond M (1984): The psychiatry of closed head injury. In: N Brooks (ed.). *Closed head injury: psychological, social, and family consequences* (pp. 148–178). New York: Oxford University Press.

Bond M (1975): Assessment of the psychosocial outcome after severe head injury. In: *Symposium on the outcome of severe damage to the central nervous system* (Ciba Foundation Symposium No. 34, Series, pp. 141–157). Amsterdam: Elsevier/Excerpta Medica.

Brooks N, McKinlay W (1983): Personality and behavioral differences after severe head injury—a relative's view. *Journal of Neurology, Neurosurgery and Psychiatry*. 46:336–344.

Brooks N, Campsie L, Symington C, Beattie A, McKinlay W (1987): The effects of severe head injury on patient and relative seven years after injury. *Journal of Head Trauma Rehabilitation* 2(3):1–13.

Diehl L (1983): Patient-family education. In: Rosenthal M, Griffith ER, Bond MR, Miller JD (eds.). *Rehabilitation of the head injured adult* (pp. 395–406). Philadelphia: F. A. Davis.

Evans RL, Bishop DS, Matlock AL, Stranahan S, Halar EM (1987): Family interaction and treatment adherence after stroke. *Archives of Physical Medicine and Rehabilitation* 68:513–517.

Glick ID, Kessler DR (1974): *Marital and family therapy* (p. 1). New York: Grune & Stratton.

Gronwall D (1986): Rehabilitation programs for patients with mild head injury: components, problems and evaluation. *Journal of Head Trauma Rehabilitation* 1(2):53–62.

Jacobs H (1987): The Los Angeles head injury survey: project rationale and design implications. *Journal of Head Trauma Rehabilitation* 2(3):37–50.

Kozloff R (1987): Networks of social support and the outcome from severe head injury. *Journal of Head Trauma Rehabilitation* 2(3):14–23.

Levin HS, Benton AL, Grossman RG (1982): *Neurobehavioral consequences of closed head injury*. New York: Oxford University Press.

Lezak M (1986): Psychological implications of traumatic brain damage for the patient's family. *Rehabilitation Psychology* 31(4):241–250.

Lezak M (1982): *Neuropsychological assessment,* 2nd ed. New York: Oxford University Press.

Lezak MD (1978): Living with the characterologically altered brain injured patient. *Journal of Clinical Psychiatry* 39:592–598.

Livingston MG, Brooks N, Bond MR (1987): Three months after severe head injury: Psychiatric and social impact on relatives. *Journal of Neurology, Neurosurgery and Psychiatry* 48:870–875.

Livingston MG, Brooks N, Bond MR (1985): Patient outcome in the year following severe head injury and relative's psychiatric and social functioning. *Journal of Neurology, Neurosurgery and Psychiatry* 48:876–881.

Livingston MG (1987): Head injury: the relative's response. *Brain Injury* 1(1):33–39.

Moos R (1972): *The family environment scale.* Palo Alto, CA: Consulting Psychologists Press.

Oddy M, Humphrey M, Uttley D (1984): Stresses upon the relatives of head-injured patients. *British Journal of Psychiatry* 133:507–513.

Panting A, Merry P (1972): The long-term rehabilitation of severe head injuries with particular reference to the need for social and medical support for the patient's family. *Rehabilitation* 38:33–37.

Romano M (1974): Family response to traumatic head injury. *Scandinavian Journal of Rehabilitation Medicine* 6:1–4.

Rosenbaum M, Najenson T (1976): Changes in life patterns and symptoms of low mood as reported by wives of severely brain-injured soldiers. *Journal of Consulting and Clinical Psychology* 44:881–888.

Rosenthal M, Geckler C (1986): Family therapy issues in neuropsychology. In: Wedding D, Horton AM, Webster J. *The neuropsychology handbook: behavioral and clinical perspectives* (pp. 325–344). New York: Springer.

Rosenthal M, Muir C (1983): Methods of family intervention. In: Rosenthal, M. et al (eds.) *Rehabilitation of the head injured adult* (pp. 407–419). Philadelphia: F. A. Davis.

Whyte J (1986): Preface. Attention and Memory. *Journal of Head Trauma Rehabilitation* 1(3):ix.

17

Systematic Care for Persons with Head Injury

Mark V. Johnston, Ph.D., and Larry Cervelli, B.S., O.T.R.

The New Medico Head Injury System, Northampton, Massachusetts, U.S.A.

The last 15 years have witnessed striking changes in care of persons with traumatic brain injury (TBI), including the advent of categorical head injury rehabilitation programs and subsequent explosive growth in the number of such programs, increased research and publications, and the founding and growth of advocacy groups such as the National Head Injury Foundation (NHIF). These developments have been accompanied by an evolving awareness of the inadequacy of traditional, fragmented TBI service delivery and by increasingly clear perception of the need for a more complete and better coordinated continuum of care.

This chapter will identify problems produced by current fragmented approaches to care delivery. It will then sketch characteristics of a more systematic approach and attempt to identify what an ideal system might look like by examining related care systems, particularly the developmental disability (DD) care system. Financial factors and requirements for improved cost-effectiveness of service delivery will then be treated. Research proposals will be presented at the end.

CURRENT PROBLEMS

Perhaps the most striking feature of current service delivery for head-injured persons in this country is its nonsystem character. Prominent systematic problems include:

1. Absence of a coordinated spectrum of care. There is a large and expanding group of disabled TBI survivors and an increasing realization

that services are required for years following onset. A large number of persons will not recover functional independence or community reintegration. Required services are not just medical but also include rehabilitation, education, recreation, vocation, and long-term supportive care.

2. Enormous inequities in funding. While some head injury survivors have funds for millions of dollars of intensive acute and rehabilitative care, other equally blameless accident victims are thrown on the mercy of the overburdened Medicaid system, which may or may not provide rehabilitative services. There is no uniformity in insurance policies, leaving the TBI survivor at the mercy of a policy he or she has never read.

3. Perverse incentives. Patients frequently must be treated in hospitals or at least in institutions to justify reimbursement, when less expensive community settings can be equally or more therapeutic. Insurance policies emphasize treatment for physical problems, despite the fact that the primary long-term disablers of head injury survivors are cognitive and social-behavioral (e.g., Brooks, 1984). Treatment facilities have to provide the care that third-party payers will reimburse, not what the head-injured person needs.

4. Trauma centers continue to save lives, despite the fact that many survivors will be left cognitively disabled and dependent for the rest of their lives. On the basis of ethical norms and laws rooted in experiences unrelated to the burden of care for severely permanently disabled cases, there is no one to take responsibility for the costs of such decisions, which fall on overstressed families and the welfare system.

5. Fragmentation of service delivery. Few head injury survivors receive long-term case management support. The burden of service coordination falls on overstressed families.

6. Lack of consideration of societal costs. Fragmentation of payment sources means that nobody is responsible for overall expenses to society. Cost control efforts focus on palming off costs to someone else rather than on improving cost-effectiveness: insurance companies, preferred provider organizations (PPOs), and health maintenance organizations (HMOs) try to write exclusionary policies with caps on liabilities, thereby shifting burdens to government and families; treatment professionals in alliance with patients and families try to maximize services to the patient, regardless of already low or nonexistent profits of medical insurance companies and competing priorities for the already inadequate government welfare budgets.

Other systematic problems include absence of uniformly enforced national accreditation standards; regulatory and payment expenses that in many cases exceed expenditures for direct patient care; lack of agreement on the relative efficacy of different treatment approaches; and absence of agreed upon standards for payment, documentation, and measurement of client progress, among others. A more systematic approach to head injury care is needed to solve or ameliorate these problems.

Expected System Outcomes

The goal of a system of care is that each service recipient should achieve the maximum possible recovery at the lowest possible financial cost.[1]

Maximum recovery naturally means different things to different readers. To the authors, this means maximum possible recovery of health, functional independence, cognitive and behavioral skills, and personal empowerment. The person's skills will be synthesized into a role that allows the resumption of life that is satisfying to the individual and useful or not burdensome to family and society. After attaining maximal medical and physical recovery, individuals will be placed in structured environments that require use of preserved skills and facilitate development of compensatory skills. This does not mean therapy forever, but rather structuring a therapeutic lifestyle. The satisfaction of the individual with his or her role in life seems essential to minimize searching for the ideal job, shopping endlessly for more therapy, or avoiding participation in practical daily living activities. The premorbid state will usually not be achieved, but the authors' experience has shown that even very severely head-injured persons can attain a stabilized, satisfactory adjustment to disability, requiring crisis management little more frequently than nondisabled persons. Targeted interventions to meet the individual's and family's physical and social needs can prevent catastrophic and expensive crises.

Families and caregivers, too, have needs. A head injury care system will reduce the number of individuals disabled by a single head injury. Families will have the resources needed to avoid dissolution under unrelenting burdens of care of the disabled family member or sustained financial problems. Families will be able to experience their disabled family member in a nonoppressive relationship.

At the community level, head-injured individuals will be experienced as citizens with special needs who partake of supportive services in a reasonable fashion. The costs of providing an array of helpful services to disabled head-injured persons will not be regarded differently from those of other protected groups such as children or the elderly. Social, vocational, avocational, and medical services will be accessible to head-injured persons of all age groups and all levels of disability and eco-

---

[1]Parts of this section are adapted from L. Cervelli, *Community Re-entry and Systematic Care for People with Head Injury,* edited by M. Rosenthal and E. Griffith (1989).

nomic capability. The productivity of the individual—vocationally, socially, or avocationally—will be valued.

Comprehensive System Characteristics

The ideal TBI system encompasses all needed services (Berrol, Cervelli, Mackworth, Mackworth, and Rappaport, 1982). Evacuation from the injury site, emergency room services, and intensive care unit treatment are delivered by specialists specifically trained in diagnosis and management of TBI and basic recording standards such as the Glasgow Coma Scale. The ideal TBI system encompasses acute medical care; acute and subacute medical rehabilitation; outpatient and at-home rehabilitation; longer-term educational, vocational, recreational, and independent living services; long-term care and supportive services. Each service element has clearly stated admission and discharge criteria. Funding to support service delivery and sensible movement across settings are coordinated by a case manager, minimizing false placements and misallocation of resources. Participants are evaluated against published service goals. Elements of the system communicate with one other effectively. Common forms, measures, and procedures make communication more efficient and prevent expensive duplicate testing of clients. At a personal level, improved communication and shared experiences and norms lead to improved cooperation and joint problem solving.

Systems for community intervention in health care ideally are (a) immediately available, accessible, and affordable; (b) flexible enough to meet special needs while still dealing with broad problem areas; (c) conducted within the person's social milieu with firm link to family and friends; (d) aimed at reducing risk of reinstitutionalization and community disenfranchisement; (e) coordinated to make the most efficient and effective use of existing community resources. Unfortunately, none of these ends is accomplished currently (Magrab and Elder, 1979).

A systems approach to TBI would actively involve virtually every human service agency within a community. The impairments, disabilities, and handicaps resulting from mild to severe head injury require all agencies to service this population. With so many agencies required to provide service, the crucial question is how to coordinate services and how to set up rewards for providing effective, coordinated services.

LESSONS FROM OTHER SYSTEMS

A lack of coordination of various service elements is a striking characteristic of the entire human service field in this country (Magrab and Elder, 1979). Intensive and systematic efforts have been made to deal with these problems for at least two decades. It should be possible to learn a great deal about how to systematically improve TBI care by study of efforts made to deal with problems of similar disabled populations.

Comparison to Spinal Cord Injury

SCI affects a population demographically similar to TBI. Both are fairly young, predominantly male, and survive for decades even after severe injury. But, whereas individuals with SCI typically have totally intact cognition and awareness, the hallmark of TBI is disturbed awareness, with more frequent and severe problems with social behavior, emotion, perception, and especially cognition.

The National Regional SCI System has focused on provision of information, education, developmental support, and funding for data collection in hospital settings combining acute medical and rehabilitative services under one roof. Development of facilities to serve a large region is appropriate given the relatively small incidence rate of SCI (about 5 per 100,000 according to Anderson and McLaurin, 1980). System development has been federally funded and administered. Data were collected and analyzed for consumption by members of the service delivery group.

However adequate the model is for SCI—and it is a good one—the model is not adequate to address the problems of most head injury survivors. The incidence of TBI is approximately 40 times that of SCI (Anderson and McLaurin, 1980). Residual deficits are not only physical and medical but also behavioral, vocational, and psychological problems. The size of the TBI population and the wide range of residual deficits requires the development of many care providers within regions. A single institution would be limited in accessibility and could not specialize in the requirements for excellence in care for very different problems. Gargantuan institutions promote institutionalization and are not optimal for community reintegration. Building a TBI system around hospitals alone would mean continued attention to medical needs and neglect of others. The current nonsystem could be accentuated.

The course of recovery of skills is different for the two groups. On average, SCI has a more rapid rehabilitation course with earlier maximum skill recovery (Berrol et al., 1982). Longer-term care providers need to be involved in TBI care systems. Even in SCI, professionals increasingly have come to realize that long-term needs cannot be met by intensive short-term efforts alone. Long-term support and follow-up are needed. These long-term needs for community reintegration are, if anything, even more obvious with TBI, where resolution of medical and physical problems does not ensure return to a satisfactory life.

Brain injury survivors have problems with generalizing what they have learned to new situations or problems. Consequently, the greater the difference between the rehabilitative treatment environment and the environment they have to perform in after discharge, the less likely are the skills gained in rehabilitation to be generalized. Acute-care hospitals and other total-care institutions are highly artificial environments, and there is every reason to believe that they are not optimal to promote generalization of treatment effects for community reintegration. Therapeutic interventions involving learning should be more useful and generalizable and probably less expensive if taught in community settings.

The Developmental Disability System

The developmental disability (DD) care system, funded through PL 95-602 and numerous amendments, has funded development and ongoing delivery of an array of therapeutic educational, residential, vocational, and case management services. Like head injury, developmental disabilities are heterogeneous, probably even more so than head injuries since the primary problem may be physical or cognitive. Problems of DD clients may be physical or neurologic and as diverse as cerebral palsy and Down syndrome. Like TBI, problems are of long duration; and at the neurophysiologic level, problems are virtually permanent.

The assumption that nothing can be done but care for developmentally disabled persons in a maintenance facility has become discredited. Fifteen years ago the predominant service mode was institutional care. As a consequence of citizen advocacy, litigation, and knowledge of high-quality noninstitutional services (e.g., in Scandinavia), the DD system has shifted the bulk of its resources away from institutional care toward community care models. The potential benefits of deinstitutionalization—superior service to the client without additional cost—are generally acknowledged today.

Characteristics of the DD system applicable to TBI include the following:

1. Services are planned and directed at state, regional, and local levels. Services are funded by the state and federal governments, and funding is channeled through state-wide DD councils composed of regional representatives, which include consumer representatives. The state body establishes state-wide service priorities through input of regional boards. Local services are developed and coordinated through a regional center that maintains linkages with primary service vendors.

2. Financial support is for a wide array of medical and nonmedical services not otherwise fundable and may be for acute or subacute problems.

3. Most costs are actually born by federal entitlement programs (Medicaid, Social Security Administration, etc.), but the DD system acts to coordinate these benefits and to direct them in ways most appropriate

to the client. The DD system has independent funding for service provision, but these are smaller than other entitlement funds.

4. Advocacy for DD patients is spearheaded by local citizen groups, but DD agencies are legally empowered to act to protect individuals in a broad range of circumstances and settings. In some states, DD officials act as ombudsmen to solve critical or unusual problems faced by individuals or by the DD system.

5. Educational funds ensure that professionals are specifically trained to deal with problems common to DD clients.

6. Program monitoring and quality assurance functions are performed in a branch of a service agency not directly responsible for operations or in a completely different or superior agency. Independent quality evaluation is much more possible in DD than in the medical system, where quality assurance and program evaluation personnel are directly responsible to a physician or administrator whose program they evaluate.

7. The DD system also has its own research funding and independent research capability.

The appeal of this model to TBI is that it addresses a large target population, coordinates service development on a regional level, and ties many service providers together. By allocating its own funds, it has the ability to reward superior services and provide performance feedback to service providers.

Psychiatric Care and Mental Health

Care delivery in both TBI and mental health must deal with individuals whose problem is "in their head." It is now generally realized that TBI is a problem and syndrome in itself and that most TBI individuals are ill served by placement in psychiatric institutions. Nonetheless, lessons can be drawn from the extensive experience of the mental health industry, a far larger, older, and better-established field than TBI care.

An obvious role for mental health professionals is to act as a resource for TBI case managers. Certain TBI individuals benefit from selected psychiatric and pharmacologic interventions. Professionals skilled in behavior modification have proven their ability to help brain-injured individuals with certain behavioral and social problems. In some communities, mental health practitioners will be the only accessible professional help, and the job of a TBI care system will be to educate the mental health practitioner in the problems of TBI and to direct clients to that practitioner.

There are a number of studies of the costs and effectiveness of different approaches to psychiatric and mental health that bear on the questions of the organization of TBI care. It is, for instance, instructive to note that it is now clearly established that mental health care tends to have a cost-offset effect on utilization of inpatient medical care (Mumford, Schlesinger, Glass, Patrick, and Cuerdon, 1984), though the magnitude of the reduction is frequently unclear.

ECONOMIC FORCES AFFECTING SYSTEM PERFORMANCE

Funding drives any service delivery system. A care system is organized—or disorganized—by funding.

Current Funding Policies Are Frequently Not Appropriate to TBI

In many respects the problem of funding for TBI is part and parcel of the larger problem of inadequate funding for catastrophic injuries of all types. Problems specific to TBI include the need for reliable funding for community reentry services (post-acute rehabilitation) and for therapies directed at cognitive and social-behavioral problems rather than at physical problems. Even when a person has adequate coverage for rehabilitation—and many do not—insurance policies may stipulate payment only for strictly medical problems, physical therapy, and very limited occupational and speech therapy services. The focus now is on physical problems. The primary problems of TBI survivors—cognitive and social-behavioral deficits—are seen as psychiatric or psychological problems, which are frequently not covered. Coverage only for hospital care ensures that rehabilitation will occur in the most expensive possible setting—or will not occur at all.

Cost-Effectiveness

In today's political climate of shrinking welfare dollars, simple appeals for more money for head injury victims may fall on ears already deafened by cries from a hundred other needy groups. Service delivery approaches demonstrated to be cost-effective are more likely to be politically attractive. Cost control is an unavoidable reality.

Much lip service is given to cost-effectiveness, but very little research is actually done on the cost-effectiveness of different approaches to head injury care (Johnston and Keith, 1983; Johnston, 1989). Consumers of TBI services are the losers in this, for without information on the cost-effectiveness of services, they are likely to have to pay too much for what benefits they do get. Without better information on cost-effectiveness, insurance companies and government have no way of containing costs except denial of services on the basis of simplistic categories. Costs will be controlled bruskly if expenditures cannot be prioritized humanely.

PROPOSALS FOR SYSTEM IMPROVEMENTS

This section will make a number of research proposals to improve the organization of care for TBI and to improve its effectiveness and cost-effectiveness.

Balance Funding between Research and Direct Funding of Service Provision

A system of care for head injury needs to directly fund provision of services, or it is likely to have little effect on care by existing providers. Without direct funding, significant changes in our current nonsystem are unlikely. Even research would be inhibited, for without direct funding it is more difficult to access a study population, and one is limited to study of the existing nonsystem.

Are funds available for direct service provision? In an era of declining welfare budgets, available funds are likely to be extremely limited, but this does not mean that no money is available. In Massachusetts, consumer advocacy has resulted in the State-wide Head Injury Project, which is spending $5.6 million dollars this year on direct service provision for head-injured persons with severe behavioral disturbances. Advocacy by the NHIF has resulted in federal initiatives in TBI research, of which this paper is a small part. Money can be made available by redirecting funds now being spent on TBI by agencies that are not specifically skilled in TBI. Substantial monies can be made available with sufficient political pressure, especially if that pressure is combined with evidence that changes in the system of care for TBI can not only benefit TBI individuals and their families but also reduce costs to society.

On the other hand, to spend all available funds on direct service provision would be unwise. Without research and program evaluation, the limited funds that are likely to be available will disappear into the yawning gulf of hundreds of thousands of individuals' needs. When we go back to legislators for funding for a second year, they will ask for numeric evidence that the money they spent the past year had an impact on the social costs of TBI. Without research and program evaluation, we will not have that evidence. Opponents of welfare expenditures will have the argument they need to deny further funding.

Research is essential not only to deal with government officials but also to educate the insurance industry, the public, and even health care professionals regarding the particular needs of head-injured individuals.

Without research, long-term improvement in the effectiveness of a TBI care system, with adequate cost control, is unlikely.

Yet all new funding for TBI should not go for research. To do so would smack of an attempt to study the problem to death rather than to deal with the needs of TBI individuals and their families. New government expenditures need to be balanced between research and direct service provision.

Cost-Effectiveness Research Needs to Be a High Priority

There will always be shortages of funds to help disabled persons, and it will always be important to know how to prioritize our efforts so that we may do the greatest good for the greatest number of individuals. Hence we propose that cost-effectiveness research be a priority. This need not imply that less money is available for research targeted primarily at improved treatment effectiveness. It does mean that relevant costs need to be measured or at least estimated as part of any effectiveness study.

Utilize Augmented Measures of Cost

In current research and practice, the standard measure of cost is length of stay (LOS) or total direct care expenditures. This ignores system costs—costs of rehospitalization, institutionalization, and long-term care; costs of lost earnings by the brain-injured individual; costs of lost earnings by family members (which can be substantial); and so on. In the authors' opinion, TBI rehabilitation is unlikely to ever justify itself by reduction in direct medical care expenditures alone, but rehabilitation is very likely to be justifiable in terms of benefits to society as a whole. By measuring the full range of costs attributable to TBI, we will be able to identify rehabilitative programs and treatments that are most cost-beneficial to society and to distinguish them from interventions that are not economically justifiable.

Research to Develop Better Payment Systems for TBI

Research that identifies a better payment system for TBI can yield substantial benefits in terms of cost control or cost savings while lessening inappropriate denial of payments.

Current attempts at cost control in TBI are fairly crude and poorly related to cost-effectiveness. Cost control attempts in hospitals currently center on limitations on maximum LOS or expenditures. This ignores special needs of individuals who require more or less care. Alternatively, the greatest resources are devoted to individuals in greatest need or with the most severe impairments, which ignores individuals' responsiveness to treatment. Great resources may, for instance, be devoted to the care of very severely impaired individuals who require total care, while monies may be unavailable for simple job modifications or supported employment programs that are likely to return other, less impaired individuals to work. From an economic standpoint, the criterion for resource allocation should be likely patient responsiveness to treatment rather than need in the sense of severity.

Cost control can in principle be based on improvement per dollar or per day or on other criteria more related to cost-effectiveness. For any such approach to work, payers would need to know what rate of improvement they can expect for their dollar over what time period. If they do not see such response to rehabilitative treatment, they would be within their rights to end funding or request a change of setting. Empirical data are needed so such decisions can be made on a systematic and realistic rather than a haphazard basis.

Research is needed to discover factors that drive TBI costs as well as patient outcomes. This research is essential if we are to discover the outlines of what a more suitable payment system for TBI needs to involve. Such cost-related research can fairly easily be incorporated into currently proposed longitudinal studies that track the progress of TBI individuals for years after their initial hospital admission. It is important that cost-related research be targeted toward administratively practical problems and solutions in order that results will be of real applicability (e.g., by utilizing simple, nonfalsifiable measures rather than measures that are only feasible in a research situation).

Prospective payment systems are attractive to the government and third party payers because they have proven ability to control costs. A prospective payment system needs to give clinicians sufficient options so that they have the ability as well as the incentive to prioritize their efforts. However, no prospective payment system is currently suitable for TBI. Current prospective payment systems are fairly crude and are open to charges of achieving savings by forcing premature discharge of patients. A prospective payment system may come. We must begin to gather data now to ensure that the payment system is tailored to the needs of head-injured individuals.

A study of new payment systems might bundle payment for rehabilitation with payment for long-term and support services to encourage a rational distribution of resources between the two.

Develop a Model Policy for Coverage of TBI

What is needed is not a ticket for unlimited coverage for TBI, which is unrealistic, but specific guidelines to help insurance personnel know how and what to cover and when to deny coverage for TBI services and what sort of documentation to ask for and expect. The cost-effectiveness of these guidelines warrants empirical investigation. What is essential is that guidelines for TBI coverage balance the needs of head-injured patients and families for increased care against the needs of payers to contain costs.

Develop Cost-Effective Community Reintegration and Support Services

Research is needed to identify what types of community reintegration and long-term support services are more versus less cost-effective.

Models for such a study can be found in the literature on alternatives to mental hospital treatment. An instructive example is the study of Stein and Test (1980) and Weisbrud, Test, and Stein (1980). In this experiment, treatment professionals in a psychiatric hospital ward were retrained to provide care to discharged patients in the community. Patients were randomly assigned to augmented follow-up and support care by this team—the "Training in Community Living" (TCL) program—or to traditional poorly coordinated outpatient care. Results showed a general pattern of superior functioning as well as greater expressed satisfaction with life situation by individuals in the experimental group. Direct costs of the augmented follow-up and support care were greater than ordinary outpatient services (about $800 per case on average). However, a reduction in rehospitalization and increased earnings among TCL subjects ($1,200 per case) more than recouped the augmented support costs. There is every reason to believe community follow-up and support services can also save money in the long-term care of chronically disabled TBI patients. Study of case management strategies and alternatives to institutionalization for TBI is another way of framing the question here.

Regardless of the intervention studied, it is already known that targeting of services is essential, or the cost of the intervention will exceed the savings. A system that allocates services entirely according to patient severity and ignores client responsiveness is unlikely to show improved cost-effectiveness, though it may meet certain needs of individuals served (Johnston and Keith, 1983; Johnston, in press). Community reintegration and support programs will need to target their interventions at reasons for rehospitalization, causes of institutional care and high support costs, and remediable causes of unemployment (by both brain-injured individual and caregivers) if they are to demonstrate cost-benefits.

Develop Uniform Measurement and Documentation Standards

Development of shared standards of documentation and clinical outcome measurement is a major means to prepare the grounds for a truly systematic approach to TBI. A uniform vocabulary will improve the efficiency and organization of the care system. Currently, a great deal of staff time is spent on documentation; and despite such expenditures, third-party payers frequently have poor information about whether to approve continued payment or not. Providers are not certain about what needs to be documented and fear loss of reimbursement if they are too frank about patients—or if they do not document compulsively and redundantly. What is needed are shared standards for measurement of functional outcomes, disability reduction, and so on. These standards need to be tied to reimbursement, for common documentation standards are likely to occur only if funding sources require them.

Work is needed to develop better outcome measures at the program or regional systems level. Global scales such as the Glasgow Outcome Scale are too gross and perhaps too unreliable to detect the effects of rehabilitative interventions. Work is needed to develop better measures of functioning in community, residential, and leisure activities, of cognitive functioning in daily life, and of social-behavioral problems. Work is not needed to develop new measures of physical disability, as good measures are already available (e.g., Fuhrer, 1987). The reliability and validity of both existing and new measures need to be quantitatively established.

Better measures of *handicap* are also needed. Handicap is defined by the World Health Organization (1980) as the disadvantage that a person experiences as a consequence of a disability or impairment. Handicap depends not just upon the objective impairment or disability of the person but also upon the environmental consequences of impairments and disabilities to the individual, upon the roles the individual needs to play in society, and upon the individual's values. The current lack of reliable standard measures of handicap is not just a technical lacuna: Even if a client improves functionally, a treatment program may still have mistargeted its efforts toward life domains of lesser importance. An example would be expensive services directed toward total elimination of physical medical problems which ignore emotional and social behavioral problems that distress the family to a far greater degree and are more likely to cause a breakdown in the family, with consequent reliance on institutional care and government to care for the individual with TBI. It is technically possible to measure handicap with TBI clients (Haffey and Johnston, 1989), but the reliability and validity of such measures needs to be established before they can be standardized.

Though work needs to be done to develop more reliable and valid outcome measures, such work must not impede study of the effectiveness and cost-effectiveness of current programs. The benefits of a system of care for individuals with TBI should be readily and publicly observable and hence relatively easy to measure. If the benefits of a treatment program are observable only by professionals using technical physiological or neuropsychological tests, that program has not proven itself in practical terms.

Publish Consumer Reports on TBI Services

Currently there is no objective way by which the family of a brain-injured person, a case manager, or a referring physician can compare the costs or outcomes of one service program for TBI individuals to another. Data comparing the costs and outcomes of one program to an alternative are generally unavailable. Even if numeric outcomes are described, the data are presented in terms that make it impossible to compare one program to the other.

The crucial problem is not primarily an insufficiency of effort toward data collection. Program evaluators and quality assurance personnel in hospitals and rehabilitation programs currently gather a great deal of data in the attempt to perform evaluative and quality control. However, the reports they generate are not public but remain confidential to staff in the facility. Moreover, the program evaluator or quality assurance coordinator is hired by the administrator or physician whose program is being evaluated. Current quality assurance and program evaluation systems in hospitals frequently have difficulty demonstrating utility or program changes commensurate with the increased documentation and administrative cost imposed by these systems. The fact that the data are always internal limits the uses.

Objective evaluation requires evaluation by another. No one can objectively evaluate himself or herself or the boss. Public use of part of the data collected by program evaluation and quality assurance would make these activities more useful. One way of doing this would be to create consumer reports for TBI programs.

The idea of consumer reports on medical and rehabilitative facilities is as radical today as *Consumer Reports* was in the 1930s—and just as appropriate. How is the prospective consumer to know where to go or what the costs are likely to be? Individual consumers experience satisfaction or dissatisfaction, but their experiences are not cumulated to affect the system of head injury care. The NHIF now has an extensive listing of treatment programs for TBI, but these listings do not provide data on relative costs and quality of programs. If prospective consumers could look through the report and see which programs were much below average in consumer satisfaction or unusually high in costs, they would be in a position to ask more pointed questions of the TBI care industry. It is entirely feasible to collect by mail information on consumers' experiences with TBI treatment facilities—their satisfaction with different aspects of care, approximate cost or length of stay, whether they were deceived, whether their goals were met, and whether they improved appreciably or not.

To be sure, it is important that any such consumer report on TBI care protect professionals: Satisfaction is likely to be lower for facilities specializing in more difficult cases with poorer prognosis. One cannot expect any such consumer reports to identify subtle differences in treatment quality or efficacy. Development of a fair format is a small research and development project in itself. But it should be fairly easy to identify the poorest programs, to spotlight any programs that systematically mislead consumers (e.g., via misleading marketing claims), and to generally increase the quantity of publicly available information about TBI treatment programs.

An Independent Research Capacity for TBI

TBI needs its own research office or at least a separately identified research agenda in the federal agencies such as the National Institute on Disability and Rehabilitation Research, Office of Special Education and Rehabilitation Research, National Institute of Mental Health, and others. TBI is a specific and complex syndrome, and progress in TBI research is not likely without the sustained effort by many devoted researchers over many years.

Methodological Proposals

Progress in TBI systems research will be speeded by certain methodological improvements.

1. More rigorous study of effectiveness. Professionals have devised numerous treatments that appear to help TBI individuals and their families, but the effectiveness of these treatments has never been rigorously demonstrated (e.g., Cope, 1985; Johnston, 1989; Johnston and Keith, 1983). Rigorous study of effectiveness is required if we are to know which treatment strategies have substantial, lasting benefits and which are little more than placebos with short-run effects.

2. Improved experimental designs. Much rehabilitation research in the past has utilized descriptive or preexperimental methods. While these yield understanding, such studies cannot tell us which interventions are highly effective and which are relatively worthless. We hope that the day is past when a study can describe patient improvement and blithely ascribe this improvement as due to the author's treatment program without stable baseline or control group data.

An outstanding reason for the limited methodological quality in rehabilitation and disability research is that it must be conducted on living human beings in natural settings. Randomized experiments are usually not ethical or feasible in such settings. Solutions to this problem have been devised. Specialists in experimental design have devised clever quasi-experimental design that, in certain circumstances, can be as rigorous or logically compelling as the randomized design, but which lacks the ethical and practical limitations of randomization. Strong quasi-experimental designs include certain "single subject" designs, interrupted time series, multiple time series, and regression discontinuity designs (e.g., Cook and Campbell, 1979). Purely statistical designs are usually much weaker than the preceding designs, and pre-post comparison designs are technically preexperimental designs. Quasi-experimental designs are much more complex and tricky to apply than randomized designs. Experts in experimental design need to be involved in the design and approval of TBI research and demonstration projects.

3. The design of data systems. A great deal of useful descriptive and prognostic data can be gained by a nationwide data system. However, no information on effectiveness or cost-effectiveness is likely to result if the data collection occurs only in very similar facilities (e.g., high quality hospitals), as there is no control group. To gain information about effectiveness, a uniform data system needs to be set up across very different treatment settings which, however, treat similar patients.

CONCLUSIONS

A real system of care for head-injured individuals should include (a) direct funding of services not otherwise fundable, (b) state and regional protection and advocacy, (c) consumer representation on oversight boards, (d) case management and liaison with other service systems, (e) a wide range of potentially fundable services, (f) education, and (g) independent research and program evaluation capacity. A system of care for TBI should not restrict itself to one subgroup or treatment setting but should encompass the entire spectrum of head-injured individuals. To restrict the system to one type of treatment facility would slight the needs of disabled TBI persons who are not optimally served in that setting. Painful prioritization of limited resources is likely to be necessary in the proposed system; but by targeting resources to areas where the benefits to head-injured individuals and society are likely to be greatest, holes in the current nonsystem can begin to be plugged. The costs and benefits of attempts to implement a system of care for head-injured persons need rigorous study.

Acknowledgment: We would like to thank John Scibak, Ph.D., and William Haffey, Ph.D., for contributions of insight and fact to development of this work. Financial support for preparation of this work was provided in part by New Medico Associates, Inc.

REFERENCES

Ackoff R (1980): The systems revolution. In: M Lockett, R Spear (eds.). *Organizations as Systems*. Milton Keynes, England: Open University Press.

Anderson DW, McLaurin RL (eds.) (1980): Report on the National Head and Spinal Cord Injury Survey. National Institute of Neurological and Communicative Disorders and Stroke. *Journal of Neurosurgery* 53: Supplement.

Berrol S, Cervelli L, Cope N, Mackworth N, Mackworth J, Rappaport M (1982): Head Injury Rehabilitation Research Project: Final Report, 1982 (grant no. RSA 13-P-59156/9-03). San Jose, CA: Santa Clara Valley Medical Center.

Brooks N (1984): *Closed Head Injury: Psychological, Social, and Family Consequences*. Oxford: Oxford University Press.

Cervelli L (1989): Community re-entry and systematic care of people with head injury. In: M Rosenthal, E Griffith (eds). *Rehabilitation of the adult and child with traumatic brain injury,* 2nd ed. Philadelphia: F. A. Davis.

Cole JR, Cope DN, Cervelli L (1984): Rehabilitation of the severely brain injured patient. *Archives of Physical Medicine and Rehabilitation* 66:38–40.

Cook TC, Campbell CT (1979): *Quasi-experimentation*. Chicago: Rand McNally.

Cope DN (1985): Traumatic closed head injury: status of rehabilitation treatment. *Seminars in Neurology* 5:212–218.

Fuhrer MJ (ed) (1987): *Rehabilitation outcomes*. Baltimore: Brookes.

Granger CJ, Gresham GE (eds.) (1984): *Functional assessment in rehabilitation medicine*. Baltimore: Williams & Wilkins.

Haffey WJ, Johnston MV (1988): An information system to assess the effectiveness of brain injury rehabilitation. In: R Wood, P Eames (eds.). *Models of brain injury rehabilitation*. London: Chapman and Hall.

Haffey WJ, Johnston MV (1989): A functional assessment system for real world rehabilitation outcomes. In: Tupper D, Cicerone K (eds.). *The Neuropsychology of Everyday Life*. Boston: Martinus Nijhoff.

Johnston MV (1989): The economics of head injury. In: M Miner, K Wagner (eds.). *Neurotrauma, No. 3*. Boston: Buttersworth.

Johnston MV, Keith RA (1983): Cost-benefits of medical rehabilitation: review and critique. *Archives of Physical Medicine and Rehabilitation* 64:147–154.

Magrab P, Elder T (eds.) (1979): *Planning for Services to Handicapped Persons*. Baltimore: Brookes.

Mumford E, Schlesinger HJ, Glass GV, Patrick C, Cuerdon T (1984): A new look at evidence about reduced cost of medical utilization following mental health treatment. *The American Journal of Psychiatry* 141:1145–1158.

Stein LI, Test MA (1980): Alternative to mental hospital treatment. I. Conceptual model, treatment program, and clinical evaluation. *Archives of General Psychiatry,* 37:392–397.

Weisbrod BA, Test MA, Stein LI (1980): Alternative to mental hospital treatment. II. Economic benefit-cost analysis. *Archives of General Psychiatry,* 37:400–405.

World Health Organization (1980): *International classification of impairments, disabilities, and handicaps*. Geneva: World Health Organization.

V

Community Integration
Issues

18

Community Integration After Traumatic Brain Injury: Infants and Children

Ellen Lehr, Ph.D.

Center for Cognitive Rehabilitation, University of Medicine and Dentistry of New Jersey and Rutgers University, New Brunswick, New Jersey, U.S.A.

DEFINITION OF TERMS AND DELINEATION OF THE PROBLEM

The terms in most common usage describing the needs and problems of individuals with traumatic brain injuries after discharge from acute medical and acute rehabilitation settings include *community reentry* and *community reintegration*. While these terms may be appropriate for those individuals who have indeed been separated from their families, schools, jobs, and friends because of relatively long hospitalizations, they do not seem as apposite for individuals with mild or moderate injuries who have not left their communities in any real sense. In fact, the primary issue becomes one of how to enable the individual after less severe traumatic brain injury to recover and adapt in his or her own setting, despite changes subsequent to injury.

The time frame of acute and rehabilitation care is often easily circumscribed. It is clearly defined by admission and discharge dates, with longer follow-up focused on specific concerns. The goals and limitations of acute and rehabilitation programs are usually stated in terms of medical stability and rapid recovery of basic functioning. In community integration, the time period is potentially life-long or, in other words, the length of the effects of TBI for any individual.

The focus of community integration is obviously not one that only

considers the injured individual, but one that involves the complexity of
the social, educational, and vocational systems that comprise daily life.
In fact, it is in this complexity that noninjured individuals take for granted
that many of the major problems occur for individuals after TBI. Their
capacity for understanding and handling the normal routines and challenges of daily life may be reduced temporarily or permanently. Also,
their world can no longer be easily limited to the restricted and manageable environment that is designed for the care of postinjured people.
Because there are limited community-based services and programs specifically designed for individuals after TBI, and services for other diagnostic groups may very well be appropriate, the complexity of service
provider systems is also compounded.

This chapter will focus on research directions and policy implications
in the context of the current state of knowledge and experience with
community integration for infants and children after TBI.

SPECIFIC ISSUES FOR INFANTS AND CHILDREN AFTER TRAUMATIC BRAIN INJURY: A FUNCTIONAL SYSTEMS APPROACH

For children, integration into the community must be integrally tied
to the developmental aspects of both the short- and long-term effects of
traumatic brain injuries. Taking into account their often rapid and more
complete physical recovery (Brink, Garrett, Hale, Woo-Sam, and Nickel,
1970; Brink, Imbus, and Woo-Sam, 1980), as well as their extended period of recovery (Klonoff, Low, and Clark, 1977), much of children's
progress after TBI will take place while they are expected to be functional members of their families, neighborhoods, and schools. The combination of factors including early return to the community or no separation at all, the interaction of development and recovery, and the
prolonged nature of gains after injury are common to most children after
TBI, whether they have had mild, moderate, or severe injuries. Because
of their more adequate physical recovery, cognitive and psychosocial/
emotional/behavioral issues are usually paramount, but at the same time
they are often underestimated (Levin, Ewing-Cobbs, and Benton, 1984).

Although the entire section on community integration will be organized according to a developmental framework, this concept will be central in this chapter on children. For adults, the focus of community-
based intervention is often on returning to preinjury levels of function.
However, for children, redoing, maintaining, and fostering their development are essential parts of recovery and functional integration into
their families and communities. Their care can also take on a preventive aspect, not only in terms of limiting repeat injuries but also in po-

tentially preventing or ameliorating sequelae of injury that may emerge well past the initial period postinjury.

That children are not simply small adults is a guiding premise of this chapter. Much of the work on evaluation and intervention of TBI has been with adults and cannot necessarily be applied directly to children after TBI (Fletcher and Taylor, 1984). Not only are children qualitatively different from adults but their brain organization and function are known to be quantitatively different as well (Luria, 1966). The effects of TBI on children, whose brains are at varying stages of development, cannot be assumed to be the same as in the adult, or indeed even in children at different periods of development (Black, Shepard, and Walker, 1975). Even the mechanisms of injury and the effects of injury on the developing brain have been shown to be different from those in the adult brain (Boll and Barth, 1981), even though these are not clearly understood especially during infancy and early childhood (Raimondi, Choux, and DiRocco, 1986).

Interestingly, age effects of TBI have seldom been the focus of study during the rapid developmental periods of infancy and childhood. In order to clarify the effects of age, not only age at injury needs to be taken into consideration but also the relationship of age to speed of recovery, to patterns of deficits, and to the ultimate extent of impairments in all areas of functioning including physical, cognitive/learning, and behavioral/psychosocial/emotional aspects (Rutter, Chadwick, and Shaffer, 1983).

Research studies have also rarely divided their subjects according to neurodevelopmental substrata, even though it is well known that major neurological/neuroanatomical changes are occurring throughout infancy and childhood. Instead, researchers have divided subjects according to arbitrary measures, for example, the age divisions of the test batteries utilized or the age midpoints of their samples. The effects of injury, both immediate and long-term, are likely to be related to the neurodevelopmental processes that are paramount throughout each period (Shapiro, 1985). During infancy, this primarily involves the effect of injury on cell migration and the organization of the brain. For toddlers, the effect of injury on cell migration is less crucial than the effect on rapid cortical myelinization of the primary and secondary association cortices. In the preschool and primary school age periods, injury has the potential of interrupting and interfering with the rapid connection and myelinization of the tertiary association cortices. And in the middle school age period, the effects on myelinization of the frontal/limbic structures become paramount.

The delayed appearance of cognitive, psychosocial, and emotional sequelae is unique to childhood (Bolter and Long, 1985; Goldman, 1971; Johnson and Almi, 1978; Teuber and Rudel, 1962). This is not only an aspect of recovery as it can be in adults but also is an integral part of development. It is obvious that the effects of injury on higher problem-solving areas in academic and psychosocial areas will not become apparent until the child becomes old enough for their expected appearance. However, it is not clear if any of these delayed effects can be avoided or ameliorated through early and/or ongoing intervention. Since delayed effects can become apparent long after the onset of injury and after immediate medical/rehabilitation management has ended, community-based personnel must be aware of the potential for emerging deficits possibly many years after injury.

Only those infants and children who have sustained traumatic brain injuries after birth will be included in this discussion. Accidental injuries, many of which involve traumatic brain injuries, are the leading cause of both death and disability in childhood (Gross, Wolf, Kunitz, and Jane, 1985; *Monthly Vital Statistics*, 1982). In the United States, the incidence of head injuries in childhood has been estimated at approximately one million per year or at a rate of 200 per 100,000 children (Annegers, 1983). However, the etiology of TBI in childhood may vary, from those related to motor vehicle accidents, falls, and other accidental injuries to those subsequent to violence or abuse, the so-called "nonaccidental" traumatic brain injuries. Because of the wide variation in the etiology of traumatic brain injuries in the pediatric age range and because the needs of individual children vary greatly, this complexity will be organized by examining needs according to (a) the age of the child at the time of injury, (b) the severity of the injury, and (c) the length of time that has elapsed since injury, that is, the acuteness of the injury.

Age at injury. Age will be divided into three groups, (a) infants/toddlers (birth to 2 years of age), (b) preschool- and primary school-aged children (3 to 7 years of age), and (c) school-aged children (8 to 12 years of age). The issues and research needs can be quite different across these age periods. However, the focus on development and redevelopment is similar.

Severity of injury. All levels of severity will be included, from mild injuries to the most severe injuries. The common factor is that all of these injuries have compromised brain function to some degree.

Acuteness of injury. The period of time since the onset of injury is a critical one in planning and understanding the community integration needs of a child after TBI. Those services that are required and appropriate shortly after injury may be unnecessary and inappropriate after several months or years. Consideration of long-term, sometimes life-long, needs will be especially important since they are currently rarely met by medical or traditional pediatric rehabilitation programs and the responsibility for them devolves directly on the community.

In order to organize the presentation of the multiple needs in the area of community integration for children after traumatic brain injury, both in the areas of research and of service, the body of this chapter will be divided according to functional systems. As much as possible this will be presented in a way that corresponds to existing community and funding systems to increase the utility and ready application of recommendations.

EDUCATIONAL SYSTEM

Cognitive/Learning Issues

Although there are well-known cognitive sequelae of TBI, especially in adolescents and adults, less is known about the cognitive effects of TBI in infants and children. The younger the child, the less is known about the short-term and long-term effects on both current and potential cognitive abilities. For example, less is known about younger than older school-aged children, and the least is known about infants, toddlers, and preschool-aged children. This is despite the fact that a relatively large number of young children sustain TBI. In those epidemiological studies that have included children, the early childhood period is often second in incidence rate, being less frequent only than the older adolescent and young adult period (Hendrick, Harwood-Hash, and Hudson, 1964; Klonoff, 1971; Mannheimer, Dewey, and Melinger, 1966). The younger the child the greater the potential of having TBI interfere most significantly during the most extensive period of development. Therefore, research on the effects of TBI in young children will necessarily need to be longitudinal in design and continued over an extensive time period.

In adults, TBI is known to affect new learning to a much greater degree than acquired skills and abilities (Boll and Barth, 1981). If this is true also for children, it would obviously have significant implications for the multitude of capacities that have not yet developed and the acquisition of the large number of skills that have not yet been mastered. However, we know very little about cognitive processes subsequent to TBI that could interfere with new learning in children. If basic processes of attention, concentration, memory, reasoning, and other cognitive areas are altered or diminished after TBI, this could have a significant impact in limiting the amount and changing the way that children learn after injury. Although the development of cognitive abilities in both basic and higher level areas is an active area of research on normal children's learning (Elkind, 1967; Feuerstein, 1980; Vygotsky, 1978), little of this has been applied to children after TBI.

Current State of the Research

In infants and young children, it has been postulated that the major effect of TBI on cognition and learning is one of reduced general capacity, rather than specific areas of deficit (Rutter, 1982). At times, this has been interpreted as brain insult having little effect on young children's functioning. However, most of this research has not followed the children for extensive periods of time to assess the effect of TBI on the rate and degree of learning or to assess the possibility of delayed cognitive effects in specific areas of higher cognitive processes that would not be expected to appear until middle childhood. The classic research that has found a better outcome at younger ages has been done with animals (Kennard, 1942), as well as with young children with surgical interventions such as hemispherectomies (Kinsbourne, 1974) and acquired expressive aphasia (Alajouanine and Lhermitte, 1965). Recent work with infants and toddlers after TBI has been less optimistic, even about their survival and immediate functional recovery (Lange-Cosack, Wider, Schlesner, Grumme, and Kubicki, 1979; Raimondi and Hirschauer, 1984). Since development is so highly integrated during this age period, it is also especially difficult initially to separate cognitive from behavioral/psychosocial/emotional effects.

Although much of the research on TBI effects in childhood has included a wide age span, often combining children as young as 5 years of age with older children and adolescents in the same group, some indications of cognitive effects can be extracted, especially for those children sustaining moderate and severe injuries. In children after approximately 5 years of age, the patterns of language impairment subsequent to left hemisphere injury are similar to acquired aphasia in adults (Alajouanine and Lhermitte, 1965). However, language deficits appear to be less severe, less consistent with site and extent of injury, and resolve more rapidly and completely than in adults (Boll and Barth, 1981).

With a loss of consciousness exceeding 24 hours, intellectual deficits are frequent, serious, and persistent (Levin and Eisenberg, 1979; Klonoff and Paris, 1974). Functioning on intelligence tests, especially the Wechsler tests, indicates greater reduction in ability for children after TBI than in adults. The pattern of Verbal IQ > Performance IQ (Klonoff, Low, and Clark, 1977), especially in the rapid recovery period immediately after injury, is consistent with the findings from the adult literature. However, this effect is demonstrated even after generalized injury, and lateralization effects appear to be less pronounced than in adults (Boll and Barth, 1981). Timed visualspatial and visuomotor tasks tended to show greater and more persistent impairment than verbal tasks (Bawden, Knights, and Winogron, 1985; Rutter, Chadwick, and Shaffer, 1983). In children, cognitive deficits may persist longer than in adolescence (Levin, Eisenberg, Wigg, and Kobayashi, 1982). Although memory is likely to be impaired after head injury, it has been difficult to accurately and fully assess memory function in children (Levin and Eisenberg, 1979).

The cognitive effects of mild injuries in children are much less clear and more controversial (Boll, 1983). Rutter and his associates (Rutter, Chadwick, and Shaffer, 1983) have asserted that there is no dose/response relationship between the cognitive functioning preinjury and postinjury in children with mild injuries. They argue that the cognitive difficulties the children demonstrated postinjury were related to preinjury difficulties and not directly subsequent to TBI. However, research in this area is so meager that their assertions should not be accepted without further corroboration, especially through research involving children with no known cognitive/behavioral difficulties prior to TBI.

Although some children recover or improve in cognitive functioning relatively quickly, others may experience prolonged improvement, even after relatively mild injuries (Klonoff, Low, and Clark, 1977). The course of positive changes, greater than would be expected from the normal rate of development, has been documented for at least 2 1/4 years in severely injured children (Chadwick, Rutter, Brown, Shaffer, and Traub, 1981) and at least 5 years in less severely injured children (Klonoff, Low and Clark, 1977). Unfortunately, there have been very few studies that have followed the same group of children over an extended period, and those studies that have been completed are confounded by sample loss over time.

Cognitive recovery/improvement in children after TBI is not likely to be a unitary phenomenon and is probably affected by multiple variables, including age, developmental level, sex, preinjury functioning levels, severity of injury, and specific injury characteristics and complications. The complex nature and relationship of these variables has not been appreciated in most of the previous research on children after TBI (Boll and Barth, 1981). It is probable that children after TBI do not form a discrete group, even when divided roughly by age and injury severity. Rather, a subgroup approach, similar to the one being developed with children with learning disabilities (Rourke, 1985; Rourke, Bakker, Fisk, and Strang, 1983), or the development of discrete neuropsychological classification systems, similar to those utilized with adults after TBI, will be more useful in designing research and intervention. However, classification and understanding of children after TBI will probably be more complex than either of these two populations.

The effect of cognitive sequelae on academic performance is not clear, though there are indications that scholastic achievement is significantly affected by relatively mild (Klonoff, Low, and Clark, 1977) as well as moderate and severe injuries (Ewing-Cobbs, Fletcher, and Levin, 1985; Heiskanen and Kaste, 1974) and may improve less rapidly than cognitive abilities (Rutter, Chadwick, and Shaffer, 1983). Most of the research on academic effects of TBI has looked only at the types of school placements and programming of children after injury, especially whether they could return to their preinjury educational setting, rather than at the effects on learning per se. Rarely have standardized, objective measures of academic attainment been used, much less on a longitudinal basis, to assess progress over several years. The effect of TBI on academic performance may be more significant for younger children, that is, those who have not mastered the basics of reading, spelling, and arithmetic prior to injury, as well as for those children who are more severely injured (Brink, Garrett, Hale, Woo-Sam, and Nickel, 1970; Chadwick, Rutter, Thompson, and Shaffer, 1981; Shaffer, Bijur, Chadwick, and Rutter, 1980). However, it has been only with very recent research that the relationship of altered cognitive processes after TBI to specific academic learning difficulties has been examined, though this has been better known clinically. Levin and Benton (in press) have suggested that difficulty after TBI in controlled processes of learning involving attention, memory, and speed of information processing interferes more significantly in mathematical calculation than in reading decoding and can coexist with "normal" IQ.

In planning appropriate cognitive/learning-based interventions for children after TBI, a careful appraisal of individual strengths and weaknesses conducted in a serial manner is essential, as there is no "characteristic" pattern at any one point in time after injury. Assessment needs to be completed as soon as appropriate (after resolution of posttraumatic amnesia) for an accurate measure of the immediate effects of injury on cognitive/learning areas, as well as to provide a baseline measure to evaluate rate and degree of recovery over time. For children who are severely injured and involved in formal rehabilitation programs, evaluation will likely be completed prior to discharge. However, because of the scarcity of professionals in clinical neuropsychology, clinical psychology, and educational specialties who have experience with TBI in infants and children, evaluations either may not be completed or data may be misunderstood. This situation becomes more critical for children who are treated in acute care hospitals, where the cognitive sequelae after TBI may not be fully appreciated.

Assessment of cognitive/learning processes after TBI in children is complex and dependent on current measurement tools, many of which are not well standardized for children and may not fully assess the range of processes that could be affected. For example, there are very few measures of memory processes in children and none of them is conceived in a developmental framework or normed adequately across the pediatric age range. Educational assessment techniques may adequately evaluate academic skills but may not evaluate the underlying cognitive processes and deficits.

Cognitive/learning intervention with children after TBI is basically an area of applied clinical expertise, with little or no formal research efforts. Although a major emphasis of adult programs has been on cognitive retraining or neuropsychological rehabilitation, adaptation of these procedures and techniques to children has only just begun and their effectiveness has rarely been studied (Light, Neuman, Lewis, Morecki-Oberg, Asarnow, and Satz, 1987). It is also unknown if the accepted educational methods and techniques utilized with children who have other cognitive or learning disorders can be applied to children after TBI. Methods and techniques developed for use with children who have learning disabilities, language disabilities, and/or attentional deficits may be appropriate, as may be procedures to foster higher level cognitive processes in normal children. However, little research has been done in this area and the basic questions remain: Is it more effective to work on a child's areas of strength or deficit? Is it better to train a child to perform a specific task or to teach him or her a general mental strategy? Are traditional teaching methods or computers more effective approaches for teaching children after TBI? (Light, et al., 1987)

Educational Programming

Because of the mandated educational programming for all handicapped children (P.L. 94-142) and the extensive range of available special education services from very severe/profound to mainstream programs, it is unlikely that a child after TBI will be homebound and totally without services for extended periods of time, as some adults might be after injury.

Since functional levels of children after TBI vary greatly, the entire range of educational services available through the public and private educational systems could be appropriate for any child (Cohen, 1986). One of the primary issues, though, involves the conflict between providing programs designed specifically for special needs unique to TBI and the continuing need for contact with normal or developmentally similar children. Although aspects of programming for children with other educationally relevant diagnoses, such as learning disabilities, behavior disorders, mental retardation, and/or emotional disturbances, may be appropriate for some children after TBI, there is a question about whether these services are able to meet their specialized needs (Ylvisaker, 1985). It is not at all clear how best to make educational programming decisions for children after TBI. However, it is well known from clinical experience that programs must be more flexible and altered more frequently than is commonly done or mandated by law (Telzrow, 1985). Guidelines and research in this area are all but nonexistent and yet are essential both in facilitating the child's continued performance in school and in aiding school personnel in appropriate planning. One exception to this is the excellent set of guidelines developed in Missouri (Kelley and Haley, 1986) to aid school personnel in the education, classification, staffing, individual educational plan formulation, and educational management of children after TBI.

Organization and provision of school-based services can be difficult to implement for children after TBI for several reasons. The first is that they do not fall neatly within any of the established educational diagnostic groupings. It is sometimes not even recognized that they are children with special needs, because for those with milder injuries, previously mastered academic skills may be quite well preserved, even though the immediate capacity for new learning may be significantly reduced or altered, only temporarily, it is hoped. Children who have sustained more severe injuries may need a variety of services that are available but cut across several program divisions. Severely injured children may be multiply handicapped children par excellence. For example, they may require physical therapy, occupational therapy, behavior management, speech/language therapy, hearing and/or visually impaired services, academic remediation, counseling, and learning disability services, among others. However, the combination of needed services may not be available in the same school program or building, forcing a choice as to which services a child will receive and which ones he or she will not.

The second reason is that children after TBI often change rapidly as the process of recovery is compounded by the pace of normal development. School programming that is appropriate for immediate return after injury may no longer be so, even after a period of only weeks or months. Flexibility in provision for rapidly changing needs, though, is often difficult to deliver on a system-wide basis. Several innovative programs have attempted to deal with this need for flexibility through the utilization of transitional school programs within the public school system (e.g., The Upton School Transitional Head Injury Program, Baltimore City Public Schools), through private special school programs usually connected to a hospital experienced in the management of pediatric TBI (e.g., Kennedy Memorial Hospital for Children, Brighton, Massachusetts, and the Rehabilitation Institute of Pittsburgh), or in after-school programs (e.g., The Neuro-Cognitive Education Project through Casa Colina Hospital and UCLA Neuropsychiatric Institute).

The third reason is the lack of awareness of school-based personnel of the needs of children after TBI. Very few educators, from classroom teachers to special education administrators, are aware of the educational management issues specific to TBI in children. Acquired neurological deficits are rarely if ever mentioned in educational textbooks or in teacher training coursework (Savage, 1987). However, with the high incidence of TBI, especially mild injuries, school personnel are very likely to have children postinjury in their classrooms and special education programs.

At this time, there are minimal to no guidelines to aid in the educational programming of children after TBI. It is important for children after injury to be clearly identified as having sustained an acquired neurological injury, rather than having to be classified according to existing groupings that may not be appropriate separately or in aggregate. After they are appropriately identified as children who have sustained TBI, then specific educational programming and services can be tailored to their immediate, ongoing, and often changing needs. Only after children are appropriately identified can educational program evaluation be attempted. Then the major issues of whether and how educational programming and services can foster recovery/improvement and help to avoid or ameliorate long-term or late-appearing deficits will be able to be addressed in a systematic and scientific manner. Research in school settings will be crucial in addressing issues of the effect and management of TBI in childhood on acquisition of learning, specifically in academic but also in cognitive and psychosocial/behavioral areas.

MEDICAL/THERAPEUTIC SYSTEM

After TBI, children may require continuing medical services in the community specifically related to injury effects and to general pediatric care. However, primary care medical personnel may not be aware of the possible sequelae and deficits, even for children who appear well recovered, that can occur immediately after TBI or following an extended period of time. Specialized services, such as physical, occupational, and speech/language therapy, as well as expertise in the management of complex physical and sensory disabilities may need to be provided in medical or rehabilitation settings. Specific expertise in the management of children after traumatic injuries may only be obtainable in medically or therapeutically oriented settings and may not be available in educational settings. The background of the therapists, both in terms of children and treatment of TBI, needs to be of primary importance.

Because of concerns in these areas, a wide range of community-based therapy services for adults, often specifically designed for individuals after TBI, has emerged within the last several years. However, these services are considerably less commonly available for children. The school system is often relied on to provide for both the educational and the therapeutic needs of children after TBI. Recently, because of their expertise in TBI concerns and management, but not necessarily because of their expertise with children, adult community-based programs are being asked to serve younger and younger children.

Adult community-based post-TBI programs focus specifically on cognitive/behavioral/social/emotional interventions, with the goal of increasing independent functioning and vocational success. The goals of community-based therapeutic programs for children after TBI would be similar, with the exception of an immediate focus on academic rather than vocational performance.

Since school programs are potentially available for most children after TBI, what would be the purpose of specific child TBI therapeutic programs? Initially after injury, many severely injured children are not capable of returning successfully to an educational setting. Their cognitive and behavioral deficits, even if sometimes transient in severity, interfere markedly with school performance in many areas. Memory, attention/concentration, reduced information processing speed and efficiency, as well as deficits in higher level reasoning and judgment all adversely affect learning in educational settings and yet are rarely the focus of direct educational interventions at a classroom level (Cohen, 1986). However, the application of learning and behavioral abilities to the mastery of academic skills in reading, mathematics, spelling, writing, and other subjects is also essential. The classroom environment itself may be a deterrent to a child's learning after TBI. The normal or even the special education class may be too large, too distracting, with lessons paced too quickly and lasting too long, with transitions occurring too frequently and rapidly.

As with adults, there are likely to be a variety of models to provide adequate therapeutic services to children after TBI. However, the models that have been developed and have been successful with adults after TBI will need to be significantly altered for utilization with children. An essential component of programs for children is the integration of therapy with educational interventions and systems.

There are also problems in devising therapeutic programs for children after TBI that are not encountered with the adult population. Since children primarily live with their families, geographic considerations limit most programs to those that can be easily reached in a manageable drive or bus ride. However, not all children after TBI can be treated in the same program. Unlike adult programs, which can provide similar services to a wide age range, varying from older adolescents to adults, programs for infants and toddlers cannot be managed in the same way as those for preschool-aged or school-aged children. And yet, there may not be sufficient numbers of children within the same age range or developmental level, functioning at approximately similar injury and disability severity levels, who live close enough together to provide adequate groupings for programs. In addition, providing services for children in strictly a TBI setting may unduly restrict their contact with noninjured peers. Taking these considerations into account, the following models for community-based therapeutic services and programs are proposed.

Proposed Models

The following models proposed for delivery of therapeutic services attempt to address the primary issues of providing services to children after TBI in a variety of formats and settings, depending on specific needs. It is important that they provide for an integration of a child's therapeutic and educational needs; for transitions between programs, without neglecting cognitive, behavioral, social, and emotional concerns; for family teaching and support; and for specialized evaluation services related to TBI effects in infancy and childhood.

Consultation service to schools. For those children who are able to return to or continue in their school programs, consultation from a team of professionals who are experienced in working with children after TBI is essential, not only for the evaluation, planning, and management of the children's needs but also for the education and support of school personnel. No one school system or even special education collaborative is likely to fully understand the range of TBI effects in children or the integration of necessary services. This is unlikely to be a one-time consultation, because a major contribution of the consultation team would be to advise the school system and teachers about alterations in programming and teaching approaches as a child recovers or improves over time. In addition, the frequent reevaluations of the child's functional level and the flexibility of program planning needed would likely be more easily provided by one identified team, rather than at the school system level.

Regional consultation teams would most likely be the most efficient in providing services to the majority of children after TBI, including those with mild to moderate injuries, those experiencing good recoveries from severe injuries, as well as those with multiple disabilities subsequent to injury. Because the team could come to the child, rather than the child traveling to the program, geographic considerations could at least be minimized if not eliminated. Another advantage of the consultation team approach is that children could receive services as close to home as possible, usually through their local school system, and yet have access to TBI professionals and expertise. If consultation services are provided through a regional comprehensive pediatric TBI program, additional therapeutic needs of both the child and his or her family could also be provided for and yet remain integrated with educational programming.

Part-time day program/part-time school program. If community-based therapeutic services are readily available, it may be possible to combine therapy and educational services for individual children, even though each program would be physically in a separate facility. For this model to be effective, a case-coordinator would need to maintain close communication and control over the child's programming in the two facilities. However, it has the advantage of being able to provide intensive therapeutic services specific to TBI needs as well as placement in a least restrictive educational setting. This model has been used successfully in helping adults after TBI return to a productive work setting, as well as with children who have significant learning disabilities.

Outpatient therapy services. Not only are specialized therapy programs needed for children after TBI but ongoing therapy services may be appropriate over an extended period of time. Even though educational needs may be able to be met within the school system, specific therapy services may need to be delivered by professionals who are experienced with the specialized needs of children after TBI. These may include physical, occupational, speech/language therapy services, as well as therapy designed to meet the cognitive, social, behavioral, and emotional needs specific to children after TBI. These services often will need to be provided in addition to a child's educational program and will closely involve the child's family.

Transitional day programs/residential programs. For those children with immediate and/or long-term significant impairments after TBI, comprehensive programs either as a transition or on an extended basis will likely be the most appropriate settings for managing both their therapeutic and educational needs. At the present time, very few of these programs are in existence. Those that do exist have often developed out of adult community-based TBI programs or pediatric rehabilitation programs. Research with adults has documented that early intervention facilitates recovery and lack of appropriate intervention may jeopardize the rate and degree of recovery (Cope and Hall, 1982). Not only does this need to be demonstrated for children after TBI but also those who would benefit from this more intensive and therefore more expensive approach will need to be clearly identified. This concern is especially critical in considering children for residential placement, which usually entails a major separation from their families and communities as well as significant funding implications. However, for a very small group of children after TBI, residential placement may present the only real possibility for amelioration of severe behavioral and emotional disorders subsequent to or complicated by TBI.

Even though each of these models probably has merit for meeting some of the therapeutic and educational needs of individual children after TBI, the delineation of which specific model would be most appropriate for which children, at which age, severity level, point in time postinjury, and with which combination of deficits needs to be the focus of programmatic research.

EMOTIONAL/BEHAVIORAL SYSTEM

Whereas cognitive effects of head injury in children are often directly related to injury severity, there is a less direct relationship of severity to behavioral and psychosocial/emotional sequelae (Rutter, Chadwick, and Shaffer, 1983). Because of the developmental characteristics that make it difficult to separate behavioral from psychosocial/emotional effects of TBI in children, these will be considered together.

Current State of the Research

The expression of what have often been called psychological or personality sequelae in adults after TBI appears to take on a behavioral character, especially in young children (Black, Blumer, Wellner, Jeffries, and Walker, 1970). Although a wide range of behaviors can occur in young children after TBI, including hypoactive apathetic behavior, one of the common patterns is an increase in frequency of temper tantrums and impulsive, aggressive, destructive behavior (Brink, Garrett, Hale, Woo-Sam, Nickel, 1970). This may not necessarily be uniquely different from preinjury behavior but may be an exacerbation of preinjury characteristics (Long, Gouvier, and Cole, 1984). For example, an active child may become markedly hyperactive after injury. The primary behavioral/psychosocial characteristic that can be directly attributed to TBI in older children is that of marked social disinhibition, which has been compared to the frontal lobe syndrome in adults (Rutter, Chadwick, and Shaffer, 1983). Otherwise, behavioral/psychosocial/emotional characteristics in children after TBI have been described as similar in nature to the problems of children in the general population who have not sustained injuries.

However, not only have behavioral/psychosocial/emotional sequelae been found to be more slowly resolving than cognitive sequelae but they also appear to increase rather than decrease with time after injury. From the work of Rutter and his associates (Brown, Chadwick, Shaffer, Rutter, and Traub, 1981; Rutter, Chadwick, and Shaffer, 1983), the incidence of new psychiatric disorders in children after severe TBI was continuing to increase $2\frac{1}{4}$ years after injury when the research follow-up was discontinued. This was true not only for children who had had difficulties prior to injury but also for those children with no preinjury behavioral or psychological difficulties. The likelihood and extensiveness of psychosocial/emotional sequelae in children after TBI appears to be related to severity of injury, presence of seizures, psychosocial adversity, and to preinjury behavioral and psychological characteristics (Rutter, Chadwick, and Shaffer, 1983). Looked at from the opposite vantage point, children who presented with behavioral problems in school were found to have had a greater likelihood of having had a past head injury (Craft, Shaw, and Cartlidge, 1972; Savage, 1985). Because of the prolonged nature of behavior/psychosocial/emotional sequelae of TBI in children, their impact is especially significant for functioning in home, school, and community settings over an extended period of time.

Compared to the work on cognitive effects of TBI in children, the information on behavioral/psychosocial/emotional effects is meager. This is especially striking considering the well-documented research in adults that psychological sequelae are often as or more impairing in terms of overall functioning than are cognitive sequelae (Lezak, 1978, 1987; Prigatano, 1987). Whether this is so for children is basically not known. It is also not clear what the expected behavioral/psychosocial/emotional sequelae of different levels of injury severity might be, of different injuries, at different ages, and at different periods postinjury. However, it is highly unlikely that the psychological sequelae of injury will be the same across the developmental periods of infancy through childhood or that they will be the same for children injured very early in life as compared to those injured after they are able to be aware and react to changes in their own functioning. In other words, very little is known about the psychological natural history of TBI in childhood, that is, how it affects and potentially interferes with psychological development throughout these critical years. One of the significant limitations on research in this area with children, as compared to the work with adults, is the absence of well-established baseline personality functioning prior to injury for comparison purposes.

Even though little is known about the behavioral/psychosocial/emotional sequelae and reaction to TBI in children, it is probable that it is a process that is affected by the age and developmental level of the child; that it alters and evolves over time both as a component of expected developmental changes and subsequent to the recovery/improvement changes after TBI; and that it is likely to be affected by the specific nature of the injury itself, posttraumatic epilepsy, as well as the preinjury personality of the child (Alexander, 1986; Kleinpeter, 1976; Rutter, 1981).

Several differences have been observed between the behavioral/psychosocial/emotional characteristics of adults and children after TBI. On a clinical level, it is interesting that many parents do not perceive their children as having experienced major alteration in personality or characterological aspects of functioning after TBI, even after severe injuries. Instead parents often describe their children as "like themselves" but in an exaggerated fashion or acting similarly to the way they behaved at an earlier developmental stage. Whether this is related to differences in parents' as opposed to spouses' perceptions, or reflects differences between children and adults, or both, is not known. However, from the work on temperament in children (Chess and Thomas, 1984), there seem to be both continuities and discontinuities in basic characteristics of personality and psychopathology during childhood. The descriptions of altered adult behavior after TBI often focus on childlike, dependent behavior, with reductions in self-control, independence, and concern for others. While these may significantly interfere with adult functioning, none of these would necessarily be inappropriate or unexpected, especially for infants and young children.

Children are also described as not experiencing the postconcussion syndrome, posttraumatic syndrome, or traumatic neurosis after TBI, as has been described with adults (Jennett, 1972). This may be an inaccurate perception, related to the developmental aspects of awareness of injury and disability effects. Even children as young as 4 or 5 years of age have been able to comprehend and react to overt changes in their functioning after injury. However, their expression of this reaction is likely to be quite different than in adults and to have a markedly behavioral character rather than a somatic or an internalized psychological one (Black, Blumer, Wellner, Jeffries, and Walker, 1970). In other words, young children are more likely to whine, cry, get angry, frustrated, fearful, sad, or withdrawn rather than to express specific complaints of headaches, memory loss, depression, and interference with their present and future functioning. By the time children are 8 to 12 years of age, though, some of the adult characteristics are likely to be present.

In research with adults, there appears to be a group of individuals who are at greater risk for accidents and injury. This seems to be related to specific behavioral characteristics including poorly focused or poorly sustained attention, impulsivity or lack of sustained control in motor action, emotional lability, higher levels of activity, risk-taking, competitiveness, aggression, and excessive tension (Bijur, Stewart-Brown, and Butler, 1986; Hakkinen, 1958; Matheny and Fisher, 1984). However, the results of research with children have been conflictual. Klonoff (Klonoff, 1971) found that an increased incidence of pediatric TBI was associated with environmental factors such as congested residential areas, lower income housing, marital instability, and lower occupational status of the father. But developmental factors, such as hyperactivity, mental deficiency, brain damage, and emotional disturbance were not associated with increased incidence of pediatric TBI. In contrast, Rutter and his associates (Rutter, Chadwick, and Shaffer, 1983) found behavioral differences between those children who sustained mild injuries in comparison with those sustaining severe injuries. Behavior characteristics were implicated directly with injury occurrence in the mild group but not in the severely injured group. Those with mild injuries were described as "less intelligent, behaviorally deviant children" who were more likely to be engaging in prohibited activities at the time of injury (Rutter, 1980). In a prospective study of accidents in the first 5 years of life, both environmental/family characteristics as well as behavioral characteristics of the children were implicated for accident repeaters (Golding, 1986). It is also not clear if children after TBI are more susceptible to further injury, although there are indications that their risk is somewhat increased. In one of the most comprehensive studies of incidence of TBI in childhood, the increased risk for subsequent injury was two times that of children who had not been injured and was equal for both boys and girls (Annegers, Grabow, Kurland, and Laws, 1980).

Research in this area is clearly critical, not only for understanding the role that behavior plays both before and after TBI but also in guiding prevention efforts. Specific research questions should focus on the following questions: Are there children who are at higher risk for TBI and, if so, who are they and why are they at higher risk? How do environmental and child behavior factors interact to increase the risk of TBI? What is the relationship of normal child development to occurrence of TBI, especially in "normally" high-risk periods such as the toddler years when physical abilities far exceed judgment? Are there parents and families who are at higher risk for having children with TBI? What intervention approaches might be successful in lowering the injury risk for these children and their family members?

Simply because the adult expression of behavioral/psychosocial/emotional sequelae and effects of TBI may not be present in children in the same way or with the same intensity does not mean that these sequelae are not present or are less important. It is probable that there are indeed significant changes in behavior/psychosocial/emotional functioning and development after injury in children. However, research in this area is unlikely to be able to rely on adult models and findings, even less so than in cognitive areas. Rather it will need to focus heavily on the processes of normal child development and child psychopathology.

In addition to the need for research on the basic nature of behavioral/psychosocial/emotional sequelae and reaction to TBI in children of different developmental levels, injury severity, injury location, and chronicity, there is also a need for research on intervention approaches with both the children and their families. Although there may be many resources for services in this area, including community mental health centers, child psychiatric programs, child development centers, and family service centers, etc., none of these resources is likely to have specific expertise in dealing with children and families after TBI. Many times, they are unlikely to even be aware that a child has had a traumatic brain injury that may be related to his or her behavioral/psychosocial/emotional difficulties. In addition, it is possible that the most effective intervention approach may be one of anticipatory guidance, that is, providing counseling/intervention services immediately after injury and prior to the appearance of difficulties. For this to occur, though, intervention services would need to be available, either directly or on referral, through the facility that manages the child after TBI, rather than waiting for difficulties to emerge. Even more so than with adults, the focus of intervention will need to be on the family, not only on the child. Services may include parent and sibling support, behavioral management, parent training, crisis therapy, and family therapy, as well as therapy specifically focused on the child utilizing play, behavioral, and/or interpretive therapy approaches. However, research on the effectiveness and timing of services will need to be a priority.

FAMILY SYSTEM

Research with adults has demonstrated that the behavioral and emotional changes after TBI are most stressful for families (Brooks, 1984; Oddy, Humphrey, and Uttley, 1978; Lezak, 1978). Whether this is similar for children is open to question and likely to be related to the age of the child at the time of injury. Very little research has been done in this area. Even for young adults, the behavioral/emotional stresses appear to be greater for spouses of individuals after TBI than for their parents (Panting and Merry, 1972; Thomsen 1974). Although this may be related to having two parents to share the burden of care, rather than one spouse, it may also be related to role changes. It may be easier for parents to adjust to the increased dependency and "immature" behavior of even their adult children, than it is for spouses (Rosenbaum and Nanjenson, 1976). The expectations of the head-injured person are likely to be quite different. For a spouse after TBI, vocational, child rearing, financial, and marital responsibilities are considerably more demanding than for an adult living with his or her parents. If this is so for adults, it is likely to be increasingly true for children, especially infants, toddlers, and preschool-aged children. From clinical experience, very few parents of young children after TBI report "personality changes." Instead, they appear to relate the child's behavior to what he or she was like at an earlier age.

It is especially critical if at all possible for children after TBI to be home with their families as soon after injury as is feasible. However, it can be difficult for families to care for children after injury until they are fully oriented and out of the confusional period. Since children often recover physically much better and more quickly than adults, they may be discharged from acute care and rehabilitation hospitals much sooner. Because of this there is a critical need to anticipate the family stresses after hospital discharge and to adequately prepare families for them. If children are treated only in acute care settings, rather than rehabilitation settings, this may not occur. Families, then, may have little preparation for possible difficulties, even if they are temporary after milder injuries or especially if they are delayed in onset.

Family issues after TBI in childhood are primarily known through clinical experience, as there is little to no formal research in the area. For the child after TBI, his or her role in the family may be jeopardized and altered as younger siblings may be more competent in comparison, even if only temporarily. Parenting of a child after TBI may be more stressful both subsequent to parents' reaction to injury occurrence and to the possible changes in the child. Parents may become reluctant to discipline, have difficulty with protecting and overprotecting their children, as well as in fostering their recovery and future development. While parents are expected to care for their children after TBI, they themselves are usually in emotional turmoil and stress, often related to the circumstances of the injury and hospitalization. Often the family is directly involved in the injury, by being in the same accident, through feeling responsible for the injury, or in extreme cases having directly caused the injury as in child abuse. For most families, the goal of family teaching and intervention is to maintain or reconstitute the family as an entity that can foster the development of all of its members, despite the stress and changes that TBI imposes on it.

SOCIAL SYSTEM

Even though the study of social perception and social cognition in children with other disorders has received increasing emphasis in recent years (Porter and Rourke, 1985; Selman, Lavin, Brion-Meisels, 1982) along with the development of specific intervention in the area of social skills training (Cartledge and Milburn, 1980; Oden and Asher, 1977; LaGreca and Santogrossi, 1980; Spivak and Shure, 1974), little or none of this research or clinical expertise has been applied to children after TBI. Yet, children after TBI are likely to be especially prone to disorders in social functioning (Oddy, 1984). This can be related not only to social isolation subsequent to the sequelae of moderate to severe injuries but also related to specific cognitive deficits after TBI. Impairments in judgment and higher level reasoning interfere not only with cognitive performance but also with social functioning. Children after TBI may not accurately perceive social cues, process complex social interaction, or be able to engage in social role-taking at the same level they were able to prior to injury.

The implications for research are clear. First, the role of TBI in social dysfunction and social learning needs to be clarified, especially in terms of the cognitive/social interface and the social/emotional interface. Then, specific intervention strategies and techniques need to be developed, applied, and evaluated to attempt to reduce social isolation, to foster catching up in social areas related to lost developmental time, and to teach specific social skills that will lead to independent social functioning as adolescents and adults.

Extreme socially unsanctioned behavior is less of a concern for children than it is for adolescents and adults after TBI. However, severe hyperactive, aggressive, and disinhibited behavior may occur in a small group of children after TBI. Substance use and abuse may become an issue in older children but rarely reaches the extent that it can in later years. However, sexual vulnerability can be a major issue for even relatively young children of both sexes after significant TBI and is an issue that has received very little attention.

COMMUNITY SKILLS/ADAPTIVE BEHAVIOR/ RECREATIONAL AND LEISURE NEEDS

Although the community-based programs that are designed for treatment of adults after TBI are vitally interested in fostering adaptive behavior and community skills to maintain or increase the independent functioning of their clients (Ben-Yishay, 1981), this has rarely been a focus of intervention with children after TBI. The effect of TBI in children on adaptive behavior, which has direct relevance in their daily life, is basically unknown. However, difficulties that significantly depart from age-appropriate levels in basic skills, such as being able to cross the street safely, making small purchases from the store, making telephone calls, etc., may greatly impinge on children's quality of life and independent functioning. For severely injured children, it is possible that adaptive behavior deficits, both in terms of regaining or maintaining their preinjury functioning level and of being able to learn new skills, could be more severe than their physical or cognitive impairments. However, in children, the immediate difference between their preinjury and postinjury levels of adaptive behavior is likely to be less striking, though not less important, than in adults. Instead, what may be most compromised is their ability to continue to learn and apply skills in this area.

Because of the possibility of compromised social and adaptive behavior skills, access to structured leisure activities is often crucial for children after TBI. They are often not able to occupy themselves profitably and can be a safety risk in unsupervised settings. This is a particular concern for preschool- and school-aged children after moderate to severe injuries, who may have quite restricted opportunities for social contact with other children, both injured and noninjured peers. However, for those children with social and adaptive skill deficits after TBI, providing for their recreational and leisure-time needs can pose significant difficulties. They can be disruptive in group settings and confusing for community recreational personnel to deal with. Their recreational needs also vary widely. Some children after TBI may be appropriate for programs designed for children with severe impairments and others for programs designed for normal children. And yet, none of these programs may be able to meet the complexity of needs of children after TBI. In order to meet these needs, several parent support groups have worked directly with their community recreation personnel to develop programs for children after TBI or have developed social programs, such as summer camps, themselves. In many geographic areas, though, there may be very limited opportunities for children to socialize in groups such as Boy Scouts and Girl Scouts, day and overnight camps, play groups, organized sports teams, or in leisure activities, such as swimming programs.

Since so little work has been done in evaluating the effectiveness of programs that focus on community and adaptive behavior skills, it is not known if intervention in these areas may in fact have a surprisingly powerful effect on children's functioning after TBI and on their family's adjustment, as well as simply occupying their time in a safe manner.

LIVING SYSTEM

Most children after TBI live at home with their families, even those children who are severely disabled and those who are in a persistent vegetative state. There can be many reasons for this, including the fact that young children are physically easier to care for than disabled adults and that parents may have difficulty comprehending the enormity of the task that they are attempting in caring for a severely disabled or comatose child. However, one of the primary reasons is that, in most parts of the country, there are very limited pediatric nursing home and pediatric chronic care facilities, much less facilities that are designed for the management of severely disabled children after TBI. Even when facilities are available, the funding for them may be nonexistent. Unfortunately, support services, such as respite care, homemakers, and home health services, are also extremely limited for children and their families.

Although the transitional living facility model that has been utilized with adults after TBI is rarely appropriate for children, those who are left with severe behavioral and emotional sequelae would often benefit from residential treatment programs. However, there are only a few programs scattered across the country that are able to manage, much less treat, this small but extremely difficult group of children. The geographic problems, much less the financial difficulties of funding the programs, though, are often prohibitive.

LEGAL SYSTEM

The issue of the individual rights of children after TBI is a crucial one. Although the right to acute care medical treatment is rarely a concern, the provision and funding for community-based services is usually significantly less available for children after TBI than for adults. Insurance companies may assert that the therapy services covered for an adult after injury are an "educational" expense for children after TBI. In contrast, educational systems may argue that at least some of the services a child needs after TBI are not educationally relevant.

Although children after TBI may be involved in litigation and/or receive settlements subsequent to their injuries, it can be more difficult to assess the long-term implications of their injuries and to ascertain appropriate compensation than for adults after TBI. Aspects of TBI in childhood, such as restrictions on potential abilities and possible delayed effects, complicate evaluation of deficits. Guardianship issues are less common for children after TBI but can be particularly complicated if their immediate families have been killed in the accident, if their families are implicated in their injuries as in child abuse, or if their families are accused of mishandling the children's financial assets.

Fewer children than adolescents or adults after TBI are likely to have contact with the justice system. However, if they do, either because of the result of their own behavior or as victims of other people's behavior, the justice system is rarely aware of the role TBI has played in the offense. Increased frequency of asocial or criminal behavior has been observed as a long-term effect of childhood TBI (Kleinpeter, 1976). Also the question of risk after TBI in childhood for later extremely violent behavior has been indicated in recent research on death row inmates (Lewis, Pincus, Feldman, Jackson, and Bard, 1986). The findings of this preliminary research have implicated the combination of neurological insult and violent environments on occurrence of severely violent behavior in adults. These findings pose significant implications for prevention, both on an individual and a societal level.

SUMMARY OF RESEARCH PRIORITIES

In general, research on the long-term effects of TBI acquired in infancy and childhood on subsequent functioning in the community needs to be conducted (a) from a developmental perspective; (b) in a longitudinal manner; (c) focusing primarily on cognitive, academic, psychosocial, emotional, behavioral, and adaptive aspects; (d) conceptualizing recovery/improvement as a process that interacts with the developmental process; (e) taking into account the multiple people and systems that are integral to a child's functioning in the community after injury (i.e., family, friends, school, therapists, etc.); (f) clearly delineating specific subgroups of children after injury at a minimum by age at injury, severity and type of injury, and acuteness of injury; and (g) carefully evaluating the effectiveness of intervention approaches, techniques, and programs for these specific subgroups of children, including the need for specialized services tailored to TBI effects, as well as appropriate utilization of existing services.

When considered in comparison with the large body of research on the effects of TBI in adults, very little is known about TBI effects in infancy and childhood. General areas of specific research need include (a) effects of TBI when sustained at different developmental periods during infancy and childhood, studied according to neurological, neuroanatomical, and neurodevelopmental changes and according to the relationship of age at injury, to speed of recovery, patterns of deficits, delayed effects, and long-term impairments; (b) specific focus on the effects of injury in infants, toddlers, and preschool-aged children because of the dearth of knowledge in this area (What are the short- and long-term effects of injury early in life? Are there specific or generalized deficits? What is the nature of delayed effects? Can they be predicted and ameliorated?); (c) effects of "nonaccidental" trauma (Are they different from the effects of accidental trauma? How should these infants and children be evaluated to assess for possible TBI?); (d) focus on the effects of mild and moderate injuries in childhood (Even though these are the most common injuries, the least is known about their effects on subsequent functioning and development in children); and (e) focus on the varying effects of severe and very severe injuries in childhood with consideration of mortality from TBI, medical/physical components, learning and behavioral/social/emotional aspects.

There are also many specific research questions that need to be addressed in order to more fully understand the effects of TBI in infants and children as well as to begin to be able to intervene more effectively to ameliorate these effects on their current and future functioning. These specific research priorities are outlined in the following sections, divided according to the functional systems approach that has been utilized in organizing this chapter. Although an attempt has been made to be as comprehensive as possible, this listing should not be considered to be exhaustive, but as an initial effort to guide research in this area.

Cognitive/Learning Research Priorities

These include the following:

1. Research is needed on the effects of TBI on cognitive processes and learning ability in children, with a focus on memory, attention, concentration, and reasoning. Is the way children learn altered after TBI? How can learning be fostered after TBI?

2. Does the course of cognitive recovery/improvement vary? Are there two groups of children, one that recovers well and rapidly and one that improves more slowly with prolonged deficits? If so, how can this be

predicted early so that appropriate intervention can be planned and implemented?

3. Do those children who are identified and evaluated and who receive intervention early do better than those who receive services only after difficulties arise?

4. There is a need to develop evaluation measures in the area of memory that are appropriate for children at different developmental stages, that assess many areas of memory functioning, and that are standardized on normal children.

5. Are traditional cognitive intervention approaches effective with children after TBI? What specific approaches need to be developed, including computer-based approaches? When is it more effective to work on a child's area of strength or deficit? When is it more effective to train a specific task or to teach a general strategy?

6. What is the interaction of cognitive abilities and academic learning after TBI in children?

Educational Programming Priorities

The following questions need to be studied:

1. How can the transition back to school after TBI be most effectively facilitated, both in terms of the child's needs and educational personnel's needs?

2. Which children require educational programs specifically designed for children after TBI? When are these programs most effective?

3. How can the appropriateness of educational programming for children after TBI be determined? Do children who are managed closely and flexibly perform better in school settings than those who return with little or no services?

4. How can educational personnel be most effectively taught to manage the educational needs of children after TBI?

Medical/Therapeutic System Priorities

1. How can the therapeutic and educational needs of children after TBI be best provided for and integrated?

2. There is a need for evaluation of the proposed models of integrated therapeutic/educational management for children after TBI (i.e., regional consultation team model, part-time school and part-time TBI therapeutic program model, out-patient therapy model, transitional day program model, and residential treatment center model). Which models are effective for which children, at what age, severity level, point in

time after injury, and how can transitions between programs be managed?

3. What is the effect on the children's recovery, improvement, and development if their management is integrated by one person (case manager) or team, instead of planned piecemeal by each agency or facility involved in their care?

Emotional/Behavioral System Priorities

1. The behavioral/psychosocial/emotional effects of TBI in children over an extended period postinjury need to be analyzed. Do they increase over time? If so, for how long a period? Are the characteristics of these effects related to age, severity of injury, type of injury? Are there delayed effects in those children sustaining injuries at very early ages? Are the effects in children with preinjury difficulties in these areas different from those in children with no preinjury difficulties?

2. The long-term impact of behavior/psychosocial/emotional effects in children needs to be studied.

3. How children understand, react to and cope with the psychosocial/emotional effects of TBI at different ages and the presence and characteristics of posttraumatic syndrome and traumatic neuroses in children needs to be analyzed.

4. Are there children who are at high risk for TBI? If so, how can they be identified? What is the interaction of child, family, and environmental variables in the occurrence of TBI in children?

5. How behavioral/psychosocial/emotional effects of TBI in children can be avoided, reduced, or ameliorated needs to be evaluated. Are anticipatory approaches prior to onset of difficulties effective in reducing difficulties in these areas? Which therapeutic intervention approaches are most effective in treating these difficulties subsequent to TBI?

6. Approaches to train community mental health personnel and other child-related professionals in working more effectively with children after TBI need to be studied.

Family System Priorities

1. The effects on the family, including parents and siblings, of having a child with TBI and how to reduce family stress and encourage family coping need to be studied.

2. The perceptions of parents of their children postinjury and how these perceptions affect the child's functioning, child rearing behaviors, and parent/child interaction need to be analyzed.

3. The effect of preparation for possible TBI effects and the process of

TBI recovery/improvement in children on parents' ability to care for and manage their children after injury and the effect of early family teaching and intervention on reduction of child and family difficulties postinjury need to be studied.

4. Are there families who are at higher risk for having children with TBI? If so, which prevention/intervention approaches might be successful in reducing the risk for injuries in these children and their families?

Social System Priorities

1. The relationship of cognitive and social effects of TBI in children, focusing on such areas as social perception and social cognition after TBI, needs to be analyzed.

2. The effect of TBI in childhood on social functioning and social development over a long-term period needs to be studied. What is the effect of TBI on social skills that have not yet been acquired? What is the effect of disruption of previously mastered social skills?

3. The effectiveness of specific intervention approaches to reduce social isolation, to foster catch-up in social areas related to lost developmental time, and to teach specific social skills that will lead to independent social functioning and reduce social vulnerability needs to be studied.

4. In-depth study of those children after TBI who develop severe socially unsanctioned behavior and analysis of TBI factors and preinjury factors in these children are needed.

Community Skills/Adaptive Behavior/Recreational Priorities

1. The effects of TBI in childhood on the acquisition and implementation of adaptive behavior and community skills and the development of intervention programs for those children with significant deficits in adaptive behavior areas need to be studied.

2. How to best provide for the recreational/leisure needs of children after TBI requires study.

Living System Priorities

1. Which children are best managed in residential facilities and the effectiveness of these programs for intervention of severe, multiple deficits subsequent to TBI needs to be evaluated.

2. The effectiveness of respite care programs for families with children who have severe impairments after TBI, both in terms of family factors and cost-effectiveness, needs study.

Legal/Justice System Priorities

1. How to provide for appropriate identification and management of children after TBI who become involved in the legal system and whether this approach more effectively deals with their severe difficulties needs study.

2. Approaches to alert legal and justice system personnel to the needs of children after TBI who come within their jurisdiction need to be developed.

REFERENCES

Alajouanine T, Lhermitte F (1965): Acquired aphasia in children. *Brain* 88:653–662.

Alexander M (1986): Pediatric head injury. Presentation at the Braintree Head Injury Conference, Braintree, MA.

Annegers JF (1983): The epidemiology of head trauma in children. In: K. Shapiro (ed.), *Pediatric head trauma*. Mt. Kisco, NY: Futura Publishing Co.

Annegers JF, Grabow JD, Kurland LT, Laws ER (1980): The incidence, causes, and secular trends of head trauma in Olmsted County, Minnesota, 1935–1974. *Neurology* 30:912–919.

Bawden HN, Knights RM, Winogron, HW (1985): Speeded performance following head injury in children. *Journal of Clinical and Experimental Neuropsychology* 7:39–54.

Ben-Yishay Y. (1981): Cognitive remediation after TBD: toward a definition of its objectives, tasks and conditions. In: Working approaches to remediation of cognitive deficits in brain-damaged persons. Rehabilitation Monograph (No. 62). New York: New York Medical Center.

Bijur, PE, Stewart-Brown S, Butler N (1986): Child behavior and accidental injury in 11,966 preschool children. *American Journal of Diseases of Childhood* 140:487–492.

Black P, Blumer D, Wellner A, Jeffries JJ, Walker AL (1970): An interdisciplinary perspective study of head trauma in children. In: CR Angle, EA Bering (eds.). Physical trauma as an etiological agent in mental retardation. Bethesda: U.S. Department of Health, Education and Welfare.

Black P, Shepard RJ, Walker AE (1975): Outcome of head trauma: Age and post-traumatic seizures. In: R Porter, D FitzSimmons (eds.). Outcome of severe damage to the central nervous system. Ciba Foundation Symposium, 34. Amsterdam: Elsevier, Excerpta Medica.

Boll TJ (1983): Minor head injury in children: out of sight, but not out of mind. *Journal of Clinical Child Psychology* 12:74–80.

Boll TJ, Barth JT (1981): Neuropsychology of brain damage in children. In: SB Filskov, TJ Boll (eds.): *Handbook of clinical neuropsychology*. New York: John Wiley & Sons.

Bolter JF, Long CJ (1985): Methodological issues in research in developmental neuropsychology. In: LC Hartlage, CF Telzrow (eds.). *The neuropsychology of individual differences: a developmental perspective*. New York: Plenum Press.

Brink JD, Garrett AL, Hale WR, Woo-Sam J, Nickel VL (1970): Recovery of motor and intellectual function in children sustaining severe head injuries. *Developmental medicine and child neurology* 12:565–571.

Brink JD, Imbus C, Woo-Sam J (1980): Physical recovery after severe closed head trauma in children and adolescents. *Journal of Pediatrics* 97:721–727.

Brooks N (1984): Head injury and the family. In: N Brooks (ed.). *Closed head injury.* Oxford: Oxford University Press.

Brown G, Chadwick O, Shaffer D, Rutter M, Traub M (1981): A prospective study of children with head injuries: III. psychiatric sequelae. *Psychological Medicine* 11:63–78.

Cartledge G, Milburn JF (1980): *Teaching social skills to children.* New York: Pergamon Press.

Chadwick O, Rutter M, Brown G, Shaffer D, Traub MA (1981): A prospective study of children with head injuries: II. cognitive sequelae. *Psychological Medicine* 11:49–61.

Chadwick O, Rutter M, Thompson J, Shaffer D (1981): Intellectual performance and reading skills after localized head injury in childhood. *Journal of Child Psychology and Psychiatry* 22:117–139.

Chess S, Thomas A (1984): *Origins and evolution of behavior disorders: from infancy to early adult life.* New York: Brunner/Mazel, Publishers.

Cohen S (1986): Educational reintegration and programming for children with head injuries. *The Journal of Head Trauma Rehabilitation* 1:22–29.

Cope N, Hall K (1982): Head injury rehabilitation: benefit of early intervention. *Archives of Physical Medicine and Rehabilitation* 63:433–437.

Craft AW, Shaw TA, Cartlidge MEF (1972): Head injuries in children. *British Medical Journal* 3:200–203.

Elkind D (1967): Cognition in infancy and early childhood. In: Y. Brackbill (ed.). *Infancy and early childhood.* New York: The Free Press.

Ewing-Cobbs L, Fletcher JM, Levin HS (1985): Neuropsychological sequelae following pediatric head injury. In: M Ylvisaker (ed.). *Head injury rehabilitation: children and adolescents.* San Diego: College-Hill Press.

Feuerstein R (1980): *Instrumental enrichment: an intervention program for cognitive modifiability.* Baltimore: University Park Press.

Fletcher J, Taylor G (1984): Neuropsychological approaches to children: towards a developmental neuropsychology. *Journal of Clinical Neuropsychology* 6:39–56.

Golding J (1986): Accidents. In: NR Butler, Golding J (eds.). *From birth to five: a study of the health and behavior of Britain's 5-year-olds.* New York: Pergamon Press.

Goldman PS (1971): Functional development of the prefrontal cortex in early life and the problem of plasticity. *Experimental Neurology* 32:366–387.

Gross CR, Wolf C, Kunitz SC, Jane JA (1985): Pilot traumatic coma data bank: a profile of head injuries in children. In: RG Dacey, R Winn, R Rimel, et al (eds). *Trauma of the central nervous system.* New York: Raven Press.

Hakkinen S (1958): Traffic accidents and driver characteristics: a statistical and psychological study. Helsinki: Finland's Institute of Technology (Scientific Researches No. 13).

Heiskanen O, Kaste M (1974): Late prognosis of severe brain injury in children. *Developmental Medicine and Child Neurology* 16:11–14.

Hendrick EB, Harwood-Hash DCF, Hudson AR (1964): Head injuries in children: a survey of 4465 consecutive cases at the Hospital for Sick Children, Toronto, Canada. *Clinical Neurosurgery* 11:46–65.

Jennett B (1972): Head injuries in children. *Developmental Medicine and Child Neurology* 14:137–147.

Johnson D, Almi CR (1978): Age, brain damage, and performance. In: S Finger (ed.). *Recovery from brain damage*. New York: Plenum Press.

Kelly T, Haley D (1986): *Procedural guidelines for development of individualized educational programs for students who have suffered traumatic head injury*. Jefferson City, Mo: Missouri Department of Elementary and Secondary Education (unpublished manuscript).

Kennard MA (1942): Cortical reorganization of motor function: studies on a series of monkeys of various ages from infancy to maturity. *Archives of Neurology and Psychiatry* 8:227–240.

Kinsbourne M (1974): Mechanisms of hemispheric interaction in man. In: M Kinsbourne, WL Smith (eds.). *Hemisphere disconnection and cerebral function*. Springfield, IL: Charles C Thomas.

Kleinpeter U (1976): Social integration after brain trauma during childhood. *Acta Paedopsychiatrica* 42:68–75.

Klonoff H (1971): Head injuries in children: predisposing factors, accident conditions, accident proneness and sequelae. *American Journal of Public Health* 61:2405–2417.

Klonoff H, Paris R (1974): Immediate, short-term and residual effects of acute head injuries in children: neuropsychological and neurological correlates. In: R Reitan, L Davison (eds.). *Clinical neuropsychology: current status and applications*. Washington, D.C.: VH Winston & Sons.

Klonoff H, Low MD, Clark C (1977): Head injuries in children: A prospective five year follow-up. *Journal of Neurology, Neurosurgery, and Psychiatry* 40:1211–1219.

LaGreca AM & Santogrossi DA (1980): Social skills training with elementary school students: a behavioral group approach. *Journal of Consulting and Clinical Psychology* 48:220–227.

Lange-Cosack H, Wider B, Schlesner HJ, Grumme T, Kubicki S (1979): Prognosis of brain injuries in young children (one until five years of age). *Neuropaediatrie* 10:105–127.

Levin HS & Benton AL (in press): Developmental and acquired dyscalculia in children. In: I Flehmig (ed.). *Second European Symposium on Developmental Neurology*. Stuttgart: Gustav Fisher Verlag.

Levin HS, Eisenberg HN (1979): Neuropsychological outcome of closed head injury in children and adolescents. *Child's Brain* 5:281–289.

Levin HS, Eisenberg HN, Wigg MD, Kobayashi K (1982): Memory and intellectual ability after head injury in children and adolescents. *Neurosurgery* 11:668–673.

Levin HS, Ewing-Cobbs L, Benton AL (1984): Age and recovery from brain damage: a review of clinical studies. In: SW Scheff (ed.). *Aging and recovery of function in the central nervous system.* New York: Plenum Publishing Corporation.

Lewis DO, Pincus MD, Feldman MA, Jackson MA, Bard B (1986): Psychiatric, neurological, and psychoeducational characteristics of 15 death row inmates in the United States. *American Journal of Psychiatry* 143:838–845.

Lezak MD (1978): Living with the characterological altered brain injured patient. *Journal of Clinical Psychiatry* 39:592–598.

Lezak MD (1987): Relationships between personality disorders, social disturbances, and physical disability following traumatic brain injury. *Journal of Head Trauma Rehabilitation* 2:57–69.

Light R, Neumann E, Lewis R, Morecki-Oberg C, Asarnow R, Satz P (1987): An evaluation of a neuropsychologically based reeducation project for the head injured child. *The Journal of Head Trauma Rehabilitation* 2:11–25.

Long CJ, Gouvier WD, Cole JC (1984): A model of recovery for the total rehabilitation of individuals with head trauma. *Journal of Rehabilitation* 50:39–45.

Luria AR (1966): *Human brain and psychological processes.* New York: Harper & Row.

Mannheimer DI, Dewey J, Melinger GD (1966): Fifty thousand child-years of accidental injuries. *Public Health Reports* 81:519.

Matheny AP, Fisher JE (1984): Behavioral perspectives on children's accidents. *Advances in Developmental and Behavioral Pediatrics* 5:221–264.

National Center for Health Statistics (1982): Advance report, Final mortality statistics. In: *Monthly Vital Statistics Report,* Vol. 31, No. 6, Supplement (DHHS Publication No. PHS 82-1120): Hyattsville, MD: U.S. Public Health Service.

Oden S, Asher SR (1977): Coaching children in social skills for friendship making. *Child Development* 48:495–506.

Oddy M (1984): Head injury during childhood: the psychological implications. In: N. Brooks (ed.). *Closed head injury: psychological, social and family consequences.* Oxford: Oxford University Press.

Oddy M, Humphrey M, Uttley D (1978): Subjective impairment and social recovery after closed head injury. *Journal of Neurology, Neurosurgery, and Psychiatry* 41:611–616.

Panting A, Merry P (1972): The long-term rehabilitation of severe head injuries with particular reference to the need for social and medical support for the patient's family. *Rehabilitation* 38:33–37.

Porter JE, Rourke BR (1985): Socioemotional functioning of learning-disabled children: a subtypal analysis of personality patterns. In: BR Rourke (ed.). *Neuropsychology of learning disabilities: essentials of subtype analysis.* New York: The Guilford Press.

Prigatano G (1987): Personality and psychosocial consequences after brain injury. In: MJ Meier, AL Benton, L Diller (eds.). *Neuropsychological rehabilitation.* New York: The Guilford Press.

Raimondi AJ, Hirschauer J (1984): Head injury in the infant and toddler—coma scoring and outcome scale. *Child's Brain* 11:12–35.

Raimondi AJ, Choux M, DiRocco C (eds.) (1986): *Head injuries in the newborn and infant.* New York: Springer-Verlag.

Rosenbaum M, Najenson T (1976): Changes in life patterns and symptoms of low mood as reported by wives of severely brain-injured soldiers. *Journal of Consulting and Clinical Psychology,* 44:881–888.

Rourke BR (ed.) (1985): *Neuropsychology of learning disabilities: essentials of subtype analysis.* New York: The Guilford Press.

Rourke BR; Bakker DJ; Fisk JL, Strang JD (1983): *Child neuropsychology.* New York: The Guilford Press.

Rutter M (1980): Raised lead levels and impaired cognitive/behavioral functioning: A review of the evidence. *Developmental Medicine and Child Neurology* 22(Suppl).

Rutter M (1981): Psychological sequelae of brain damage in children. *British Medical Journal* 3:200–203.

Rutter M (1982): Developmental neuropsychiatry: concepts, issues, and prospects. *Journal of Clinical Neuropsychology* 4:91–115.

Rutter M, Chadwick O, Shaffer D (1983): Head injury. In: M Rutter (ed.). *Developmental neuropsychiatry.* New York: The Guilford Press.

Savage RC (1985): *A survey of traumatically brain injured children within school-based special education programs.* Rutland, VT: Head Injury/Stroke Independence Project, Inc., pp. 1–6.

Savage RC (1987): Educational issues for the head-injured adolescent and young adult. *The Journal of Head Trauma Rehabilitation* 2:1–10.

Selman RL, Lavin DR, Brion-Meisels S (1982): Troubled children's use of self-reflection. In: FC Serafica (ed.). *Social-cognitive development in context.* New York: The Guilford Press.

Shaffer D, Bijur P, Chadwick O, Rutter M (1980): Head injury and later reading disability. *Journal of the American Academy of Child Psychiatry* 19:592–610.

Shapiro K (1985): Head injury in children. In: DP Becker, JT Povlishock (eds.). *Central Nervous System Status Report, 1985.* Bethesda: National Institute of Neurological and Communicative Disorders and Stroke.

Spivak G, Shure MB (1974): *Social adjustment of young children: a cognitive approach to solving real-life problems.* San Francisco: Jossey-Bass.

Telzrow CF (1985): The science and speculation of rehabilitation in developmental neuropsychological disorders. In: LC Hartlage, CF Telzrow (eds.). *The Neuropsychology of Individual Differences: A Developmental Perspective.* New York: Plenum Press.

Teuber HL, Rudel RG (1962): Behavior after cerebral lesions in children and adults. *Developmental Medicine and Child Neurology* 4:3–20.

Thomsen IV (1974): The patient with severe head injury and his family. *Scandinavian Journal of Rehabilitation Medicine* 6:180–183.

Vygotsky LS (1978): *Mind in society: the development of higher psychological processes.* Cambridge, MA: Harvard University Press.

Ylvisaker M (ed.) (1985): *Head injury rehabilitation: children and adolescents.* San Diego: College Hill Press.

19

Adolescent Community Integration

Jeanne Fryer, Ph.D.

*Community Rehabilitation Services, Rehab Systems Co.,
Annapolis, Maryland, U.S.A.*

COMMUNITY INTEGRATION AFTER TBI

Current views of rehabilitation are increasingly focusing attention on problems associated with environmental adaptation (Frey, 1984). Rehabilitation may be viewed as "a process of integrating persons with physical or mental impairments into community life. In cases of an acquired injury this process is one of re-adaptation to community living" (Frey, 1984). The aims of this integration effort are to assist individuals in obtaining the roles, rights, and responsibilities that define life in the surrounding community. This view of rehabilitation clearly identifies community integration as a part of, indeed the goal of, the rehabilitation process.

In order to facilitate community adaptation, we need to understand the abilities, interests, and behavior patterns of persons with impairments, as well as the demands placed on them by their particular environments. We then must work toward improving this relationship through enhancing the abilities and skills of the person as well as through environmental modification. In the end the most we can do is to assist individuals "to mobilize their own resources, decide what they wish and are able to be, and achieve goals through their own efforts and their own ways" (Jacques, 1970).

Successful neurorehabilitation may be defined as return to a state of independence or interdependence in which the person is productive (work/school/avocation) and contributes to family or interpersonal life (mutually satisfying personal relationships) (Prigatano, 1987). Thus the ultimate consequence of rehabilitation following head injury is community integration—a place to live, productive work and leisure activity, and meaningful social interaction.

The real issue as the individual who has experienced a traumatic brain injury and his or her family and significant others move through the rehabilitation process is integrating into the community in meaningful ways. This is an ongoing process of adaptation, an interaction between the person and the environment. There is a vast difference between living in a community and being socially integrated into that community. In order to prepare people for life and work in integrated settings, it is necessary to provide them exposure to and experience in dealing with the demands and expectations of ordinary environments (*Rehab Brief,* 1985).

What abilities, skills, or information levels are necessary for successful integration (or conversely what barriers prevent meaningful reentry), and what services are required to facilitate and maintain this process? These are the current issues of concern with respect to community integration.

In this chapter a review of the systems that exist both internal and external to the individual that work together to make up the fabric of "community" will be addressed. Participation in, connection with, or support from at least a subset of these systems is required for successful community integration. Discussion of each system will present current information and pose questions that need to be addressed in order to enhance our understanding of successful community integration for survivors of traumatic brain injury in the adolescent age range.

SPECIFIC ISSUES FOR ADOLESCENTS AFTER TRAUMATIC BRAIN INJURY—A SYSTEMS APPROACH

Adolescents and young adults are the highest risk group for sustaining a traumatic brain injury resulting in a multiplicity of physical, cognitive, emotional, and social problems (Levin, 1979; Levin et al., 1983). Annual incidence estimates of brain injury have ranged from 180 per 100,000 to 295 per 100,000. In teenagers the rates for males are about 1.3 to 2.0 times greater than those for females. Highest incidence rates for both boys and girls occur between 15 and 19 years (Rivara, 1986).

Adolescent development is characterized by physical maturation (particularly developing sexual maturity), a drive for independence, and personal identity. Firm gender identity is gained through socializing and competing with peers. Most normally developing adolescents are in the formal operational stage of cognitive development (Piaget, 1983) establishing skills in self-evaluation with accompanying self-doubt (Eisert and Kahle, 1982).

An inability to move through this developmental process and resolve issues of sexual maturity, ego identity, and autonomy can result in a lack of purpose, inability to find intimacy with others, and self-defeating behavior (i.e., substance abuse) (Erickson, 1963).

As TBI affects the physical, emotional, and social functioning of individuals, these normal developmental challenges of adolescence are all at risk and are greatly affected by a traumatic brain injury. Emerging executive skill behaviors are particularly vulnerable. How these skills re-emerge after a traumatic brain injury and the long-term consequences of residual impairments are questions of particular importance in adolescent community integration.

Cognitive and psychosocial disturbances are the most commonly cited residual deficits after traumatic brain injury and are the major cause of long-term disability (Brooks, 1983; Prigatano, 1986; Thomsen, 1984; Lezak, 1987). In age-controlled studies this same pattern seems to be true for adolescents.

Studies of long-term consequences of TBI (Oddy, 1984; Lezak, 1987) are consistent in reporting psychosocial issues as the factors that interfere most with community integration (successful adaptation, i.e., residential independence, productive activity, meaningful relationships) and create the greatest family burden (Ben-Yishay, 1986; Brooks, 1987).

In a 10 to 15 year follow-up study of severely brain-injured individuals, Thomsen reported that the problems that were the biggest deterrent to reentering a normal lifestyle centered around personality disturbances. From the individual's point of view the single biggest problem 10 to 15 years following traumatic brain injury was social isolation (Thomsen, 1984). Lezak (1987) reports similar findings.

This is particularly noteworthy when considering community integration issues with respect to adolescents. Socialization, peer esteem, group participation, and ego identity are major developmental issues in adolescence. When this process is disrupted how do we go about enhancing normal development (habilitation) while involved in a rehabilitation process focused on restoring and compensating for impaired functions? The issue is of course a broader one involving the developmental framework from which rehabilitation needs to be structured for children and adolescents.

Results from a survey of adolescents in the public school system (Fryer, 1987) indicate that the preferred activity of those teenagers surveyed is "go out with friends." This was true for reentering TBI students as well as non-TBI students. In responding to "What is important to you?" "image" was number 1 for non-TBI students, followed closely by "the future," "relationships," "having close friends" (but particularly boyfriend/girlfriend), and "do well in athletics."

For reentering TBI students, "fitting in" was the major concern followed by "having friends." Responses to "What worries you?" differed somewhat in the two groups, but only in emphasis. Non-TBI individuals worried about "what you look like," "how other people see you," "what your parents think or pleasing your parents," "getting into college," and "getting into fights—getting hurt." Reentering TBI individuals worried about "being weird," "not being understood by friends," "not having friends," "not understanding themselves," "feeling alone," "feeling depressed" (periodically feeling as if they can't cope with the situation).

It is clear from these results that a major concern for adolescents is self-validation through interaction with a close group of peers and valued others. It is also clear from this survey as well as other evidence (Kozloff, 1987) that strengthening this network is a major goal for successful adolescent community integration.

The most important functional systems for adolescents are the family system and the educational system. It is from this base that knowledge about and experience with other systems that constitute the community at large emanate. The community that an individual with a head injury reenters includes recreational pursuits, friends, intimate relationships, work or productive activity as well as home and family. For adolescents these activities are found mainly through school. Peer relationships are the most important issue (as discussed above) for adolescents themselves. Community integration from the adolescent's point of view is socialization. As adolescents strive for independence, personal identity, and autonomy, with the attendant risks involved in this endeavor, a secure base to work from is crucial.

Educational System

Cognitive/Learning Issues

Cognitive deficits and related psychosocial issues have been identified by researchers and clinicians as the greatest obstacles to integrating into satisfying vocational and social lives after TBI. Most of the research in this area is reviewed in Brooks (1984), Levin, Benton, and Grossman (1983), Prigatano et al. (1986), and Ylvisaker and Gobble (1987).

There has been little work done specific to adolescents. Vocational and social issues as well as many other systems within the community are centered in the school system during the critical transitional years of adolescence.

Cognitive impairments that commonly persist among head-injured adolescents include, in varying combinations and degrees of severity, "impaired attention and perception; inflexibility in attending, thinking and acting; slow and inefficient processing of information; difficulty processing large amounts of information; difficulty learning/remembering new information, rules and procedures; inefficient retrieval of old information and words; poorly organized behavior, verbal expression and problem solving; impulsive and socially awkward behavior and impaired executive functions, such as self-awareness of strengths and weaknesses, goal setting, planning, self-initiation or self-inhibiting, self-monitoring and self-evaluating" (Szekeres, Ylvisaker, Cohen, 1987). Even though the evidence clearly points to a syndrome (pattern) of cognitive impairments the need for a flexible approach to intervention cannot be stated clearly enough.

Within commonly occurring patterns of cognitive deficit and broad guidelines of typical stages of recovery (Rancho Los Amigos Levels of Cognitive Functioning Scales, 1981) individual differences are as varied as the individual survivors of traumatic brain injury.

These individual differences result from the difference in the types and severity of brain injury; pretraumatic difference in personality, intelligence, and educational achievement; and from differences in the support systems that are available to the individuals, the coping styles they have, and rehabilitative interventions after injury.

The residual cognitive impairments that many students are left with after traumatic brain injury are not compatible with traditional educational goals—the integration of basic processing abilities while learning academic subject matter (Cohen, 1986). Thus the development or redevelopment of basic cognitive skills may have to precede or accompany academic learning.

It is likely that students will need continued therapy, particularly cognitive retraining, in addition to specialized classroom interventions.

A whole continuum of interventions may be necessary from training in basic cognitive skills, through modified academic training, through training specific to functional activities.

In order to ensure the appropriate level of service as well as to ensure continuity and appropriate timing of services, it is critical to begin educational reentry while the adolescent is still in a hospital or rehabilitation program.

Appropriate assessments are a critical factor in providing suitable reentry services. Testing must be used to have students demonstrate what they know as well as what they don't know and, most importantly, how they process information. Testing done by individuals experienced in the area of TBI is necessary in order to make meaningful interpretations.

Two issues must be stressed in discussing successful educational community reentry. I.Q. and achievement test scores are not necessarily a measure of students' ability to function in mainstream classes. Special support services are almost always indicated after TBI. The degree of support can vary from a full-time, self-contained special education setting to a counselor/tutor, who contacts the student in mainstream classes several times a day to check on problems and provide help with assignments (Cohen, 1986).

High school students need to be as carefully integrated into the social structure of the school as into the academic structure.

Underlying cognitive problems observed in many head-injured adolescents—memory, attention, focusing and sustaining attention over time, distractibility—all effect social functioning as well as academic functioning.

Effects of cognitive training for adolescents have received little attention in the literature. Research is needed to assist in the creation of interventions for specific deficits at different stages of recovery (Ewing-Cobb, 1985).

School Reentry/Educational Programming

There is little literature on effective systematic transitions from medical rehabilitation into community systems (school, work, social networks, recreation, etc.) (Lezak, 1987; Ben-Yishay, 1986; Prigatano, 1986; Fryer, 1987).

However, from available reports and personal contact it is clear that students who have experienced traumatic brain injury have not integrated well into the school system as it exists (Savage, 1986).

Many TBI survivors return home and to school with few if any support systems and little if any information on head injuries for their families and the schools to which they return. This lack of information is a major impediment in successful school integration.

Educational systems need to give careful consideration to several issues in order to facilitate reentry for the student who has experienced TBI.

Savage (1986) has identified 5 key questions that need to be addressed:

1. Do the teachers who will be working with these students have knowledge about TBI and the associated problems?
2. What kinds of special services and programs will the student need?
3. Who should be a part of the basic educational team for this student?
4. What kinds of intervention strategies are necessary to help the student reenter the academic and social milieu of the school?
5. What types of long-range plans are necessary to ensure a transition of services?

With the passage of P.L. 94-142, schools became responsible for educating all children with handicaps. This places the major responsibility for adolescent community integration with the school. Vocational training as well as socialization and recreational activities along with academic preparation are provided through the educational system for adolescents.

Research and clinical experience are demonstrating that schools need to be aware of the following recommendations when a head-injured adolescent reenters the educational system (Savage, 1987):

1. "The transition from the hospital (or rehabilitation center) to the school must involve both parties. Specialists from the medical area and educators from the school system need to meet before the student reenters school. Information about the student needs to be shared and recommendations need to be made to ensure proper transition of services for the head-injured student.

2. Teachers and staff in the school need in-service training about head injury and all of its ramifications. Literature, videotapes, teaching suggestions, and so forth need to be shared with everyone involved.

3. The school needs a team approach for the head-injured student to best continue his or her recovery. Head injury reeducation is much too complicated to be left to one person, and the splintering of instruction without overlap only creates additional problems for the head-injured student.

4. The needs of the head-injured student require the careful integration of all domains: cognitive, affective, and psychomotor. Since the head-injured student's problems are pervasive and complicated they need to be rebuilt in conjunction with one another.

5. The school needs to be cautious in determining educational placement. Head-injured students should not be categorized as mentally retarded, learning disabled, or emotionally disturbed. Exclusive placement into these programs does not meet the special needs of the head-injured student, and such inappropriate placement may further complicate already existing problems.

6. The school needs to recognize that the majority of head-injured students experience common problems with concentrating and paying attention for long periods of time; retrieving facts/skills; learning new material; and organizing, abstracting, and adapting thinking. They usually lose some basic academic skills and thinking processes; experience high levels of frustration, fatigue, and irritability; and demonstrate inappropriate behaviors. In addition, head-injured students usually have problems reassociating with peers.

7. The school will need to use teaching methods that concentrate on cognitive processing as academic skills are learned. Focus needs to be

on the interaction between teacher and student, not necessarily on the material itself.

8. The school must project the head-injured student's needs on a long-term basis, not just year to year. As 5-year plans are constructed, vocational, rehabilitation, and other agencies need to be involved to maintain transition services as the student moves from school to community (IEP process)."

Community college programs in a number of states, particularly California, have been responsive to the needs of young adults with traumatic brain injury. These programs are discussed in Chapter 20, Adult Community Integration.

Vocational System

The world of work is a major milestone for adolescents. Transition into this world is a major goal of the adolescent years. At best this is a process fraught with decision, breaks from perceived security, and challenges of freedom and independence. Facilitating a smooth transition into this world for an adolescent with traumatic brain injury can be a rocky course. Will's article (Will, 1984) on Bridges affords a structure which is applicable for TBI as well as other disability areas. The greatest concern for this population is appropriate assessment so that realistic goals can be established and a network of services can be established to provide the support needed to facilitate movement from school into productive activity (work).

Head-injured adolescents, like their nondisabled peers, experience the normal stress of development from dependent child to independent adult (Havinghurst, 1972). Since employment involves the individual's need for independence and a feeling of responsibility, it is a source of major anxiety. Severely head-injured adolescents must additionally learn to compensate for the cognitive and psychosocial deficits that could dramatically reduce their chances for successful employment (Gobble, 1986).

The focus of vocational development should include the roles of a family member, unpaid worker, and citizen and participation in avocational pursuits as well as preparation for paid work (Gobble, 1985).

For the adolescent who has experienced a TBI, self-awareness and realistic goal setting are critical issues in vocational preparation.

Careful assessment, both of the individual *and* of available productive work activities within the community are necessary. It does not do much good to prepare an individual for employment or avocational pursuits if the possibility for placement does not exist (Szymula and Schleser, 1986). Therefore, exploration and assessment of realistic placements is a critical factor in successful transitions into productive activity.

Residual impairments that may exist as a consequence of TBI (as discussed above) make it imperative that individual assessments address the following cognitive and psychosocial areas: initiative in goal setting; interpersonal skills, including communication; self-direction in daily living activities; problem-solving ability; learning ability for new skills and tasks; perceptual skills; memory; attention span; selective attention; attentional flexibility; orientation to person, place, time, and task; organizational ability; and emotional ability (Gobble, 1985).

Physical and occupational therapists should provide detailed descriptions of gross and fine motor functioning and potential. The work evaluation can then fit the individual's current functioning level. This initial evaluation should demonstrate the person's ability to integrate cognitive and motor skills with vocational tasks.

Realistically examining skills and matching them with an appropriate occupational choice is the goal of a good assessment. For TBI youth it may actually also be part of the treatment intervention as self-awareness remains such a difficult area for many adolescents after TBI.

Individuals must be made aware of their adaptability to work demands. In any given job the worker may be required to do any of the following: to maintain attention on a repetitive short cycle job; move flexibly from one task to another; meet precise standards, requirements, or duties on the job; follow directions from a supervisor and also independently organize a task; make judgments, generalizations, or decisions; perform under stressful conditions where working speed and sustained attention are required; communicate effectively with other individuals in a work setting (U.S. Dept. of Labor, 1972).

In building a realistic appraisal of work abilities other areas of vocational behavior must also be addressed. These include self-direction and motivation, effective interpersonal and communication skills, application of academic knowledge, management of personal and self-care needs, self-reliance in transportation, and mobility in the community.

Vocational goals for adolescents are somewhat different from those for adults. Traditionally they have been viewed as exploration of career options, ability to make tentative career choices, and the development of critical vocational skills (Gobble, 1986). However, for disabled adolescents a high priority should be placed on preparing for job placement.

Therapeutic intervention to achieve these goals includes: determining specific behavioral competencies to be acquired by the individual; reviewing the effectiveness of compensatory strategies by the individual in other (nonwork-related) situations; selecting teaching strategies that incorporate task analysis and allow for the acquisition, proficiency, and maintenance of behaviors; programming for generalization into the work environment (Gobble, 1985); and identifying work opportunities for placement.

Much of this is accomplished within the educational setting. It is therefore imperative that the educational and vocational system work closely so that there is not a duplication of services and, most importantly, to provide for smooth transitions from school to work.

Social System

The social context within which the adolescent and his or her significant others exist influences the behaviors which are a consequence of the physical, cognitive, emotional, and social sequelae of traumatic brain injury.

Successful adaptation to the environment is based on a balance of biological, psychological, and environmental forces that allows an equilibrium to exist (Trieschmann, 1987). The environment repeatedly presents challenges and stress. Trieschmann presents a model of adaptive health that stresses the interaction of these influences. Table 19-1 presents a catalogue of variables that interact and influence all of our lives (Trieschmann, 1987, p. 47). The dynamic balance among these variables

Table 19-1. *Behavior (B) as a Function of the Interaction of Psychosocial (P), Organic (O), and Environmental (E) Variables*

Psychosocial variables (P)	Organic variables (O)	Environmental variables (E)
Take responsibility for self	Intelligence and cognitive ability	Income
Will to live		Transportation
Social skills	Endurance	Architectural and geographic barriers
Style of coping with stress	Strength	
Locus of control (I-E)	Perceptual motor coordination	Access to knowledgeable health professionals
Self-confidence		
Judgment	Aptitudes	Educational and vocational resources
Problem-solving ability	Amount of physical impairment	
Education		Financial disincentives
Work history	Sensory abilities	Family and interpersonal support
Job skills	Bladder and bowel control	
Cultural and ethnic groups		Socioeconomic status
	Respiratory function	Availability of physical assistance (if needed)
Gender	Pain	
Creativity	General health status	Behavioral supervision (if needed)
		Payment for medical care
		Role models

From Trieschmann (1987), p. 47.

(POE) produces a healthful state allowing an individual to function meaningfully as a wholly integrated member of a social system.

Social networks play an important part in an individual's ability to obtain the resources, both material and nonmaterial, to cope with the crisis of a head injury and the long recovery process associated with it (Kozloff, 1987).

The head-injured youth looks to family, kin, friends, and neighbors for confirmation of his or her worth and value and for feedback about his or her behavior. The reaction of the members of the individual's social network and the social validation he or she receives have an effect on his or her self-image, self-esteem, motivation, and capability.

Kozloff's recent study of social networks demonstrates that as time from onset increases, network size decreases and network density increases. Patients in her study reported a decrease in their social relationships and a feeling of isolation from their peers. This came about not only by the changes imposed by injury but also by rejection by peers because of the consequences of these changes. These included sexual disinhibition, inappropriate laughing (emotional lability), and verbal and physical abusiveness. As a result of isolation some individuals reported involvement in transient peer relationships. These lack the strength, durability, priority, and commitment of more enduring relationships. They therefore are not effective in providing emotional or task-oriented support. At best these transient relationships offer no feedback or support. At worst the head-injured persons are taken advantage of by new friends. Some individuals resume their previous pattern of drug and alcohol abuse or begin these activities with old and new aquaintances (Kozloff, 1987).

The people who do remain in the head-injured person's networks are mostly family who know each other. The family attempts to compensate for the individual's lack of peer relationship and the limitations imposed by injury by spending more time with him or her. As fewer nonrelated people attempt to meet the head-injured person's needs, families serve multiple functions for the head-injured person.

TBI persons whose behavior was not in keeping with peer group norms were considered a "burden" by friends who were used to a relationship of mutual aid and support rather than one in which they functioned as caregivers.

This evidence points to the need to include members of the individual's social network in the recovery process.

It is particularly important to train peers to understand the needs of the person with a traumatic brain injury. Peer training at school and building a strong support group could be one of the most effective transitions in community integration for adolescents.

Behavioral sequelae that interfere most with adequate social function are decreased attention, noncompliance, deficient social judgment, and depressed thought processes (Ylvisaker, 1986). Social functioning is also related to possible deficits in social perception, learning rate, information processing, and the capacity to abstract and generalize social rules. For example, an individual may be unable to distinguish between two similar social situations to which two very different sets of rules apply. He or she may be slower in learning which social behaviors are appropriate and which are unacceptable. Or the individual may have difficulty in rapidly processing all of the social and environmental cues required to make a correct social response (Ylvisaker, 1986). Socially disinhibited behavior is the biggest deterrent to smooth community integration after TBI for adolescents.

Those intervention strategies that focus on improvement of ability to mediate behavior, reduce impulsivity, and deal with parental expectations appear to be the most promising.

Specific social skill training may be a useful intervention. However, in many cases it is an understanding of the social situation that is actually impaired. Social cognition must be dealt with directly through structuring the environment so that the person can gain an understanding of the entire social context. More research needs to address the issue of the development of social cognition in addition to social skill training, particularly in the area of self-cuing techniques.

Socially Unsanctioned Behavior

Socially unsanctioned behavior is a most disturbing occurrence after traumatic brain injury in adolescents. Examples such as substance abuse, criminal activity, extreme behavioral problems—that is, disinhibition, sexual acting out, and violent (aggressive) behaviors—have been frequently reported. Tendencies toward some of these behaviors may have existed prior to the head injury. Substance abuse (alcohol or drugs) is certainly implicated in many occurrences of TBI. Up to 50% has been reported in the literature (Reilly, Kelly, and Faillace, 1986). Even without a history of substance abuse, problems in this area may develop after head injury. New peer influence, reduced control, and impaired social judgment all contribute to this behavior. Little is known about effective treatment in this area.

Sexual acting out can be a case of extreme disinhibition. Promiscuity can be a symptom of reduced self-esteem, as well as poor social judgment. Sexual inappropriateness is a frequent deterrent to community integration for adolescents. More information is needed as to intervention strategies and long-term sequelae.

When behaviors are outside the boundaries of acceptable community standards, confrontations with the law will occur. A lack of social cognition; impaired social skills; reduced frustration tolerance; lack of self-esteem; and impaired judgment, self-regulation, and problem solving may all contribute to behaviors that result in criminal treatment. There is increasing evidence that many individuals in jails have a history of traumatic brain injury.

Certainly more research is indicated in this area. Can early intervention make a difference? What is appropriate intervention? How can we safeguard others while providing services to the TBI survivor? Prevention efforts through the criminal justice system may be useful.

A major question to investigate is "When is changing the behavior, managing the behavior, or changing the environment more appropriate?"

Socially unsanctioned behaviors frequently result in institutional settings, jails, psychiatric hospitals, and so forth, at a great financial cost to society and a great cost both financially and emotionally to individual families.

The issues they raise are difficult ethically and practically, but they cannot be ignored.

Emotional System

Emotional well-being after traumatic brain injury is a very serious issue with adolescents. In the survey cited above (Fryer, 1987) all of the traumatically brain-injured adolescents interviewed felt a sense of depression based on feeling socially isolated and misunderstood. These feelings are not unique to the adolescent with a head injury; however, with impaired information processing and memory skills, the ability to work through these feelings is greatly reduced. Prigatano (1987) reports work done by Goldstein (1952) which emphasized how problems of abstract reasoning or impairment of the abstract attitude predisposed patients to behave impulsively and socially inappropriately. He also discussed the "catastrophic reaction" which occurs when patients become overwhelmed with their deficits. This phenomenon is extremely important in the clinical management of adolescents with traumatic brain injuries and, as Prigatano (1987) suggests, needs further evaluation.

Personality changes in adolescents have not been well documented.

Bond (1975) reported the importance of memory and personality disorders as correlates of impaired social functioning in assessing psychosocial outcome after severe head injury. Weddell, Oddy, and Jenkins (1980) reported a high correlation between personality change and memory disturbance.

Helping TBI adolescents accept the trauma and adjust to their new circumstances is a major challenge in community integration.

Attempts to establish personal identity and autonomy and the resulting rebellion against adult authority are normal developmental issues and conflicts of adolescents. Peer support in dealing with these issues is characteristic of this age group. Cars, alcohol, and drugs often become symbols of autonomy and rebellion. Normal strivings and conflicts are only intensified after a TBI with denial, depression, and acting out as typical responses (Barin, 1985).

These responses have been classified as psychoreactive or as organic. They may be either or both. Prigatano has developed a particularly useful schema for understanding personality disorders after brain injury (Table 19-2).

Table 19-2. *Schema for Typical Personality Disorders after Brain Injury*

Reactionary problems	Neuropsychologically mediated problems	Characterological styles
Anxiety	Impulsiveness	Obsessive or superorderly behavior
Depression	Socially inappropriate comments or actions	Hardworking attitude
Irritability	Emotional lability (includes poor tolerance of frustration)	Congeniality and friendliness
Mistrust of others		Social deceptiveness (psychopathic tendencies)
Hopelessness	Agitation	Desire to maintain satisfying interpersonal relations
Helplessness (i.e., more demanding attitude)	Paranoia	
Anger	Unawareness of deficit (or severity)	Encouragement or discouragement of family support
Social withdrawal	Childlike behavior (giddiness or insensitivity to others)	Distrustfulness
Phobias	Misperception of the intentions or actions of others	Feeling of not getting "enough" help from others and therapists
	Apparent lack of motivation	Avoidance of insight into self or discussion of personal topics
	Hypoarousal	Enjoyment of upsetting others
		Enjoyment of a dependent role
		Defiant attitude (challenging therapist to go ahead and treat them if they can)

From Prigatano (1986).

Helping to explain to families, friends, and others who will be in contact with the person why the person is behaving as he or she does is extremely helpful in facilitating adequate coping. By reducing confusion, distress may be lessened and tolerance developed.

Of course it is of utmost importance to increase the TBI individual's awareness and understanding of deficits; it is this lack of awareness that has been identified as the single greatest barrier to community integration (Prigatano, 1986; Ben-Yishay, 1987; Lezak, 1987). Although this work was not specific to adolescents, the evidence we do have through clinical observation points to the fact that as with adults those adolescents who develop realistic attitudes regarding the effects of their injuries show better outcome with regard to community integration.

Continued denial leads to acting out behaviors. Poor judgment, both for safety and social concerns, makes this very dangerous. Girls may be very vulnerable sexually since they may no longer feel attractive. Driving is a major issue for adolescents over the legal driving age (Barin, 1985).

Loss of self-esteem is chronic with brain-injured adolescents. Perceptions of intelligence, competence, career possibilities, and physical attractiveness are altered. Self-doubts increase and depression may follow.

Adolescents may become suicidal after continued failures. Little research has been done in this area, but teenage suicide is a problem with nondisabled youth and there is every reason to believe it is of great concern with brain-injured teenagers.

Adequate preparation of parents is especially important in the treatment of adolescents. "In no other age group will the problem of emotional lability have such an impact on the family or will the behavior problems be so blatant, dangerous or difficult to control" (Barin, 1985, p. 372).

Legal System

Legal issues for adolescents with traumatic brain injuries rarely involve constitutional rights. Rights to privacy and self-determination to decide medical treatment are assumed by the child's parents as his or her natural guardians. When a child turns 18, however, he or she is presumed competent to give consent; and if this is not the case, parents are not automatically the legal authorized representatives. If the young adult is not considered competent, a guardian must be appointed by the court, where it will be decided if the individual is incompetent and whether the proposed guardian is appropriate (Kolpan, 1986).

A parent may serve as a guardian in a lawsuit, but may not give consent to proposed treatment until he or she has been legally appointed guardian if the child is 18 or over (Kolpan, 1986). There is a range of conservatorship and guardianship options available for those youths with impairments in social judgment as well as more severely injured individuals. These should be explored on an individual basis as there are pros and cons for each option, dependent on the individual family's social and financial conditions.

Structured settlements and long-term life planning are particularly important for moderately as well as severely injured adolescents as the impulsivity and social vulnerability frequently associated with TBI can lead to a lack of judgment in the use of alloted resources.

Many adolescents after TBI have contact with the criminal justice system. Impulsivity, poor social cognition, impaired cognitive functions, (i.e., memory, processing speed), and impaired language and perceptual functions all contribute to situations that may result in unlawful acts. Frequently TBI youth are victims, either of their own vulnerability (taken advantage of) or of actual aggressive acts against them. They are also agents of self-initiated illegal actions due to impaired judgment and problem solving.

Example: Legal System

Jerry was in the county jail where it was reported he had attempted suicide. Testing was requested by the court. At 14, Jerry had been hit by a car while crossing the street. He sustained a traumatic brain injury. Diffuse damage was noted with particular damage to the frontal lobes and the right parietal area. Jerry was in the hospital for 12 days. He was released to his mother's home. Jerry did not return to school due to a left-sided hemiparesis, balance problems, visual problems, and generally not being able to "keep up." Over the years Jerry had various episodes with the police. He would wander off and get lost, pick up something from the store and forget to pay, and so forth. He lived with his mother, who was separated from his father. An older sister had just left the home. Jerry stayed at home all day while his mother worked. He watched TV or wandered in the neighborhood. He had no friends and did not participate in any activities outside the home. Sometimes his mother worked at night and then he was alone during the night. Jerry frequently used the phone, making random calls. When a little girl answered, he said he wanted to see her and play with her; her mother got on the phone and arranged a place to meet Jerry. She met him there with a police officer. Jerry was arrested and, at 18, put in jail to await trial. Based on thorough neuropsychological test reports and testimony, along with numerous educational meetings between the attorneys and the neuropsychologist, the judge ruled that Jerry be placed in a TBI residential rehabilitation program rather than be sent to jail.

It is most important to train the criminal justice system about TBI so that appropriate actions can be taken to facilitate community integration, rather than inappropriate incarceration.

Recreational/Leisure

Evidence points to the fact that the way a person spends his or her time is severely altered after traumatic brain injury (Fryer, 1984; Lezak, 1987). Families report that the injured person is unwilling or unable to participate in activities. Individuals themselves report social isolation (Thomsen, 1984; Lezak, 1987; Kosloff, 1987).

In a 5-year follow-up study, Fryer (1984) reported the characteristics that distinguished those individuals who perceived themselves as having successfully adapted after traumatic brain injury from those who did not were a strong belief system (religion, family, etc.); perception of productive activity; a mentor relationship through the rehabilitation process and continuing into the community (this was not necessarily the same individual throughout the process, but there was a continuous flow); and participation in a structured recreational program. These TBI individuals represented a variety of living settings (skilled nursing facility, group home, family, interdependent, independent) and a variety of work settings (competitive employment, supported employment, sheltered employment, part-time employment, volunteer, avocational, school, daycare setting). Living settings and work activity were not necessarily matched with belief in successful recovery, or adaptation. If the person was involved in activity he or she perceived as meaningful, felt safe and comfortable in his or her living setting, and had continuous social interactions, self-perception (corroborated by significant others) was that of successful community integration. The single factor that all those who reported successful adaptation had in common was a structured recreational activity.

This information is very helpful in understanding successful community integration.

Services that encourage ongoing friendships are not easily accessible to head-injured teenagers. It is necessary to educate peers about the consequences of head injury and appropriate ways to handle situations and integrate friends into existing social situations. It is also necessary to coordinate community services—educational, vocational, and social (mental health, maternal and child health, etc.)—so that education about head injury can be presented and services that are meaningful to these individuals can be provided. Recreational programs can be provided through community services such as the Y.M.C.A. or community parks and recreational programs, if education with respect to the special needs of TBI youth is provided and adjunct services are coordinated when required.

Family Systems

Traditionally when an adolescent is discharged from an acute or sub-acute rehabilitation program he or she goes home with family.

Family burden has been documented (Thomsen, 1984; Brooks, 1986; Bond and Brooks, 1979). However, the unique effects of an adolescent, particularly with respect to siblings and changing roles in the family, have not been directly addressed.

Research (Kozloff, 1987) has shown that the family becomes the major source for financial, emotional, and task-oriented support for the head-injured individual, and that this increases over time. Ultimately the head-injured person and his or her family become socially isolated. All of their time and energy is devoted to the survivor's recovery or to the resulting consequences of the injury, and they have little opportunity or energy to maintain outside relationships. Siblings eventually express jealousy and disapproval of the central role in the family played by the head-injured person and withdraw their support (Kozloff, 1987). Gothlieb (1981) and Barrera (1981) report that friends, parents, and siblings tire of their change in roles, the infringement on their time, and the alteration in the structure and content brought about by the head injury. How head-injured individuals and their significant others cope with these changes depends to a great extent on the patterns of interaction, role expectations, and history of conflict resolution that characterized their relationships before the injury (Kozloff, 1987). At best, family harmony is precarious during adolescence. The added stress of the behavioral manifestations subsequent to head injury can be an insurmountable barrier without support services.

American society values individual rights and responsibility. The "American ethic" places responsibility for action on the individual or family structure. Patterns emerge for dealing with the head injury based on the family's basic beliefs and values about conflict resolution which are embedded in its cultural framework. Some deny that the individual has limitations (some may blame others) while others, at first denying the limitations, eventually acknowledge them. "Families who reached out for help from significant others, hospital personnel, and community organizations immediately after the trauma are most often the ones who have in the past requested and received professional services" (Kozloff, 1987).

In Kozloff's study it was the woman who ultimately became the head-injured son's sole source of task-oriented and emotional support. Household social standing decreased significantly from preinjury to postinjury, and this was often related to the fact that the mother stayed home to care for the head-injured child.

Lack of communication among professional caregiver, the individual, and his or her family about the head-injured survivor's prognosis and the resources available for long-term management is frequently cited as a major family concern (Kozloff, 1986). This speaks clearly to the need for a coordinated case-management system of services. Families need education with respect to TBI, information with respect to available services and support systems, and guidance on managing their family members' needs.

The types of support services needed by families at different points of reentry should be identified.

One of the most needed services for families is respite care. Opening up options for head-injured youth for camping experiences, time away from home in productive, meaningful programs, would offer families needed respite as well as prepare the young person for leaving home. Building independence skills and fostering autonomy are much more difficult with disabled teenagers. Programs within the community could address these issues.

A major concern for families is "What happens to my family member if I am not here to take care of him or her?" This becomes a larger societal problem of how do we care for those in the society unable to care for themselves. Of course the goal of successful community integration is that this concern can be addressed through the coordination of services matched with individual needs so that adaptive community living is possible.

Community Survival Skills/Adaptive Behavior/ Activities of Daily Living

Impairments in functional community skills have great impact on the adolescent's ability to integrate into the community. Rarely are these skills addressed directly with teenagers. There has been some effort to instruct educators (Cohen, 1986; Savage, 1987; Ylvisaker, 1986–1987) to incorporate strategies to remediate cognitive deficits which underlie community survival skills. However, there has been little in the literature to demonstrate the effectiveness of this approach. Outcome data (Fryer and Haffey, 1987) has shown that for some individuals it is more productive to teach community skills through teaching compensatory strategies for the functional activities themselves. It is likely that this may also be the case for adolescents. More research needs to be done in this area. We need more data on the "proper match" between treatment goals and individual deficits.

Identifying the barriers to reentry, developing strategies to eliminate these barriers, and working specifically on these strategies has proved effective in individual cases.

Example

Eddie suffered diffuse brain damage with particular damage noted in the frontal lobes and right parietal lobe as a result of a motorcycle accident at the age of 16. He was in a coma for 5 days out of his 36-day hospital stay. He was discharged home to mother and two younger brothers. Eddie had been a B-C student at school, a good athlete, popular with both boys and girls, and active in student affairs. Upon returning to home and school, he had trouble remembering, trouble following through with plans, and began to act out aggressively in class. His friends began to avoid him. After many physical fights he was suspended from school. He started drinking with some kids he had not known before. He decided to quit school, get a job, and live on his own. At this point he was referred to a head-injury program for testing. Assessments demonstrated that Eddie was unable to monitor his behavior in relationship to the immediate environment. His ability to learn new information was compromised by his impairment in organizing information. He was not taking care of daily grooming due to short-term memory problems. His impulsiveness led to an inability to control his emotions and to socially inappropriate behavior. Eddie needed specific intervention in how to structure information internally and externally. He needed to deal directly with self-awareness and realistic goal setting. He also needed to develop compensatory memory strategies. Eddie entered a brain injury day treatment program. The social worker went to the school and worked with a group of his peers to teach them about head injury and also specific ways to handle the impulsive behaviors that Eddie might exhibit. The social worker and the special educator from the brain injury program did in-service training with the high school teachers.

The brain injury program special education teacher taught Eddie strategies for organizing information and specifically for following through on assignments. She worked with the teachers at the school to structure Eddie's assignments in manageable ways. The speech pathologist worked with Eddie to develop compensatory memory strategies. Eddie's mother met with the team and organized a plan for Eddie to follow at home so that he could follow a structured routine and yet have some feeling of autonomy.

The recreation therapist from the brain injury program introduced Eddie to a weight lifting program at the Y.M.C.A. Soon Eddie was participating in a volleyball program he found, with the help of the recreation therapist, at the Y.M.C.A. He also started tutoring some younger children who came to the Y.M.C.A. for after school care. The recreation therapist also organized some outings with Eddie's friends. Eddie wanted very much to start driving again. The occupational therapist worked with him on driving skills. She and the social worker together worked with Eddie and his mother to plan practice sessions and guidelines with respect to driving. Eddie's case manager from the brain injury program worked with Eddie's school to develop an IEP for him, which included continued work at the brain injury program, to continue work on community survival skills (activities of daily living) which might not be dealt with directly at school, as well as transitioning into an academic program with supports built into it at school. The IEP plan was completed for the duration of the school year and included a 5-year plan with vocational goals. The vocational rehabilitation counselor helped plan Eddie's vocational program. He helped assess Eddie's present and potential work skills in regard to specific vocational training programs. Eddie's plan was to graduate with his peers but not formally receive a diploma so that he could remain in school until age 21 to complete his vocational technical school program and be placed in a job. The case manager at the brain injury program would continue to facilitate training for transition from his mother's home to independent living. The brain injury day program staff worked with the community county health department to prepare staff for crisis intervention if necessary for Eddie and his family, as well as ongoing counseling for Eddie's mother to help her cope with the new pressures Eddie's brain injury placed on the family.

Funding

Major funding issues for adolescent community integration revolve around coordination of efforts and smooth transitions. With the passage of P.L. 94-142 and subsequently P.L. 98-199 schools were given the responsibility for educating all children with handicaps in the least restrictive environment. If the child fits back into the school comfortably, perhaps integrating into one of the existing special education programs, this does not present a problem. If, however, the child does not find his or her niche within the school system, how are services funded? Clearly there must be coordination between educational services, rehabilitation services, and vocational services. Schools may provide services to children until they are 22. Providing opportunities for young adults to use this opportunity for vocational preparation should be offered through management of coordinated services.

If the child requires rehabilitation services before reentering school or in conjunction with school they may be funded in a variety of ways.

Insurance usually covers medical rehabilitation. Creative cooperative efforts may be worked out among responsible payers (insurance, schools, vocational rehabilitation) to provide needed services for the adolescent. This, however, requires information about the needs of head-injured individuals as well as education with respect to head injury in general for each party as well as a plan for coordination of services both generally and specifically.

Medical System

Although in outcome studies to date cognitive and psychosocial factors have been clearly identified as the issues that are the greatest barriers to successful community integration, the physical sequelae of TBI cannot be ignored.

Impaired mobility, when it exists, remains a substantial barrier to community integration. There are still many unanswered, even unstated questions with respect to effects of age on a once injured system. How will an organic system injured before it is fully developed progress through later stages of development and interaction with the environment? Endurance, disrupted sleep, subtle visual problems, and other sensory impairments, that is, touch, taste, hearing, as well as chronic pain, are all issues that persist and have been particularly noted in mild head injury. These conditions need to be followed from a medical perspective within the community.

The issues of a health care model versus a sickness treatment model expressed so eloquently by Roberta Trieschmann (1987) stress the concept of a systems approach to interventions. Biological-organic function needs to be addressed with ongoing interventions within an adaptive environment, encouraging functional independence to work around or compensate for altered biological function. Rather than waiting for medical crisis the challenge becomes facilitating a balance among psychosocial, biological-organic, and environmental influences. Health becomes a function of the interaction of these variables.

Definitions of health implying wholeness and perfection become static and arbitrary. Biologic-organic factors need to be treated as one factor in the balancing act leading to health. The personal, spiritual, and environmental influences all have similar influence in the equation (Trieschmann, 1987).

What are the implications of this viewpoint for community integration?

Ongoing health care needs to be provided within the community. Resources for preventing complications and the comprehensive management of chronic disability need to be as valued as those for treating acute episodes.

Specific information about consequences of traumatic brain injury needs to be widely disseminated within the medical community.

Psychopharmacological issues are as important in community integration as they are in acute medical care and rehabilitation. Continued research in biochemistry, as well as efficacy studies with respect to specific pharmacological interventions, are critical to management of traumatic brain injury beyond the acute stage of recovery. Facilitating successful adaptation after a traumatic injury is greatly enhanced by stabilizing behavior and maximally increasing organic function.

Therapeutic Services

Traditional therapeutic services (occupational therapy, physical therapy, speech and language therapy, recreation therapy, social services, psychology services) are often required after an adolescent has been released from a medical rehabilitation program. In the case of TBI, these more traditional services need to be integrated into a categorical brain injury program. This provides for a comprehensive approach which may need to include cognitive training and social skill training to prepare the child for or enhance participation in a school program. Frequently an adolescent will need a period of therapeutic services before returning to school as well as additional rehabilitation services while in school, as discussed above under community survival skills.

Living Setting

Adolescents, as well as younger children, generally live at home with their families. After traumatic brain injury, families are eager to have their children at home with them and frequently do not understand the burden a disabled child can place on family functions. If the child has been developing normally, there is the increased stress of comparing current function with pretrauma function.

Without carefully orchestrated plans for support services, families are frequently left to manage alone. As a followup to the survey done with TBI youth (Fryer, 1987), a brief interview was conducted with each family. Those families interviewed expressed the greatest needs in the areas of respite care, behavioral management, and developing peer supports (friendships) for their teenaged children.

For adolescents who require specialized residential services options are very limited. Long-term medical facilities are usually not designed to provide a stimulating environment for teenagers. Residential placements designed for emotionally or behaviorally impaired youngsters do not always have an understanding of TBI necessary for developing intervention strategies for these individuals.

Learning to live independently is one of the challenges of late adolescence. With disruptive behavioral sequelae, impulsivity, poor judgment, impaired memory function, characteristic of TBI, this challenge may become overwhelming. Specific supports may be needed to address functional residential skills (budgeting, meal preparation, household chores, etc.) and community survival skills (transportation, banking, shopping, etc.). These are not typically provided to adolescents through the school system.

Specific living alternatives must also be made available for adolescents and young adults so that the natural transition to independence from family may take place. In some instances this may be an interdependent situation. Condeluchi (1987) presents a range of living settings that span from most to least supervised. Many of these options are discussed in Chapter 20, Adult Community Integration.

INTEGRATION OF FUNCTIONAL SYSTEMS

A coordinated organized system for community integration after TBI does not currently exist. Pieces of this system exist, and parts of other systems may be appropriate for providing services or supports for successful adaptation.

Community integration represents those comprehensive, coordinated services required by persons with traumatic brain injury and their families after acute medical and neurological treatment diminishes. The concept includes the educational, vocational, recreational, residential, social, emotional, and other support services that may be needed that will enable the person with TBI to live as independent a life as possible in integrated settings with nondisabled peers and relatives.

Planning for these services should begin while the person is still hospitalized, as a coordinated effort, involving family, community liaisons, representatives from community services, and other personnel concerned with the person's treatment program and community reentry process. The person *with the traumatic brain injury should be included in the decision-making process to as great a degree as possible.* Successful community integration is accomplished through a coordinated network of services and support assistance unique to each situation.

The need for and intensity of these community-based, integrated services will vary, depending upon the person's age, severity of impairments, and psychosocial and environmental factors. For younger adolescents with TBI, the services required may focus more on educational and socialization skills. For older adolescents, the focus of community integration may be more on vocational rehabilitation and independent living skills services.

Community integration is a process of social adaptation. Services that exist to facilitate this process for other groups may be appropriate for individuals after TBI if personnel is properly trained, services are coordinated in a comprehensive delivery system providing options designed for the special needs of TBI, and the system is managed and monitored through individual case management.

Considerations for a Model System

Flexibility is an essential feature of a model system because of the extensive number of unknowns. Some needed services will await new understanding or new technology. Flexibility will be required for funding, training, research initiatives, service options, and all other parts of the system. Coordination of all components of the system must be designed from the outset.

Several states have recommended a statewide coordinating body such as a Head Injury Council to coordinate and oversee the entire head injury system (Maryland, California, Massachusetts, Michigan). In order for this type of coordinating body to be effective it must have appropriate authority and staffing.

Along with *flexibility* and *coordination* (with operational and regulating authority), a *case management* system should be developed. The complex and rapidly changing service delivery system needed to deliver services after TBI make this activity essential. Case managers could be expected to provide a broad range of services including data collection (incidence and severity of new head injury, current need for services), basic training for families, advocacy for head-injured individuals, coordination of head injury training programs for service providers, and timely referral for all services (DHMA Maryland Task Force, 1987).

It is clear that the complicated, diverse long-term needs of traumatic brain injury require sophisticated case management. An interesting policy question is who does case management. The most logical source of case management is the payer of services. It should be in the payers' best interests to provide the "best product" to their clients, thus assuring the best services for the TBI survivor and family. The best examples of this are private insurers' catastrophic management plans and worker's compensation case management systems. On the other hand, when there are limited (or unlimited) resources, efficient case management becomes less of a priority and inefficient and ineffective allocation of resources can occur. One perspective of case management is as a monitoring system. There is a question, then, as to whether the case manager should be within or outside of the system.

The family is ultimately the case manager. As Kozloff (1987) points out, "The greatest responsibility for the head injured is assumed by the family rather than the community." Providing the family with support to stay together is then a major service need.

As discussed earlier, the survivors of traumatic brain injury require a variety of services to assure community integration. Specialized services need to be provided due to the unique and complicated needs of the brain-injured individual. However, many of these services may be provided in established service delivery systems.

Examples of this are the educational system, vocational rehabilitation system, and mental health system. With adequate *training* and *staffing* these well-established delivery systems could provide community services for TBI. In order for specialized programs to develop, TBI needs to be recognized as a category for service delivery. Comprehensive *assessment* is a priority issue in TBI rehabilitation. Appropriate placements, prognosis, and long-term service needs are dependent on timely, relevant, meaningful assessments performed by a well-qualified professional team. Continued research needs to be conducted in this area.

There is a great need for networking rehabilitation services for TBI. Each person is a unique individual and needs a unified approach to rehabilitation. All the service needs discussed earlier need to be integrated into a coordinated delivery system, so that individual plans can be created from options presented, thus avoiding duplication of and gaps in service delivery.

A long-term relationship between the brain-injured individual and family and case manager may be crucial if the head-injured individual is to be convinced to follow recommendations and remain in his or her program.

Prevention must be addressed as part of a coordinated system of traumatic brain injury services (DHMA Task Force, 1987). For teenagers it is particularly important to have prevention programs available through schools, driver's education programs, and vocational programs, perhaps also through the criminal justice system. Prevention of repeat head injuries should be a very high priority in the management of all head-injured individuals. Avoidance of substance abuse should also be a central theme. *Training* for all service providers on an ongoing basis is necessary for adequate community services to support community integration after traumatic brain injury.

Research needs to be a priority in a traumatic brain injury system. Many questions remain unanswered in this field. Merely providing more services will not solve all the problems.

Data on incidence and severity need to continue to be collected. Many states have instituted Trauma Registries. However, these data are not uniformly collected. Comprehensive needs assessment surveys should be conducted as part of an ongoing research effort to document needs of the head-injured individual and his or her significant others at different phases of recovery. These data should help to identify the intervals of time at which professional assistance should be made available and the types of interventions best suited to the population being served. In addition, an analysis of the people likely to be most successful in providing support and the methods that would be most constructive in doing so should be undertaken (Kozloff, 1987).

There is also a need for efficacy and outcome studies on the issues discussed earlier as well as many others. These are complicated and expensive studies and should be done under the guidance of careful researchers.

Funding is always an issue in developing and maintaining a comprehensive system of care and services to support successful community integration. Adequate staffing to operate coordinating functions and case management is necessary. Reimbursement needs to be available for the broad array of services within the public and private sectors. These funds represent investments designed to keep traumatically brain injured individuals out of long-term institutions to retain intact families, to decrease lifelong public income subsidies, and to return individuals with a TBI to self-directed lives and when possible to the paying labor force (DHMA Task Force, 1987).

Post-acute rehabilitation programs, community reentry programs, and community support services all need to be designed to support the individual in pursuing quality of life. For most people this means a degree of control over their environment and a sense of productivity.

Community integration services may include post-acute rehabilitation. This includes:

1. Outpatient services such as physical therapy, occupational therapy, psychology, social services, etc.
2. Categorical brain injury day programs, with focus on cognitive retraining, socialization, and vocational training.
3. Transitional residential programs, with focus on community skills, cognitive retraining, vocational training, and behavioral management.
4. Residential school programs with a behavioral focus.

Community integration services also include services that exist in the community:

1. Educational programs: public schools (mainstream), special education, and community colleges.
2. Vocational rehabilitation: prevocational training to include socialization skills, behavior management, and cognitive training; vocational training.
3. Mental health programs, including client counseling, family counseling/education, and support groups.
4. Avocational programs, such as fitness programs (exercise), community interest groups, and recreation.

Community integration also needs to include services to support self-directed living situations:

1. Home health, including the services of an R.N., O.T., P.T., or aide.
2. Supervised living arrangements.
3. Interdependent living.

The specific service and support needs for adolescent community integration which emerge from a review of the interactive functional systems presented earlier are as follows: peer support, appropriate educational intervention, work preparation and placement, recreational activities, family support and respite, independent living skills, community survival skills, and long-term living arrangements. Coordination of service needs, matching service needs to service delivery, and preparation of service providers in regard to traumatic brain injury are key issues in successful community integration.

In order to gain understanding and give direction to our efforts in integrating individuals who have experienced a traumatic brain injury meaningfully into the community, research is crucial. Research issues have been posed as part of the discussion of each system above. Following is a summary of research issues with respect to adolescent community integration from which specific hypothesis may be generated for study. Developing standardized assessment measures and the use of a uniform data bank are overiding issues.

ISSUES FOR FUTURE RESEARCH

Educational System

Cognitive retraining research issues include: (a) efficacy of interventions for specific deficits at different stages of recovery; (b) recovery curves correlated with developmental curves; (c) the impact of organic impairment within the developing brain with respect to social adjustment over an extended period of time; and (d) generalizability of task-specific learning.

To ensure successful school reentry, the following should be investigated: (a) effectiveness of specialized educational programs; (b) patterns of transitions—comparing different models, gathering data on creating a "good match" between program goals and individual characteristics; (c) effectiveness of teacher/family training; (d) and ways to train and involve peers in the reintegration of youth into the social system.

Vocational System

The following should be explored: (a) assessment techniques; (b) matching clients with services; (c) cost-effectiveness of models of vocational services—what service, for whom, and when; and (d) effectiveness of staff training.

Social System

Social research should investigate: (a) increasing strength and durability of social systems; (b) the impact of residual impairment on developing social cognition; (c) the impact of disability on developing self-concept within the social network; (d) efficacy of substance abuse treatments; (e) long-term effectiveness of behavioral interventions; and (f) effectiveness of targeting at-risk populations for specific prevention interventions.

Emotional State

Areas for study should include: (a) personality disorders as a consequence of TBI (descriptive data, development of interventions, efficacy of treatment, outcome variables) and (b) psychopharmacology.

Recreation/Leisure

The effect of leisure activity on outcome should be systematically studied.

Family Roles

The following issues should be investigated: (a) the family adaptation process; (b) differential effects on siblings, parents, and family status; and (c) support services—types of services needed at different times in recovery/adaptation process.

Therapeutic Services

Specific research questions with respect to efficacy of treatment for different severity levels at different times in the recovery process need to be addressed—i.e., when and for whom is a residential-treatment model more effective than a day-treatment model. Also, clearer descriptions of entrance and discharge criteria need to be developed for specific programs based on outcome data.

Community/ADL Skills

The receiving community is as important a factor in community integration as is the physical, cognitive, and emotional status of the individual. Creative ways to prepare and train the community for community reentry need to be developed and researched.

REFERENCES

Barin J (1985): Counseling the head injured. In *Head injury rehabilitation: children and adolescents,* ed. M Ylvisaker. San Diego: College Hill Press.

Ben-Yishay Y, Silver S, Piasetsky E, Rattok J (1987): Relationships between employability and vocational outcome after intensive holistic cognitive rehabilitation. *Journal of Head Trauma* 2:35–48.

Boll TJ (1983): Minor head injury in children—out of sight but not out of mind. *Journal of Child Psychology* 12:74–80.

Bond MR (1975): Assessment of the psychosocial outcome after severe head injury. In: *Outcome of severe damage to the central nervous system.* New York: Elsevier–North Holland Publishing Company.

Brooks DN (1983): Personality and behavioral change after severe blunt head injury—a relative's view. *Journal of Neurology Neurosurgery and Psychiatry* 46:336–344.

Brooks DN, Campsie L, Symington C, Beattie A, McKinlay W (1987): The effects of severe head injury on patient and relatives within seven years. *Journal of Head Injury Rehabilitation* 2:1–13.

Cohen R (1986): Education re-integration and programming for children with head injuries. *Journal of Head Trauma Rehabilitation* Vol. 1, No. 1.

Condeluchi A, Cooperman S, Seif B (1987): Independent living: settings and supports. In: *Community re-entry for head injured adults,* ed. M Ylvisaker, EMR Gobble. San Diego: College Hill Press.

Maryland State Department of Health and Mental Hygiene, Task Force on Closed Head Injuries, 3/03/87. Unpublished.

Erikson E (1963): *Childhood and society.* New York: W.W. Norton & Company.

Ewing-Cobb L, Fletcher J, Levin HS (1985): Neuropsychological sequelae following pediatric head injury. In: *Head Injury Rehabilitation: Children and Adolescents,* ed. M Ylvisaker. San Diego: College Hill Press.

Fletcher JM, Ewing-Cobb L, McLaughlin EJ, Levin HS (in press): Cognitive and psychological sequelae of head injury in children: implication for assessment and management. In: B Brooks, D Hoelzer (eds.). *The injured child.* Austin: University of Texas Press.

Frey WO (1984): Functional assessment in the 80's: a conceptual enigma, a technical challenge. In: *Functional assessment in rehabilitation,* ed. AS Halpern, MJ Fuhrer. Baltimore: Paul Brookes Publishing Company.

Fryer J (1984): Five-year follow-up study of a cognitive training program. Presented at the 8th Annual Post-Graduate Course on the Rehabilitation of the Brain Injured Adult, Medical College of Virginia, Williamsburg, VA, June 1984.

Fryer J (1987): A three-county survey of traumatic brain injured high school students. Unpublished.

Fryer J, Haffey W (1987): Cognitive rehabilitation and community re-adaptation: outcomes from two program models. *Journal of Head Trauma* 2:51–63.

Gobble EMR (1985): *Career development head injury rehabilitation in children and adolescents,* ed. with M. Ylvisaker. San Diego: College Hill Press.

Goldstein K (1952): The effects of brain damage on the personality. *Psychiatry* 15:245–260.

Hagen C (1981): Language disorders secondary to closed head injuries: diagnosis and treatment. *Topics in Language Disorders* 1:73–87.

Havighurst RJ (1972): *Developmental tasks and education.* New York: McKay.

Jacques ME (1970): *Rehabilitation counseling: scope and service.* Boston: Houghton-Mifflin.

Kozloff (1987): Networks of social support and outcome from severe head injury. *Journal of Head Trauma* 2:14–23.

Levin HS, Benton AL, Grossman RG (1983): *Neurobehavioral consequences of closed head injury.* New York: Oxford University Press.

Levin HS, Grossman RG, Rose JE, Teasdale G (1979): Long-term neuropsychological outcome of closed head injury. *Journal of Neuropsychology* 50:412–422.

Lezak MD (1987): Relationships between personality disorders, social disturbances and physical disability following traumatic brain injury. *Journal of Head Injury Rehabilitation* 2:57–70.

Oddy M (1978): Stresses upon the relatives of head injured patients. *British Journal of Psychiatry* 133:507–513.

Piaget J (1983): Piaget's theory. In: KW Kessen (ed.), *Handbook of Child Psychology,* vol 1: *History, theory and methods.* New York: John Wiley & Sons, pp. 103–128.

Prigatano G (1986): *Neuropsychological rehabilitation after brain injury.* Baltimore: Johns Hopkins Press.

Rehab Brief Volume VIII, Number 7, 1985. Prepared by PSI International, Inc. 510 North Washington Street, Falls Church, Virginia 22046.

Reilly K, Faillace (1986): Role of alcohol use and abuse in trauma, advances *Psychosomatic Medicine* 16:17–30.

Rimel R, Jane J (1983): Characteristics of the head injured patient. In: *Rehabilitation of the head injured adult,* ed. M Rosenthal. Philadelphia: F.A. Davis.

Rivara FP (1984): Childhood injuries III, epidemiology of non-motor vehicle head trauma. *Developmental Medicine and Child Neurology* 26:81–87.

Rosen CD, Gerring JP (1986): *Head trauma: educational integration.* San Diego: College Hill Press.

Ruegamer LC, Kroth R, Wagonseller BR (1982): *Public Law 94-142: putting good intentions to work.* Champaign, IL: Research Press.

Rutter M (1981): Psychological sequelae of brain damage in children. *The American Journal of Psychiatry* 138:1533–1544.

Savage R (1987): Educational issues for the head injured adolescent and young adult. *Journal of Head Trauma Rehabilitation* 2:1–10.

Szekeres S, Ylvisaker M, Cohen S (1987): *A framework for cognitive rehabilitation therapy in community re-entry for closed head injured adults,* ed. M Ylvisaker, EMR Gobble. San Diego: College Hill Publications, Little, Brown, and Company.

Szymula G, Schleser R (1986): A reappraisal of vocational evaluation from an ecological systems perspective. *Rehabilitation Literature* 47:224–229.

Thomsen IV (1984): Late outcome of very severe blunt head trauma: A 10–15 year second follow-up. *Journal of Neurology, Neurosurgery and Psychiatry* 47:260–268.

Tobis, Pari, Sheridan (1982): Rehabilitation of the severely brain injured patient. *Scandinavian Journal of Rehabilitation Medicine* 14:83–88.

Trieschmann RB (1987): *Aging with a disability.* New York: Demos Publications, p. 47.

United States Department of Labor (1972). Handbook of Analyzing Jobs. (Reprint 13) Menomonie, WI: University of Wisconsin, Stout, Stout Vocational Rehabilitation Institute.

Weddell, Oddy M, Jenkins (1980): Social adjustment after rehabilitation: A two-year follow-up of patients with severe head injury. *Psychological Medicine* 10:257–263.

Weiner R (1985): *P.L. 94-142—impact on the schools.* Arlington: Capital Publishing Company.

Will, M (March/April 1984): Programs for the handicapped, clearinghouse on the handicapped. Department of Education, Office of Special Education and Rehabilitative Services, Office of Information and Resources for the Handicapped, Washington, DC.

Ylvisaker M, Gobble EMR (1987): *Community re-entry for head injured adults.* San Diego: College Hill Publications.

20

Adult Community Integration

Harvey E. Jacobs, Ph.D.

Department of Psychiatry and Biobehavioral Sciences,
Neuropsychiatric Institute, UCLA Medical Center, Los Angeles,
and Casa Colina Hospital, Pomona, California, U.S.A.

Community integration may be a relatively new topic in traumatic brain injury rehabilitation, but it has a long history among other populations of persons with disabilities (Beard, Malmud, and Rossman, 1979; Bernstein, Ziarnik, Rudrud, and Czajkowski, 1981; Dalrymple, Richards, and Frieden, 1985; Fairweather, Sanders, Maynard, and Cressler, 1969). The concept of community integration has existed at least informally since the first persons suffering disability attempted to return to their premorbid lifestyle, probably in some cave. In many historical periods, community integration was the responsibility of the person with the disability. The individual tried the best he or she could to eke out some level of self-sufficiency. Some people were fortunate enough to befriend others or institutions such as churches for their basic sustenance. In other periods, society provided at least some level of public assistance for persons with disabilities, typically at a substandard level of living.

A central issue in community integration is what type of community the person should integrate into. In the early 1800s crucial concepts of Pinel's moral treatment focused on independent communities away from the daily stressors of the "normal" population. In concept, here was a community where persons with psychiatric disabilities could live, farm, and follow a fulfilling community existence separate from the rest of society. "Prayer, good manners and occupied hands and minds . . ." were considered key elements for rehabilitation. Idleness was considered a contributing factor to psychiatric disability, and a full complement of activity and productivity were leading prescriptions of the time. The importance of functional work and personal gain was also recognized by other psychiatric contemporaries such as Freud, Kraepelin, and Rush. Over time, however, the promise of Pinel's moral community and other "holistic" treatment communities deteriorated as concept met reality. Many of these separate societies gradually evolved into the massive institutions that were to remain well into the twentieth century (Jacobs, Donahoe, and Falloon, 1985).

Landmark changes in public advocacy and human rights legislation since the 1950s paved the way for a different concept of community integration, this time with disabled and nondisabled people as equal members within one society. Perhaps best exemplified among persons with developmental disabilities, but also replicated by others, significant gains have been made over the past three decades in helping many people become active members of society, with all *rights* and *responsibilities* (Ruegamer, Kroth, and Wagonseller, 1982).

This time, treatment, living arrangements, and daily life patterns are being incorporated into "normative" society, resulting in changes both for persons with disabilities and for the general public. Cut curbs, accessible buildings, rights to education, rights to decide about the receipt of treatment, and many other issues are evidence of some of the changes that are beginning to occur.

Community integration also exists for persons with traumatic brain injuries within this social framework. Vocational rehabilitation systems, public education programs, hospitals, social service agencies, legal services, and other programs have never *excluded* persons with traumatic brain injuries from their services. The problem has been a *lack of distinction* regarding the unique needs presented by this population.

Attempts to equate presenting problems of this population, which often superficially relate to other types of disabilities, have not always been successful (Musante, 1983). For example, to the untrained professional lethargy may indicate amotivation or malingering instead of problems with arousal or attention. The client may subsequently be denied benefits based on an assumption of noncompliance rather than a treatable neurobehavioral deficit. Aggressive behavior disorders may be treated through neuroleptic medications because of apparent psychiatric manifestations, although these medications may actually be counterindicated for brain injury. Poor executive functions may be seen as indifference rather than an inability to make a difference. As a result, many persons with traumatic brain injuries fall through the cracks of service delivery systems because of improper assessment of presenting needs and inadequate knowledge about proper treatment approaches by those who provide the services (Fawber and Wachter, 1987).

The purpose of this chapter is to review some of the critical issues related to community integration for adults who have experienced traumatic brain injuries. These include education, work, social interaction, emotional reactions, recreational and leisure activities, community skills, funding, medical services, therapeutic services, living settings, legal issues, and family involvement. Unfortunately, there is no substantial base of literature for review because of the relative infancy of this area in brain injury rehabilitation. Hence, information was collected from available literature on postacute outcome and contact with selected professionals and programs in the field. Although the incidence of minor and moderate traumatic brain injury surpasses that of severe traumatic brain injury, the chapter focuses more on severe injury by virtue of the greater research and publication in this area. The following section provides a general overview of each of the areas noted above followed by recommendations on future needs and systems.

CRITICAL ISSUES RELATED TO COMMUNITY INTEGRATION

Adult Education

Because the average age at incidence of traumatic brain injury is 22 years, the majority of this population have completed their formal education at the time of their injury. In the Los Angeles Head Injury Survey, of the 25% who were in school at the time of their injury, 33% returned to school postinjury (Jacobs, 1987a). However, these figures do not take into consideration the amount of time lost between injury and return to school, changes in the course of study or class work, or decreased performance that may be noted postinjury. It is assumed that persons with minor and moderate traumatic brain injuries have relatively better outcomes.

Educational systems are not formalized for adults in the manner available for those under 22 years of age (Rosen and Gerring, 1986). With no legislation such as PL 94-142, adults must rely on a patchwork of systems and programs to continue their education. Private adult educational systems are not well established. Most frequently they consist of individual therapists (or programs) who work with the individual and a local school to facilitate class attendance and course requirements. The cost of such programs is determined by the combined costs of the school program and therapist fees.

Public education systems such as community colleges, adult education programs, and universities may offer a potpourri of services including general counseling for students with disabilities, specialized courses, programs that help individuals enter mainstream courses, or entirely specialized curriculums. The scope and magnitude of services vary across the country.

One of the earliest recognized full curriculum programs developed for this population was at Coastline Community College, in Costa Mesa, California. Developed out of the college's Office of Handicapped Student Services, the program offers a two-year curriculum designed to help persons with acquired brain injuries develop functional daily skills and possibly attain competitive community employment. In this program, students work through a series of seven areas, including cognition, communication, psychosocial adaptation, academic preparation, psychomotor skills, independent living, and vocational training. Approximately 100 persons are served by the program per year, at a cost to each student of $50 per semester. The remaining costs are covered by the State of California. Encouraged by the popularity of the program, other community colleges in California have adopted portions of the program into their services. The entire curriculum has also recently been published (Cook, Berrol, Harrington, Kanter, Knight, Miller, and Silverman, 1987).

Educational programs are often used for other reasons besides formal degree matriculation. Within the limited sample of the Los Angeles Head Injury Survey, less than 10% of those in school postinjury completed a degree. In some cases, educational settings are used as a prevocational assessment before placing the individual in a job (i.e., the ability to participate in prolonged course work may be a good measure of how a person may respond at work).

A second use for adult educational systems has been as a high-level day activity placement for those who are not job-ready and present no significant behavior problems. In such settings, the person may learn new skills and participate in a variety of academically and cognitively oriented tasks appropriate to their abilities. A school versus day treatment setting can also help to improve self-esteem and increase opportunities for socialization that may not otherwise exist. On the other hand, expectations that the school will result in a formal degree and job potential may not be well founded. Many families and persons who experienced a traumatic brain injury find a sense of loss and lack of direction after their participation in the time-limited educational program has ended and there is no subsequent placement or marketable degree. More work is needed to address the availability, eligibility requirements, and goals of postinjury educational programming.

Vocational

Work is a central element of most adult life and plays a significant role in our daily roles and functions (Weiss and Reissman, 1961). The importance of work on well-being has also been noted among nondisabled populations in which the incidence of physical and mental illness, asocial behavior, marital problems, and other stressful life events have been correlated to job loss (Catalano, Dooley, and Jackson, 1981; Dooley and Catalano, 1980; Jahoda, Lagrsfeld, and Zeisel, 1960).

The ability to work is also perceived as an important indicator of rehabilitation outcome (Anthony, 1979; Anthony, Buell, Sharratt, and Althoff, 1972; Anthony, Cohen, and Vitalo, 1978). In order to find and keep a job, the individual must be able to execute a broad range of social, community, vocational, and personal management skills that ensure stable patterns of behavior. Deficits or lapses in any of these areas can result in job loss. In this manner, work is a test not only of a person's vocational competence but of his or her overall social abilities.

Employment offers additional advantages. The work environment may provide social support networks and sources of leisure and recreational contacts. Job-related income is often the only way to cover the costs involved in community tenure. Finally, work helps the person transform his or her social status from a dependent to a contributor.

Unfortunately, returning to work is elusive for many persons who have experienced a traumatic brain injury. Those with adult injury onset face the challenge of trying to return to work. Those who experienced their injuries before entering the work force face a different experience of working for the first time. Hence, the field faces two challenges: (1) helping persons with work experience return to a job (rehabilitation) and (2) teaching persons with no experience how to work (habilitation).

Research findings have generally reported overall low levels of vocational activity postinjury, with some distinction relative to the severity of the injury. Between 20% and 43% of all persons with severe traumatic brain injuries return to competitive community employment, although frequently at a lower job level than preinjury (Jacobs, 1987a, 1988; Levin et al., 1979; Mikula and Rudin, 1983; Weddel et al., 1980; Thomsen, 1974). Perhaps twice as many persons with moderate or mild head injuries return to work, depending on the criteria used for vocational outcome (Ben-Yishay, Silver, Piasetsky, and Rattok, 1987).

Helping persons with traumatic brain injuries return to work requires comprehensive and continual coverage. Traditional approaches of assessment, training, and placement are frequently insufficient to ensure vocational success. Generic vocational assessments and interest inventories need to be supplanted with functional assessments and in vivo evaluations in simulated and real work settings that are tailored to the challenges faced by this population (Fawber and Wachter, 1987).

The concept of successful outcome following 60 days of job placement is also insufficient for this population. Many persons with a traumatic brain injury are able to remain employed for several months before problems develop. Part of this may be due to the subtle and discrete nature of "high-level" sequelae that many people face. Although many persons can perform most of the basic tasks required to enter a job, they begin to develop "cracks" over time that threaten job tenure (e.g., perceptions among co-workers, poor social skills, variable rates of performance, incidents that by themselves are not critical but add up over time, etc.). Cognitive, emotional, or behavioral sequelae may make it more difficult for the person who experienced a traumatic brain injury to manage these issues. Too often, the person is unaware of the impending situation until it is too late to rectify it.

Supported work models and job coaching may help promote job longevity or rebuild the self-esteem of a worker who is returning to a lower-level job (Fawber and Wachter, 1987; Musante, 1983). Training in job maintenance, social, interpersonal, independent living, daily problem-solving skills, and a host of other skills contribute to outcome. For example, the person who is technically proficient but cannot work with his or her co-workers is not likely to be retained. Similarly, stellar performance on the job can be undermined by marital problems at home, a poor living situation, financial difficulties, or other "extra-curricular" issues.

The challenges faced by those beginning work differ from those who are returning to work, owing to a greater emphasis on training and initial skill development. Unlike the experienced worker, the new worker has no personal or historical reference on which to base his or her behavior, or to understand the mores of the work place. Many have had little opportunity to develop prevocational skills (e.g., getting to work on time, cooperating with co-workers, proper grooming, etc.) or to practice any technical skills learned in the classroom. If the person presents no technical skills of market value he or she may be relegated to unskilled and transitory work, if work is an option at all. Hence, prevocational and technical skills training is just as important as job placement for this unseasoned population. Success in training will be at least partly dependent upon the individual's cognitive, emotional, behavioral, and other postinjury abilities.

Vocational service delivery systems may also vary with the treatment services that the person can afford. Those covered by workmen's compensation insurance may be provided with intensive private vocational rehabilitation services in addition to services that are available to the general public. Services may be provided to the individual until he or she is able to return to work or is considered permanently disabled.

Persons with accident and health insurance policies or public aid are less likely to receive comprehensive vocational rehabilitation since these services are usually not considered medical in nature. Preliminary vocational services can sometimes be provided through occupational therapy during the course of inpatient or outpatient treatment, but are usually limited in value and do not provide critical on-the-job programming.

Sometimes it is possible to convince insurance companies that extra-contractual funds spent on vocational rehabilitation will be cost-effective in preventing future injuries; the argument is that a person who is involved in a productive and structured setting such as work is less likely to be re-injured. However, the persuasiveness of such an argument has not been adequately substantiated.

Those without private funding must rely on public programs, which are generally focused around state vocational rehabilitation programming. Although a number of states have become increasingly responsive toward the needs of persons with traumatic brain injuries, far too many clients continue to "fall through the cracks." Part of this problem may be traced to systems that are overburdened with case loads and cannot provide the individual attention that this population requires. Inadequate knowledge and training of counselors in traumatic brain injury is another factor. A third issue is a frequent emphasis on positive case closure. Vocational counselors may be less willing to take on cases that are too time consuming if their productivity is measured in absolute numbers of persons placed. Job placement and job maintenance are frequently two separate factors requiring different forms of assistance.

Changes in the direction and focus of agencies can also influence service delivery. For example, in recent years, some vocational rehabilitation programs have reportedly changed their emphasis from helping those in the greatest need to helping those who have the greatest chance of returning to work. This is based on the assumption that fixed resources can be more "profitably" used among those who are closer to entering the competitive job market. The "cost" of such planning is to decrease opportunities for those who require more assistance or a vocational alternative to full-time competitive employment.

In summary, the ability to help individuals return to work, or economic self-sufficiency, is a cornerstone of rehabilitation efforts in this country and has frequently been used to justify its cost (Berkowitz and Berkowitz, 1983; Wright, 1980). Preliminary work in this area for persons who have experienced a traumatic brain injury has been equivocal and inconclusive. The need for more work in the design and validation of work rehabilitation programs is evident, but so is the need for increased training of those who provide these services, program availability, services networking, funding mechanisms, and assessment of vocational competence among persons with traumatic brain injuries who are attempting to enter the work force.

Simple prediction of vocational potential based on a one-time screening is unlikely to be useful for many individuals, given the complexities of work. In-vivo work performance evaluations may be more effective given the diversity of skills and situations in which the individual needs to be evaluated over time (Ben-Yishay, Silver, Piasetsky, and Rattok,

1987). This approach has proved highly successful for other populations of persons with disabilities (Jacobs, 1987b).

Ultimately, not everybody who experiences a traumatic brain injury will be able to enter competitive employment and a wide range of options from supported employment to day activity need to be explored. Program cost is but one issue to address, in conjunction with other factors including clinical effectiveness, entitlement, and social contribution.

Social

Literature over the past 20 years has noted that social, behavioral, and cognitive sequelae may have a greater influence on long-term outcomes than physical sequelae. Surveys have reported that 21% to 38% of the population are socially isolated (Caveness, 1966; Levin, Grossman, Rose, and Teasdale, 1979; McKinlay, Brooks, Bond, Martinage, and Marshall, 1983; Weddell, Oddy, and Jenkins, 1980), and many other individuals face decreased opportunities for socialization and a loss of friendships.

Lack of socialization affects both the individual and those around the individual. Social isolation frequently follows changes in emotional lability, financial resources, mobility, or an inability to keep up with established peer groups. Behavioral changes such as disinhibition, poor judgment, temper tantrums, and poor social skills all contribute to decreased friendships. Reduced comprehension of social mores and social perception may also affect opportunities for interpersonal interaction.

Without traditional outlets for socialization such as work, school, or community activities, persons with traumatic brain injury have few opportunities to develop new social networks. Many become dependent upon immediate care providers for this support, increasing already extended levels of family burden and obligation above acceptable or even manageable levels. This can result in burnout and erosion of the basic support networks that the individual needs to participate in the community. In the absence of pro-social opportunities, the individual may also turn to drugs, alcohol, or negative peer groups for sources of attention and support.

"Programmed" opportunities for socialization through community groups, outings, camps, or other programs for persons with disabilities barely scratch the surface of need or acceptability for this population. First, the limited number of programs do not meet the diversity of interests and abilities. Second, many of these programs include persons with developmental or psychiatric disabilities because they are similar in age to the traumatic brain injury population. However, many persons who have experienced a traumatic brain injury prefer not to be labeled as disabled, feel that association with other populations of persons with disabilities connotes the stigma that these populations may carry, and they may not be capable of acknowledging their own deficits.

Most community programs also focus on services for persons with developmental or psychiatric disabilities due to the relative tenure of these populations in the community. Limits in funding often preclude services for other needs. Addressing this situation requires education and adjustment for both the individual with the head injury and the community program. Both must adjust within their capabilities and resources. Perhaps most important, it is necessary to recognize each individual for his or her abilities and contributions to society, rather than any deficits or diagnosis.

Social skills training can also be effective in helping persons reestablish social competence. Social skills training procedures have been remarkably successful with a variety of different populations (Bellack and Hersen, 1979; Bellack, Hersen, and Turner, 1976; Wallace, Nelson, Liberman, Ferris, Lukoff, and Falloon, 1980), but work is still early relative to the present population (Gajar, Schloss, Schloss, and Thompson, 1984). A key issue in social skills training involves the ability of the participant to generalize the skills taught in the classroom to real-world (community) situations. This requires in-vivo (real-situation) training as well as concept-based training strategies that have only recently begun to be addressed by the field. In addition, many persons who have experienced a traumatic brain injury may not be aware of their deficits or be willing to try to solve problems that they do not perceive.

In summary, decreased socialization represents one of the most frequently identified problems among persons who have experienced a traumatic brain injury. This impact can be noted throughout a wide range of life areas, both for the individual and for those who compose his or her social network. Most adult social networks are in a constant flux as jobs change, interests change, or people move. New opportunities for socialization are provided by the constant flow of new people and topics that most of us encounter during the course of the "normal" day. A wide range of posttraumatic sequelae can interfere with these opportunities, thereby decreasing and potentially destroying the delicate social network that most of us weave. Programmed opportunities for socialization and social skills training may provide partial solutions to personal stagnation. However, a holistic approach is needed to fully address this problem. This involves recognizing the interdependent roles that each component of adult life plays in contributing to the overall quality of life for a person living in the community.

Emotional

There are frequent reports of adverse emotional and behavioral reactions following traumatic brain injury. Lishman (1966) noted that 86%

of those surveyed experienced psychiatric or emotional problems, which was comparable to the 84% noted in Thomsen's (1974) study. In the Los Angeles Head Injury Survey (Jacobs, 1987a, 1988), at least 90% of the participants studied experienced at least one behavioral disorder postinjury and approximately 25% experienced severe behavior disorders that significantly interfered with daily life. Similar levels of emotional or behavior disorder have been noted by Najenson et al. (1980) and Lezak et al. (1980). The specific issues of greatest incidence have included anxiety, depression, withdrawal, aggressive behavior, temperament, decreased initiation, poor self-control, and attention seeking.

Data on the levels and frequency of behavioral or emotional dysfunction among persons with mild or moderate traumatic brain injuries are not conclusive, owing in part to less research among these populations. In addition, only those with presenting problems come to the attention of the treatment community. This leaves a possibly large "silent majority" of persons with mild or moderate traumatic brain injuries absent from representation or analysis.

Many different factors may be responsible for postinjury emotional reactions. First, changes may occur as a result of neurological damage. For example, persons with frontal lobe damage may be likely to react more impulsively now than before their injury. Temporal lobe dysfunction is frequently ascribed to temper outbursts, rage to hippocampal disturbances, and so on.

A second factor may relate to emotional reactions toward postinjury dysfunction. Hence, a person who has a short-term memory disorder may become frustrated when he or she cannot remember what to do next. Or, a person with poor stamina may become depressed when he or she does not have the strength to participate in an outing with family or friends. In both cases, it is the person's emotional reaction to a disability that causes the change in behavior.

Emotional factors of adjustment following a catastrophic event are also relevant (Fink, 1967). Accommodation and adaptation to perceptions of mortality, priorities, and future expectations often undergo substantial metamorphosis following a brush with death. The person's perceived social role and outlook on life frequently change. The reconceptualization of these basic personal values may require substantial time and support. Posttraumatic stress reactions may also be evident postinjury, as well as states of learned helplessness (Seligman, 1975). These issues frequently require intervention if the individual is to assume responsibility for his or her daily affairs.

Since many individuals experience their traumatic brain injury in late teen or early adult years, emotional maturity may also not be adequate to meet the presenting challenges. Inadequate ego integrity and self-perception may also contribute to postinjury emotional outcome. Loss of friends and social support can also lead to emotional problems in a classic vicious cycle. Aberrant emotional behavior on the part of the person with the head injury causes others to distance themselves, and this decreases support to the person as well as feedback about his or her behavior. This in turn may result in more acting out, which in turn increases the social distancing by others, and so on.

Issues of denial, accommodation, and acceptance may too simplistically describe the process of emotional adjustment that occurs following a traumatic brain injury. Problems of denial may more often be issues of inadequate information or knowledge. Acceptance may be an unrealistic goal of the rehabilitation community, as few persons may ever accept their decreased abilities, but many accommodate to them. The focus on disability must also be supplanted with a focus on individual ability since it is what a person can do that distinguishes him or her in society, not what he or she is incapable of accomplishing.

Recreational/Leisure

As previously noted, the opportunities for socialization following traumatic brain injury are challenged by many factors. Although accessibility and physical endurance are key variables, transportation, finances, cognitive and neurological abilities, social skills, networking, initiation, and related issues may be more problematical. For example, those who do not drive postinjury have fewer opportunities to engage in activities away from home. Similarly, limited funds due to unemployment may restrict the forms of recreation that are available to the individual.

Changes in functional abilities postinjury can also preclude participation in more demanding avocations. Poor social skills may exclude the participant from group activities as well as the social networks that provide these opportunities. Poor initiation or self-deprecation may result in the person's not planning or joining activities. In the Los Angeles Head Injury Survey 54% of those surveyed did not independently initiate participation in recreational programs, but 69% would engage in activities that were prearranged. Families reported that many individuals stayed out of public activities because of physical problems or poor self-image.

With a lack of external opportunities for leisure and recreational activities, many persons turn to their families and primary caregivers for support, with mixed results. Family recreation may be limited, caregivers may become overburdened with this added responsibility, and family members need personal recreational time of their own. Formalized recreational programs such as Saturday Clubs, where people congregate one weekend day, provide a relatively new alternative while also providing respite for family members. Camps, friendship matching boards, special-event clubs, and general community programs involving city services, churches, and schools are also sporadically available. Programs specifically designed for people with disabilities have varied success relative to the individuals involved, program curriculum, and individual interest. Available programs are often in short supply or do not match the personal interests of the participants. In other situations, the individual may choose not to associate with persons from other disability groups or even other persons with traumatic brain injuries because of a perceived stigma of being classified as disabled.

Regardless of the origin of any type of recreational program, diversity and "normalization" are key factors in facilitating successful socialization for this population. A brain injury does not define a person; it defines only a specific aspect of that individual. As a population, persons with brain injuries represent a diverse group of individuals with diverse interests and expectations. Recreational and leisure programming must be able to meet these needs in order to be successful.

Community Skills/Adaptive Behavior

There are at least two approaches to community skills training following traumatic brain injury. One approach involves helping the person return to premorbid levels of community competency. A second focus involves helping the person learn new skills that are relevant to their new status, especially if significant disabilities are present.

As with other life areas, postinjury levels of community competency will be affected by the sequelae that the person with the traumatic brain injury experiences. Problems with physical or emotional stamina, judgment, perception, and other factors adversely affect ability as well as opportunity. Persons who cannot arrange or conduct their own local transportation are unable to travel to the community resources they seek. Poor problem solving or overreaction to stressful situations also takes its toll, especially when one is trying to respond to the "red tape" involved in most public programs. The ability to return to one's "old self" is dependent on the ability to remediate these deficits.

Because not all deficits can be remediated, the individual may also find himself or herself in a new world that requires different skills to meet daily community challenges. Part of this challenge can be met by learning how to adapt to postinjury abilities and deficits. Both therapeutic and prosthetic approaches can help facilitate this change. Learning how to obtain services that one can no longer provide for oneself is also critical. Consumerism, advocacy, and accessibility take on new meaning following a traumatic brain injury. Few people learn the skills required to advocate and access rights for persons with disabilities prior to a catastrophic injury, but they are expected to demonstrate these abilities after the injury. Unfortunately, development of these competencies is expected to occur in the face of probable emotional, behavioral, and learning deficits. Families and other direct care providers frequently assume the role of advocate when the affected individual cannot. Still, it often takes years to learn the maze of tattered resources and rights for persons with the brain injury and their significant others.

For a growing population of individuals with traumatic brain injuries, new opportunities for program development and advocacy are needed. With increasing numbers, persons with traumatic brain injuries and their supporters have the potential to become a stronger political voice and become more effective in obtaining the resources required to meet their needs. Increased numbers may also present more lucrative markets for program development and service delivery in both the public and private sector. Ultimately, community competency involves the ability to manage one's strengths and resources in order to facilitate successful tenure in the community.

Funding

Funding for community integration services is sporadic and frequently dependent upon the etiology of the injury. People who are injured on the job are usually covered by worker's compensation insurance, which traditionally has a greater responsibility in helping the individual return to premorbid status, especially in the area of vocational productivity. Persons who suffered their injuries through the liability of others and successfully sue for compensation may also have at least some of the resources necessary for extensive help. However, few people receive sufficient, if any, compensation for their injuries.

Most cases are covered by accident and health insurance policies that provide medical treatment in medical-based facilities. Unfortunately, most community integration activities are considered educational or psychosocial rather than medical in nature and do not qualify for coverage. Although insurance companies may occasionally fund nonmedical services in the belief that a well-adapted and integrated person is less likely to have a second injury, or other medical complications, this has been addressed on a case-by-case basis with no general precedent in the industry.

Persons with no insurance who are dependent on Medicare, Medicaid, or other public funds often receive primary inpatient medical treatment and some outpatient medical treatment, but few other options. Limited public funds may be available for respite or day-care services, but the level of funding rarely provides the resources required for active and effective levels of community intervention. When return to work is a possibility, state vocational rehabilitation services may be used with the limitations previously noted.

Secondary sources of funding can come from public programs for persons with disabilities. For example, HUD Section 201 funds are available to develop low-cost housing programs for persons with disabilities including traumatic brain injury, but may take up to two years to receive. Some financial assistance for work-related activities is available to persons receiving Supplemental Security Income (SSI) or Social Security Disability Insurance (SSDI) compensation from the Social Security Administration (Kodimer, 1988). Impairment Related Work Expenses (IRWE) can be deducted against earned income each month in determing levels of significant gainful activity and subsequent SSI or SSDI benefits for that month. These deductiions may include a variety of prostheses, medications, and in some cases professional interventions that are directly related to the person's ability to work. Whether or not costs associated with supported employment programs or job coaching would also be allowed as an IRWE has not been determined.

Personal assistance monies, usually available to persons with physical disabilities, may be pooled in certain circumstances to provide joint services. For example, many residents in a cooperative living arrangement could pool their resources to provide the appropriate group treatment milieu required for independent community living. Whereas each member may individually receive 30 to 40 hours of attendant care per week, several clients working together can assure their group of more efficient round-the-clock coverage through pooled resources. These funding sources currently offer more promise than service since they have been used only on a limited basis.

Private alternatives for community funding are available for some individuals with sufficient resources. Long-term cooperative living arrangements have been suggested where each person with a traumatic brain injury buys into a house or program. A monthly maintenance fee covers ongoing program costs. When the person leaves, the space can be sold to someone else. Program members may range from persons with traumatic brain injuries to a mix of people with and without disabilities. Unfortunately, few people have the funds to initiate or support these programs. In some cases, this problem can be ameliorated if one person with substantial resources buys the house and provides low-cost rent to others. The "landlord" in this arrangement benefits by the fact that he or she will not become socially isolated since other people will be sharing the living environment.

Finally, blended funding of both private and public monies must also be considered. This may include supplementation of Social Security or state disability stipends with private funds, matching funds for public grants, and other sources. Regardless of the source(s) of funding, questions of personal entitlement, social responsibility, and financial capability must also be addressed when considering the overall costs and national priorities of community integration for persons with traumatic brain injuries.

Medical

Persisting physical disabilities generally preside over medical stability in community integration. It may be presumed that by the time the person returns to the community, he or she will be medically stable, with a general morbidity similar to that of the overall population. However, numerous forms of long-term physical disability are common postinjury and may require continued care. These may include decreased stamina, sensory disorders, weakness, paralysis, imbalance, vision, seizures, and similar issues. Most of these disorders are diagnosed soon after the injury and will begin to be addressed during formal stages of rehabilitation. Epilepsy is one of the few disorders that may develop years after the injury, although the chances of its occurrence decline over time (Jennett, 1983; McQueen, et al., 1983).

The continuing effects of physical disabilities will vary according to their individual nature, severity, and course of treatment. Presenting disabilities will partially determine the level of community adaptation that the individual is capable of relative to personal goals, adaptive procedures to circumvent the specific disabilities, and general living environment.

The medical community plays a much greater role than medical management in community integration, as physicians and hospital emergency rooms are frequently the first source of contact for many of the long-term problems that this population faces. Accordingly, it is important that they understand how to identify and properly refer presenting issues to appropriate services. In addition to medical considerations, the long-term neurological, neuropsychological, cognitive, and behavioral consequences of the trauma must receive preeminent consideration.

The treatment community must also take a responsible position regarding "cures" for long-standing problems. Although most persons who have experienced a traumatic brain injury and their families learn to live with presenting deficits, the hope of a cure for persisting sequelae remains at least a subliminal priority. Owing to the developmental status of the field, it is inappropriate to close the door on new or alternative treatment approaches that may hold some promise. Professionals must take responsibility for helping persons with traumatic brain injuries and their families learn how to evaluate the credibility, validity, and potential outcomes (both positive and negative) of any such services. The information must be presented in a manner that affected individuals can understand and use to make logical decisions.

Finally, many persons with traumatic brain injuries face significant challenges obtaining medical insurance for general health care. Some persons may continue to be covered postinjury through Medicare/Medicaid, or health insurance from work, family members, or group plans. However, a substantial number of people are not eligible for such support and find individual health insurance too expensive. Many insurance plans also exclude coverage for preexisting conditions, including any illness that may be related to traumatic brain injury or other neurological damage. This can deny the individual a wide range of necessary protection including treatment for a second traumatic brain injury, stroke, or other neurological disorders that may occur irrespective of the initial injury. Alternative and affordable health care plans are needed for this segment of the population.

Therapeutic

Community-oriented therapies focus on helping the person overcome fixed deficits and acquire skills necessary for improved community function (Condeluchi and Gretz-Laksy, 1987). Traditionally these services are delivered by individual therapists, transitional living centers, day hospitals, day-care programs, home programs, or residential centers. Treatment frequently focuses on cognitive, behavioral, and functional skill training orientations.

Although many people may benefit from such services, programs are often inaccessible and costly. Private therapist time is expensive and most funding sources do not cover community integration services. This has predictably hampered program growth, which in turn has resulted in a sporadic distribution of services.

An alternative approach to formal community-based traumatic brain injury programs has been to access generic community resources to meet the specific needs of the individual. Utilizing general community programs such as parks, libraries, and volunteer services, as well as more specific programs for persons with handicaps (e.g., vocational rehabilitation, medi-rides, etc.), it is possible to piece together a service delivery system to meet some of the needs of an individual. Because few of these programs were developed for persons with traumatic brain injuries, their focus and accessibility are often incomplete and may compromise the needs of the individual. For example, a sheltered workshop developed by a local chapter of the Association for Retarded Citizens may have an opening for a person with a traumatic brain injury, but the focus of the work, peer group, and potential benefit may not meet the individual's goals. Similarly, community day-activity centers more frequently service the elderly or frail than the "walking wounded." Although state vocational rehabilitation services are available to every citizen, their focus may not reflect the needs of persons with cognitive and neurological disabilities but may lean toward more commonly experienced physical handicaps.

Training staff and adapting existing services to meet new needs provide a partial solution to this problem. Where possible, inservices, support, and public advocacy may help to redirect available resources to needed problems. However, there are insufficient resources to meet existing demand. Other populations of persons with disabilities may also be competing for the same resources. Existing programs serving one population may also be unable to stretch their programs to meet different needs.

Returning to the community and remaining in the community are also two separate goals, with correspondingly different tasks. Therapeutic approaches that stress concept formation must frequently give way to functional adaptation where individuals learn how to respond to daily challenges in the community within their existing abilities and resources.

The concept of therapy itself may also not be wholly productive to community integration. Therapy typically implies some form of dependency by one person upon another to help ameliorate a problem. Functional adaptation, on the other hand, connotes personal responsibility, maximizing the independent abilities of the consumer. Within the community, treatment must change over time from the directive to a supportive process, providing a framework for individuals to develop their greatest levels of self-sufficiency, self-respect, and self-worth possible. This focus on functional abilities and adaptive change helps the individual regain independent skills while receiving support in areas of insufficient skill competency, thereby facilitating their community tenure.

Living Setting

Upon hospital discharge, most people return to live with a family member unless they present significant sequelae that are beyond the scope of family management. This smaller group of people will move into transitional living centers, nursing facilities, institutions, or other alternative residences. Regardless of the initial placement, many people face significant changes in living arrangements within months of hospital discharge for a variety of reasons.

Marital problems begin to accelerate one year postinjury, resulting in separations and divorce (Jacobs, 1987a). Temporary placements following discharge from the hospital may become permanent placements if injury-related sequelae persist or alternative living arrangements are not located. Postacute services end as funding sources expire. Living arrangements in the community change as friendships fade in lieu of the person's "new" personality. When these types of problems occur, the person will most frequently return to the home of aging parents (Jacobs, 1987a; Mikula & Rudin, 1983).

As dependent persons with traumatic brain injuries return to their families, parents begin to face the question of what will happen to the nonindependent person after they die. Independent or semistructured living settings for those with moderate to severe behavioral, physical, or cognitive sequelae are rare because of cost and unavailability. Transitional living programs are not a long-term option because of their high cost and overall mission of deinstitutionalization. Board and care facilities, nursing homes, and other institutional placements may become "the least desired" but the only available solution for a number of individuals.

Persisting needs have spawned increasing interest in the development of long-term community-based living programs that provide a low-cost and supportive environment. The primary purpose of such programs is not to provide therapeutic services but to help dependent persons live in the community, away from their families, with the greatest level of independence and self-sufficiency possible. Program costs vary according to the design of the program, but a basic goal is to provide a living environment within the monthly income of the individual. For those receiving Social Security compensation, this may be about $450 per month. Outside sources of support are used to subsidize the remaining costs.

Several notable programs meeting this challenge include Accessible Space Incorporated, of Minneapolis, Minnesota, and Project Headway, of Sylmar, California. Accessible Space Incorporated is a nonprofit agency established six years ago to provide independent living for persons with physical disabilities. The first programs were designed for persons with mobility disabilities, but over the past two years, several houses and apartment settings have been opened for persons with traumatic brain injuries. Program funding is derived from a variety of sources including state and local grants, private donations, federal funds such as HUD monies, and participant rent. Approximately 20 persons with traumatic brain injuries now participate in the program.

Project Headway was started in 1984 by four families who needed to find an alternative placement for their traumatically brain-injured sons, because of behavioral and interpersonal problems. The families purchased a home in Sylmar, California, and designed a low-level intervention program to meet daily living needs. This includes two staff members in the house at all times and limited social programming. Therapeutic services are provided by the program. Part of the costs of the program

are covered by whatever each resident can afford, usually through personal income, Social Security checks, and a small monthly contribution
from the families. The remaining program deficit, of $40,000 to $50,000
per year, is covered by a variety of fundraising programs including theater parties, rummage sales, and private donations from persons directly
contacted by the families. Two additional houses have been established
by Project Headway over the past four years.

Similar programs are gradually being developed across the country
through a variety of funding mechanisms. In some situations, one person with substantial resources may purchase a house and provide living
space for others in exchange for supportive or therapeutic services. In
the cooperative concept, several persons (or their families) buy into a
home or living program and then pay a monthly maintenance fee to
cover ongoing costs. The slot owned by the person with a traumatic brain
injury can then be sold to another person when the living environment
is no longer necessary or suitable to the individual. U.S. Department of
Housing and Urban Development monies are also being solicited in conjunction with independent living programs as another means of funding
such programs. However, these monies may be difficult to obtain and
frequently require 18- to 24-month lead times.

Despite the future promise of community-based living programs for
persons with traumatic brain injuries, their relative inaccessibility and
uncertain funding mechanisms make them generally illusive and unavailable. The most pressing challenge lies in the development of cost-
effective funding and operating mechanisms that allow dependent persons
with traumatic brain injuries to take a more self-sufficient, independent, and long-term role in their community.

Socially Unsanctioned Behaviors

Socially unsanctioned behaviors may include substance dependency
(alcohol and drugs); criminal, aberrant, or excessive behaviors; inappropriate sexual conduct; and violent outbursts. The area may be one of the
least studied and most presumed issues in community integration for
persons with traumatic brain injuries.

Some forms of socially unsanctioned behavior may be evident prior to
the injury. For example, it is estimated that half of all persons who
experience a traumatic head injury were intoxicated at the time of their
accident (Reilly, Kelly, and Faillace, 1986; Rimel and Jane, 1983; Tobis,
Puri, and Sheridan, 1982). Although one episode of intoxication does not
implicate chronic substance dependency, it is inferred that at least part
of this population may have been habitual users before injury onset.
Others, with little or no prior history of substance dependency, may develop dependencies postinjury with a variety of substances, because of

boredom, lack of social opportunities, inability to work or go to school, pain, anxiety, personality changes, or new peer group influences.

The combination of deficits incurred from substance dependency and brain injury can compound the problems of addressing these individual disorders. Poor judgment, lack of insight, impulsiveness, and other neurobehavioral deficits mix poorly with the effects of drugs and alcohol, resulting in even greater levels of unawareness and behavioral dysfunction. There are few if any substance abuse programs directed toward the specific needs of persons with head injuries (National Head Injury Foundation, 1988). Treatment generally involves the use of established detoxification programs followed by participation in Alcoholics Anonymous or other support group programs. There is little data on success rates or outcomes, and it has been noted that there may be no cure for some individuals, but rather lifelong management of the problem, requiring prolonged and intensive intervention (Falconer and Tercilla, 1985).

Social skill deficits may also lead to civil sanctions for inappropriate behavior, relative to community mores and level of dysfunction. The individual with a poor frustration tolerance who gets into arguments is likely to be ignored or shunned by others. If the behavior builds into physical confrontation, the individual will face stronger public reaction and possible professional treatment. Inappropriate sexual behavior may receive a similar reaction especially as it relates to disinhibition, impulse control, and the need for sexual gratification. "Harmless" but rude comments are likely to be ignored while stronger or more perseverative behaviors will come under community sanction and intervention. Poor social adjustment, lack of awareness of behavior and its consequences, or miscomprehension of social mores further exacerbates these problems.

As behavior becomes more aberrant, it moves into the realm of the criminal treatment system. At least one study on selected prisoners has noted that many had histories of traumatic brain injuries and other neurological insult (Lewis, Pincus, Feldman, Jackson, and Bard, 1986). While these types of studies present considerable data for speculation, the findings must be considered correlative rather than predictive, because of the selective manner in which the information was collected. For example, does having a traumatic brain injury mean that a person is more likely to engage in criminal behavior, or does criminal behavior result in a greater likelihood of experiencing a traumatic brain injury? It is clear, however, that there are a significant number of persons with traumatic brain injuries in the criminal justice system who are currently operating at an impaired level. Regardless of whether the criminal behavior or the traumatic brain injury occurred first, both are now present and may signify the need for a revised approach to their treatment and management.

Legal

Adults who have experienced a traumatic brain injury face a diverse array of legal issues. These include the rights and responsibilities as adult members in society, issues of competency, financial trusts, conservatorships, the right to decide on treatment, and interface with the legal system.

Trusts and conservatorships present the most frequent issues. Methods of preserving capital and resources that facilitate the long-term community sustenance of the individual are of eminent concern to families of dependent persons with a traumatic brain injury. Public benefits such as Social Security do not provide sufficient support for productive community tenure, and few people have the necessary capital for lifelong living programs. There is also frequent concern about the ability of the person to effectively manage daily expenses, let alone any principal sum of money that must be husbanded over a lifetime. Structured support plans and trusts can be developed through attorneys and legal aid programs, but many consumers need basic education about the purpose and availability of such opportunities before they can pursue them. Funding these plans is another obvious issue.

Conservatorship is a much thornier issue involving financial and legal competency. Many persons who have experienced a traumatic brain injury are capable of managing their affairs either independently or with some assistance. In other cases, dependent persons with brain injuries may be able to competently manage part of their life but not other aspects. An individual who is not aware of signficant deficits may also fight any motions for conservatorship. Too, some families may be over-protective and inappropriately seek conservatorship as a means of controlling their family member. Unlike the obvious deficits presented by a person in a persistive vegetative state, the person living in the community presents more subtle deficits, which can make proper adjudication of the case difficult. There are few accepted guidelines to follow in this area. Evidence of functional capacity that is acceptable to the medical and rehabilitative communities is not uniformly accepted in court (Koplan, 1988). Careful deliberation of all information is also critical when considering restrictions on the rights and responsibilities of any individual, and many jurors have insufficient background about brain injury to assess such information.

As competent adults, those who have experienced the head injury can legally make decisions to obtain or decline treatment. In most cases, treatment problems relate to insufficient services for expressed needs rather than refusal to consent to treatment. Because the right to decide on treatment is constitutionally based, the rights of the individual must be judiciously guarded. Implicit within this right to make a decision, however, is the social responsibility to assume the consequences of one's decision, a responsibility that may also (rightfully or inappropriately) be assumed by the family of the dependent and legally incompetent person.

When consent for necessary treatment becomes problematical, legal intervention is often required, invoking battles over conservatorship or involuntary treatment. Decisions that arise from this process do not necessarily offer appealing solutions. Deliberation may be prolonged and intrusive. The subsequent determination may only partly address the presenting question and may direct the individual to available but inappropriate services. For example, behaviorally disturbed individuals may be sent to a psychiatric facility where the regime of psychotropic and milieu therapy may actually exacerbate the condition. The length and obtrusiveness of the process also reserve it for the most extreme conditions. Training and intervention programs to help persons with brain injuries and their significant others mediate and negotiate realistic treatment options are needed.

In a similar manner, interface with police and the criminal justice system can also become overly complicated. As previously noted, many long-term postinjury sequelae parallel other disorders. For example, it is not unusual for a person with a gait disturbance to be pulled over for drunk and disorderly conduct (when the officer assumes that the person is walking in the community while intoxicated). The subsequent course of inquiry may further exacerbate the problem, resulting in the individual's having to return to the police station or being temporarily held until the issue is resolved. Weaving through the maze of legal procedures is difficult enough for the general populace, let alone for a person with cognitive deficits. Strident advocacy is required to ensure the most expedient form of due process in each given situation.

In summary, the right of tenure in the community is matched by the implicit responsibilities that all members of the community face. The unique community challenges that persons who have experienced a traumatic brain injury may face must be balanced through personal responsibility, advocacy, and interface with established legal systems. This challenge can be met in part though legislation and public awareness. In the community, however, each person is ultimately the primary advocate of his or her own personal rights, regardless of ability or disability.

Family

The role of family members and their reaction to severe traumatic brain injury has received considerable attention (Brooks, 1984; Brooks, Campsie, Symington, Beattie, and McKinlay, 1987; Jacobs, 1987a, 1988, in press; Jacobs, Muir, and Cline, 1986; Jennett, 1978; Lezak, 1978, 1987; Livingston, 1986; Mauss-Clum and Ryan, 1981; Muir and Haffey, 1984; Panting and Merry, 1972; Romano, 1974; Rosenbaum and Najenson, 1976; Rosenthal, 1984; Rosenthal and Muir, 1983; Rosin, 1977; Thomsen, 1974). Across studies, families are reported to constitute the major source of support, socialization, and assistance to the person with the traumatic brain injury. This support is evident across all major life areas. With few alternatives for care, advocacy, living, or other support systems, family members also often find themselves in a variety of roles that they are poorly prepared for.

Marital breakup, separation and divorce, family discord, physical and emotional illness, and financial problems are all noted to be significantly higher among family members of persons with traumatic brain injuries than in the general population. These problems continue with time rather than dissipate (Brooks, Campsie, Symington, Beattie, and McKinlay, 1987). Part of this may be related to the persistent nature of long-term traumatic brain injury sequelae and the increased involvement of family members. As options for education, work, socialization, and other needs are closed for persons who have experienced a traumatic brain injury, these individuals frequently turn to their families for support.

Most families report mild to severe financial problems immediately following the injury relative to the medical/rehabilitative services required, availability of insurance coverage, and family financial status. For example, in the Los Angeles Head Injury Survey, 28% reported that all or most of their resources were used, 34% reported moderate to mild financial drain, and 34% no change in financial status. For 3%, financial status was reported to improve because of a settlement or receipt of new services. For many these financial problems continue over time. Some people find alternative sources of income to meet their daily need, while many others learn to adapt with less.

However, there are indirect as well as direct costs to the family. In order to be able to live at home many dependent persons with traumatic brain injuries require continuous supervision. In 36.6% of the families surveyed in the Los Angeles Head Injury Survey, a family member had to continuously supervise the person with the traumatic brain injury. In half of these cases, this family member had given up a job or full-time schooling to meet this need, with the resulting loss of income and benefits to the entire family unit.

Because few persons are married prior to their injury, marital status does not significantly change for the overall population. However, the postinjury rate of divorce or separation among those who were married preinjury was higher than the national average. Traumatic brain injury affects both the person with the brain injury and the spouse, and both become different people. The person with the traumatic brain injury changes as a result of neurological damage and reaction to the experience of a catastrophic accident. The spouse may change by virtue of his or her reaction to the chain of events that follow the injury. Over time, changes in both members can begin to adversely affect the marital relationship and lead to its dissolution. Changes in marital status on the Los Angeles Head Injury Survey were particularly evident beginning one year postinjury, a point in time when most formal rehabilitation and supportive services end. Faced with continuing challenges but no continuing support, these marriages appeared to be more susceptible to failure (Jacobs, 1987a).

In the Los Angeles Head Injury Survey (Jacobs, 1987a, 1988), perceptions about the most difficult problems that the traumatic brain injury presented varied with family composition and patient sequelae. Behavioral, emotional, and cognitive problems were generally reported more difficult to cope with than physical problems, and long-term financial issues were a source of concern for everybody. Most parents worried about what would happen to their dependent child once they died. Finding a long-term placement for their disabled child occupied a significant portion of their time. Spouses expressed similar concerns whether they remained in the marriage or chose to leave. Most were still concerned about the individual's quality of life. The direct impact of the traumatic brain injury on other family members also appeared to cause significant stress in most areas of family living.

Help for family members is generally inconsistent. As with most other services for persons with brain injuries, the amount and types of support diminish after inpatient rehabilitation. Ironically, this is when family members need the greatest assistance, as they assume a greater role and responsibility for the needs of the person with the traumatic brain injury (Lezak, 1978, 1987). Support groups provide one means of continuing assistance, but this is not sufficient for many family members. Issues of advocacy, understanding the long-term nature of traumatic brain injury sequelae, finding resources, program development, funding, and personal support can be only partly addressed in monthly peer support groups.

Family members also have limited time to devote to the continuing needs of their traumatically brain-injured member. Although many families may be willing to sacrifice other individual needs at the time of the injury, the personal and communal goals of other members in the family must rebalance over time (Jacobs, in press; Jacobs, Muir, and Cline, 1986; Muir and Haffey, 1984). Hence, jobs or businesses need to be attended to, children grow up and need guidance through their development, personal interests must be pursued, and so on. Although these issues can be deferred for brief periods of time, such as at injury onset, most families cannot maintain these changes indefinitely. Accordingly, the attention and family-unit resources devoted to the person with the traumatic brain injury diminish over time.

Expectations that family members can assume total responsibility for long-term treatment are also ill-founded. Few families have the training to assume such a role or the time and ability to develop the required skills. Professional treatment teams represent decades of diverse education and experience, and it is not realistic to assume that many families can match or acquire this knowledge. It is realistic to teach family members how to ask the right questions to find the people or programs with the proper answers, i.e., to learn how to become effective case managers.

The concept of the family as a therapeutic agent is therefore a critical but limited component in long-term recovery and community integration of adults with traumatic brain injury. Family assistance must be used judiciously, within their individual abilities to contribute and within an overall framework of service delivery and support for this population. Family members may provide *some* of the needed resources for the person with the traumatic brain injury, but they present their own needs that must be addressed as well.

INTEGRATION OF FUNCTIONAL SYSTEMS

Integration of Services

There is considerable linkage between service delivery systems and personal life areas when considering community integration. For example, the fact that a person is unable to work does not simply imply decreased income. It may also mean decreased opportunities for living independently, socializing, or being a social contributor. With a decreased perception of social purpose and fewer outlets for interaction there is also an increased likelihood of despondency and depression. In a similar manner, when a person with a traumatic brain injury returns to live with his or her family, significant financial, emotional, medical, and daily life changes may also occur for family members, well beyond the simple provision of living space.

A working model of community integration must emphasize functional systems of service delivery rather than individual treatment prescriptions. It is incumbent upon programs and service delivery systems to work within the integrated nature of adult community life rather than against it. Hence, providing housing for an individual not only places a roof over his or her head but also helps to establish a new social milieu. It may also present new challenges in community transportation; changes in relationships with existing friends, family members, and former living mates; and perhaps a change in spirit that may either facilitate or hinder other life areas. Similarly, cognitive and behavioral deficits that result in poor attention and concentration will affect not only performance in school but interpersonal interaction, management of daily affairs, and personal business as well.

Successful community integration programming begins early, while the person is still in the hospital. Within weeks of admission, it is critical that initial discharge arrangements, review of funding sources, application for financial aid and other support, assessment of outside living arrangements, and evaluation of social and vocational networks begin. An early emphasis on functional skills development may also be critical to overall success. Without an early estimation of functional abilities and resources it is difficult to direct proper rehabilitation programming or consider posttreatment alternatives.

Although significant emphasis is paid to continuum of services approaches that imply a gradual transition back into the community, the actual community transition often occurs abruptly upon hospital discharge. This is when most financial resources for treatment dry up and integrated service delivery ends. Faced with few resources and limited knowledge of either continuing needs or services, community integration can become a struggle for survival rather than a planned and orderly return to self-sufficiency and social contribution.

Prosthetic versus Therapeutic

Community integration must also address the issue of prosthetic versus therapeutic service delivery. At some point in time, the focus of the person as a patient or survivor ends. The individual must be more properly noted as a person who experienced a traumatic brain injury. This distinction is important because the catastrophic episode of a brain injury does not define the person's entire future or his or her abilities. We may, however, use it to define a specific episode in the person's life and its specific effects on the *overall* individual.

Just as it is improper to consider a perpetual patient role for the person who experiences a traumatic brain injury, long-term community integration cannot assume a perpetual therapeutic or treatment role either. As therapeutic outcome diminishes, it is necessary to direct attention toward prosthetic support rather than amelioration of sustained deficits that may not be responsive to available forms of treatment. It is imperative that we work to help individuals attain prominence within their community, within their individually unique package of abilities and disabilities.

Individual Responsibility and Rights in the Community

Returning to the community must be viewed as a right, not a privilege. However, with this right come the implicit responsibilities that all members of the community face. The residual sequelae following a traumatic brain injury may require a different role for the individual post-trauma, but each competent person still retains the same social responsibilities of all adult community members. As a member of the community, each individual has the right of self-determination as well as the responsibility for the choices he or she makes. Each person has the right to secure or defer treatment as well as the obligation to find the resources to cover accrued expenses. Refusal or unavailability of treatment may not be sufficient cause for deferral of personal responsibility. Each person has the right to be viewed for abilities rather than deficits. However, this right comes from the active demonstration of such skills rather than via the expectation of respect for "potential."

Exercising these rights requires personal responsibility, advocacy, and coordination of effort among individuals. In a society where opportunities are abundant but rewards are the product of effort, individual persistence and social competence are critical in determining quality of life. Hence, returning to and remaining in the community are often two different issues. The resources and ability of the person with a traumatic brain injury to achieve each must be individually considered.

For those who are not capable of independent community tenure, the question of who is ultimately responsible for continued care remains. Although families have traditionally assumed responsibility for many dependent persons, the life span of the family unit is generally shorter than that of the dependent person. Parents die, spouses separate, siblings and children grow apart, or resources are inadequate to meet presenting needs. Questions about what level of responsibility society maintains for this individual remain unanswered, with services being provided on a take-what-you-can-get approach. This frequently results in a substandard level of living in which the individual is more aptly considered a survivor, a person who is literally hanging onto the fringes of society instead of being a contributor. Questions of whether and how much society should dedicate limited resources to persons with disabilities versus "more capable" people who might improve the quality of life for many are hotly debated but remain unresolved.

Community Case Management

In many cases, the issues faced in community integration are not amenable to cure but can be managed. Like those of any other adult member of society, the priorities, resources, and goals of an adult with a traumatic brain injury fluctuate over time and situations. However, many persons with traumatic brain injuries are not able to manage at least some aspects of their daily affairs, requiring outside assistance, such as a case manager.

For the most part, family members and significant others fill this role, although their abilities may not meet the demands of the position. Private case-management systems are often out of the economic reach of people who need them. Public case-management systems are frequently absent or inadequate in training or mission to meet the demands of vibrant but dependent people. Most public systems focus on assessment and placement rather than ongoing management. The needs of an individual in the community are also not constant, but vary, requiring the case-management system to be responsive to such fluctuations. The notion that "you cannot have a crisis today when your appointment is on Wednesday" may be comical but is unfortunately all too true. Then, too, the individual with the brain injury and the social support system must learn how to use available resources, including case-management systems, judiciously rather than continually.

Finally, it is important to respect the limitations of case management as well as its promise. Case management is a tool, not a panacea. It flourishes because of a need to match services to clients. If the necessary services do not exist, they simply cannot be provided and advocacy rather than case management becomes critical. When properly operated, case management can serve as an effective networking and brokering system to help an individual reach toward his or her potential. When improperly managed, the system may become its own bureaucracy, especially when all services have to go through the case manager.

CONCLUSIONS

The surface of community integration following traumatic head injury has barely been scratched, although there is increasing interest in the area. The concept of community integration is not new. Its formal application to this population is. It is critical to consider a functional systems approach when considering community integration, especially for this population. It is not appropriate to consider treatment or amelioration of specific problems as the key to long-term planning.

Systems of care can impact on personal systems and systems of living, with dramatic repercussions well beyond the individual's life. When properly managed, synergistic outcomes can be facilitated that strengthen the individual's role as a social contributor. This requires interacting with and respecting individuals for their abilities as well as their deficits. The label of "survivor" connotes a person who is barely hanging on to the fringes of society. The recognition of a person who experienced a traumatic brain injury acknowledges the fact that the individual is much more than the catastrophic incident faced at some point in the past.

Obviously more research and program development are needed in this field. This need is noted in each of the individual topic areas reviewed as well as in the integration of these topics into a person's daily life. Questions about cost-effectiveness, outcomes, personal rights and responsibilities, society's responsibilities, law, and ethics remain pervasive. It is also important to learn how systems developed for other populations of persons with disabilities can be used for persons with traumatic brain injuries.

Ultimately, the topic of community integration may be a constitutional issue of what rights, responsibilities, and privileges are guaranteed for each citizen, and which are available for the effort, whether this effort is provided by the individual or advocates.

REFERENCES

Anthony WA (1979): *The principles of psychiatric rehabilitation*. Baltimore: University Park Press.

Anthony WA, Buell GJ, Sharratt S, Althoff ME (1972): Efficacy of psychiatric rehabilitation. *Psychological Bulletin* 78:447–456.

Anthony WA, Cohen MR, Vitalo R (1978): The measurement of rehabilitation outcome. *Schizophrenia Bulletin* 4:365–383.

Beard JH, Malmud TJ, Rossman E. (1978): Psychiatric rehabilitation and long-term rehospitalization rates: The findings of two research studies. *Schizophrenia Bulletin*, 4:622–635.

Berkowitz M, Berkowitz E. (1983): *Rehabilitation research review: Benefit cost analysis*. Washington, D.C.: National Rehabilitation Information Center.

Bellack AS, Hersen M. (1979): *Research and practice in social skills training*. New York: Plenum Press.

Bellack AS, Hersen M, Turner SM (1976): Generalization effects of social skills training in chronic schizophrenics: An experimental analysis. *Behavior Research and Therapy*, 14:291–298.

Ben-Yishay Y, Silver SM, Piasetsky E, Rattok J. (1987): Relationship between employability and vocational outcome after intensive holistic cognitive rehabilitation. *Journal of Head Trauma Rehabilitation*, 2:23–48.

Bernstein GS, Ziarnik JP, Rudrud EH, Czajkowski LA (1981): *Behavioral rehabilitation through proactive programming*. Baltimore: Paul H. Brookes Publishing Company.

Brooks N. (ed.) (1984): *Closed head injury: psychological, social and family consequences*. Oxford: Oxford University Press.

Brooks N, Campsie L, Symington C, Beattie A, McKinlay W. (1987): The effects of severe head injury on patient and relative within seven years. *Journal of Head Trauma Rehabilitation*, 2:1–13.

Catalano R, Dooley D, Jackson R. (1981): Economic predictors of admissions to mental health facilities in non-metropolitan areas. *Journal of Health and Social Behavior* 22:284–297.

Caveness WF (1966): Post-traumatic sequelae. In: Caveness WF, Walker AE (eds.): *Head injury*. Philadelphia: Lippincott.

Condeluchi A, Gretz-Lasky S. Social role valorization: A model for community reentry. *Journal of Head Trauma Rehabilitation* 2:49–56.

Cook J, Berrol S, Harrington DH, Kanter M, Knight N, Miller C, Silverman L. (1987): *The ABI handbook serving students with acquired brain injury in higher education*. Glendale, CA: Glendale Community College/The Consortium for the Study of Programs for the Brain Injured in California Community Colleges.

Dalrymple J, Richards L, Frieden L. (1985): Independent living: An update for the mid-eighties. In: E Pan, T Backer, C Vash, S Newman (eds.) *Annual Review of Rehabilitation Volume IV*. New York: Springer Publishing Company.

Dooley D, Catalano R. (1980): Economic change as a cause of behavioral disorder. *Psychological Bulletin,* 87:450–468.

Fawber HL, Wachter JF. (1987): Job placement as a treatment component of the vocational rehabilitation process. *Journal of Head Trauma Rehabilitation,* 2:27–33.

Fairweather GW, Sanders DH, Maynard H, Cressler DL (1969): *Community life for the mentally ill: An alternative to institutional care*. Chicago, Ill: Adeline.

Falconer JA, Tercilla E (1985): *Chemical abuse and head injury*. Paper presented at the third annual statewide meeting of the Washington State Head Injury Foundation, Belleview, Washington.

Fink S. (1967): Crisis and motivation: A theoretical model. *Archives of Physical Medicine and Rehabilitation,* 48:592–597.

Gajar A, Schloss PJ, Schloss CN, Thompson CK. (1984): Effects of feedback and self-monitoring on head trauma youths' conversational skills. *Journal of Applied Behavior Analysis,* 17:353–358.

Jacobs HE (1987a): The Los Angeles Head Injury Survey: Project rationale and design implications. *Journal of Head Trauma Rehabilitation* 2:37–50.

Jacobs HE (1987b): "Vocational Rehabilitation," In R.P. Liberman and Associates (eds.) *Psychiatric Rehabilitation of the Chronic Mental Patient*. Washington, D.C.: American Psychiatric Press.

Jacobs HE (1988): "The Los Angeles Head Injury survey: Procedures and preliminary findings." *Archives of Physical Medicine and Rehabilitation,* 69:425–431.

Jacobs HE (in press): "The family as a therapeutic agent in long term traumatic head injury rehabilitation." In DE Tupper and KD Cicerone (eds.) *The Neuropsychology of Everyday Life*.

Jacobs HE, Donahoe CP, Falloon, IRH (1985): Rehabilitation of the chronic schizophrenic: Areas of intervention. In E Pan, T Backer, C Vash, S Newman (eds.) *Annual Review of Rehabilitation Volume IV*. New York: Springer Publishing Company.

Jacobs HE, Muir CA, Cline J (1986): Family reactions to persistent vegetative state. *Journal of Head Trauma Rehabilitation,* 1:55–62.

Jahoda M, Lagrsfeld PF, and Ziesel H (1960): *Die arbeitslosen von marienthal.* Allensback & Bonn: Verlag fur Demonskipie, 2nd ed.

Jennett B (1978). If my son had a head injury. *British Medical Journal,* 1:1601–1603.

Jennett B (1983): Post-traumatic epilepsy. In M Rosenthal, ER Griffith, MR Bond, JD Miller (eds.) *Rehabilitation of the Head Injured Adult.* Philadelphia: FA Davis Company.

Kodimer C (1988): Neuropsychological assessment and social security disability: Writing meaningful reports and documentation. *Journal of Head Trauma Rehabilitation,* 3:77–85.

Koplan K (1988): Neuropsychological assessment. *Journal of Head Trauma Rehabilitation,* 3:96–97.

Levin H, Grossman R, Rose J, Teasdale G (1979): Long-term neuropsychological outcome of closed head injury. *Journal of Neurosurgery,* 50:412–422.

Lewis DO, Pincus JH, Feldman M, Jackson L, Bard B (1986): Psychiatric, neurological and psychoeducational characteristics of 15 death row inmates in the United States. *American Journal of Psychiatry,* 143:838–845.

Lezak MD (1978): Living with the characterologically altered brain injured patient. *Journal of Clinical Psychiatry,* 39:592–598.

Lezak MD (1987): Psychological implications of traumatic brain damage for the patient's family. *Rehabilitation Psychology,* 31:241–250.

Lezak MD, Cosgrove JN, O'Brien K, Wooster N (1980): *Relationships between personality disorders, social disturbances, and physical disability following traumatic brain injury.* San Francisco: International Neuropsychological Society.

Lishman WA (1966): Brain damage in relation to psychiatric disability after head injury. *British Journal of Psychiatry,* 114:373–410.

Livingston MG (1986). Assessment of need for coordinated approach in families with victims of head injury. *British Medical Journal,* 293:742–744.

Mauss-Clum N, Ryan MR (1981): Brain injury and the family. *Journal of Neurosurgical Nursing,* 13:165–169.

McKinlay WW, Brooks DN, Bond MR, Martinage DP, Marshall MM (1981): The short term outcome of severe blunt head injury as reported by relatives of the injured person. *Journal of Neurology, Neurosurgery and Psychiatry,* 44:527–533.

McQueen JK et al. (1983): Low risk of late post-traumatic seizures following severe head injury: Implications for clinical trials of prophylaxis. *Journal of Neurology, Neurosurgery, and Psychiatry,* 46:899–904.

Mikula J, Rudin J (1983): *Outcome of severe head injury patients after head injury rehabilitation.* Braintree, Massachusetts: 60th Annual American Congress of Rehabilitation Medicine.

Muir CR, Haffey WJ (1984): Psychological and neuropsychological interventions in the mobile mourning process. In BA Edelstein, ET Couture (eds.) *Behavioral assessment and rehabilitation of the traumatically brain damaged.* New York: Plenum Press.

Musante S (1983): Issues relevant to the vocational rehabilitation of the traumatically head injured client. *Vocational Evaluation Work Adjustment Bulletin,* 16:45–49.

Najenson T, Grosswasser Z, Mendelson L, Hackett P (1980): Rehabilitation outcome of brain damaged patients after severe head injury. *International Rehabilitation Medicine*, 2:17–22.

National Head Injury Foundation (1988): *Substance abuse task force white paper*. National Head Injury Foundation, Southborough, MA.

Panting A, Merry PH (1972): The long term rehabilitation of severe head injuries with particular reference to the need for social and medical support for the patient's family. *Rehabilitation*, 38:33–37.

Reilly EL, Kelly JT, Faillace LA (1986): Role of alcohol use and abuse in trauma. *Advances in Psychosomatic Medicine*, 16:17–30.

Rimel RW, Jane JA (1983): Characteristics of the head-injured patient. In M Rosenthal, ER Griffith, MR Bond, JD Miller (eds.) *Rehabilitation of the Head Injured Adult*. Philadelphia: FA Davis Company.

Romano MD (1974): Family response to traumatic head injury. *Scandinavian Journal of Rehabilitation Medicine*, 6:1–4.

Rosen CD, Gerring JP (1986): *Head trauma: Educational integration*, San Diego, CA: College-Hill Press.

Rosenbaum M, Najenson T (1976): Changes in life patterns and symptoms of low mood as reported by wives of severely brain-injured soldiers. *Journal of Clinical and Consulting Psychology*, 44:881–888.

Rosenthal M (1984): Strategies for intervention with families of brain injured patients. In BA Edelstein, ET Couture (eds.) *Behavioral assessment and rehabilitation of the traumatically brain damaged*. New York: Plenum Press.

Rosenthal M, Muir CA (1983): Methods of family intervention. In M Rosenthal, ER Griffith, MR Bond, JD Miller (eds). *Rehabilitation of the head injured adult*. Philadelphia: FA Davis Company.

Rosin AJ (1977): Reactions of families of brain-injured patients who remain in a vegetative state. *Scandinavian Journal of Rehabilitation Medicine*. 9:1–5.

Ruegamer LC, Kroth R, Wagonseller, BR (1982): *Public Law 94-142: Putting good intentions to work*. Champaign, Ill: Research Press.

Seligman MEP (1975): *Helplessness: on depression, development and death*. San Francisco, CA: WH Freeman and Company.

Thomsen IV (1974): The patient with severe head injury and his family. *Scandinavian Journal of Rehabilitation Medicine*, 6:180–183.

Tobis JS, Puri KB, Sheridan J (1982): Rehabilitation of the severely brain injured patient. *Scandinavian Journal of Rehabilitation Medicine*, 14:83–88.

Wallace CJ, Nelson C, Liberman RP, Ferris C, Lukoff D, Falloon IRH (1980): A review and critique of social skills training with chronic schizophrenics. *Schizophrenia Bulletin*, 6:42–64.

Weddell R, Oddy M, Jenkins D (1980): Social adjustment after rehabilitation: A two year follow-up of patients with severe head injury. *Psychological Medicine*, 10:257–263.

Weiss RS, Reisman D (1961): Social problems and disorganization in the world of work. In RK Merton, RA Nisbet (eds.) *Contemporary Social Problems*. New York: Harcourt, Brace and World.

Wright GN (1980): *Total rehabilitation*. Boston: Little, Brown and Co.

21

Concluding Remarks

Paul Bach-y-Rita, M.D.

The National Institute for Disability and Rehabilitation Research (NIDRR) has identified TBI as a priority area, and through the Office of Special Education and Rehabilitation Services it co-sponsored a national TBI meeting to evaluate the current status of the field and to set a research agenda. In addition to professionals involved in basic research, early trauma care, hospital-based treatment, rehabilitation, and community reentry, participants included federal agency representatives, consumers and their families, and representatives of the co-sponsors of the meeting, the NHIF. Each invited participant was asked to comment on the present status of his or her research area, and to suggest future research areas. Extensive discussions with other participants during the three-day meeting were valuable in achieving the goals of the conference. Further, lunch conferences by consumers, by a perceptive family member, and by Secretary of Education William J. Bennett, and a panel discussion by federal agency representatives helped to provide the tone of the meeting.

The recent interest in TBI has brought attention to a field that spans many disciplines and interest groups, but which is still in the process of developing an identity, a data base, and a consistent approach in each of its components and at each of its stages from injury through immediate care, coma management, hospital treatment, rehabilitation, and community reentry. In the absence of a strong scientific base, many components of the TBI management community have developed programs that remain to be tested. For example, Larry Marshall, M.D., has been quoted as pointing out in his keynote address to the National Head Injury Foundation that there are now 1,400 or more software packages for cognitive retraining and none of these has been properly tested. Yet there is a need now—today—for today's traumatic brain-injured per-

319

sons. Many conference participants emphasized the need to deliver services while others emphasized the need for research and validation of treatment methodologies. Agreement between these groups on the distribution of scarce resources was not obtained. The high cost at every stage of the saga of TBI patients compounds the problems related to the determination of the distribution of those resources.

How many TBI patients are there? What is the incidence, the age distribution, the average length of treatment? What percentage of patients receive appropriate treatment by present standards (for example, Dr. Clifton noted that probably no more than 10 to 20% of TBI patients nationally are receiving the benefits of early trauma care)? How many receive rehabilitation services? These are just some of the questions that must be addressed in order to establish a data base. But the absence of a uniformly accepted nomenclature and classifications (e.g., what are the characteristics that determine whether a TBI patient should be classified as mild, moderate, or severe?) compounds the difficulties in establishing a data base.

The role of theory and of basic research in the development of treatment methodologies was emphasized by several speakers. It was noted that in the case of polio, although vast sums were spent on improved iron lungs and on improved treatment, the major breakthrough emerged from a basic science lab: the identification of the polio virus, leading to the development of a vaccine and the virtual elimination of polio. Comparable advances in neurotransmitter research, in brain plasticity research, in edema control and improved vascular perfusion research, and in several other areas could lead to significant therapeutic advances. However, the largest influence on TBI would be improved measures of prevention. Reduction of drunk driving, improved automobile construction, and injury reduction measures such as air bags, greater use of seat belts, and helmet use by motorcycle riders could lead to dramatic reduction in the incidence of TBI.

Federal agency representatives had strong words of advice for the participants. Dr. Michael D. Walker, director of the Stroke and Trauma programs of the National Institute of Neurological and Communicative Disorders and Stroke of the National Institutes of Health, emphasized the need for controlled studies, adequate definitions of methodologies, hypotheses, and articulated and carefully set endpoints. We need to do research on TBI methodologies since we do not yet know the kinds of research we should be doing. Critical to good research is nomenclature: we must be able to communicate among ourselves, and we must have adequate measurements and assessments of our approaches. Each therapy that we employ must be validated according to the usual scientific approaches. There are no shortcuts.

Dr. Walker pointed out that models are needed. We need animal models and we need human models. However, the controlled clinical trials are still essential; they are the prime tool by which we make progress in any field. The controlled, prospective, randomized clinical trial is one of the hardest things to do, but it is the linchpin of progress. Dr. Walker noted that heterogeneity is often invoked as the reason controlled trials cannot be performed, but he stated that heterogeneity washes out in the randomizing procedure. He considers that other factors invoked as barriers to clinical trials (such as spontaneous recovery) are equally invalid, and thus the trials should be developed. Many of the research methodologies used in cancer, heart disease, and stroke studies can serve as guides for TBI research. Dr. Walker sees a major problem in our becoming paralyzed by the size of the problem we have in the TBI field. Research issues must be not only prioritized but sequenced, since certain things must be done before we move on to other things. It's not good enough to have a thesis on rehabilitative activity; that thesis must then be translated into a research hypothesis, which will in time be built around the methodology with defined endpoints that can show the difference. Researchers must maintain the flexibility to move wherever the science tells us we should move. Flexibility is required not only from the research community but also from federal agencies. He emphasized that the brightest ideas come from the community rather than from centrally established research agendas.

Dr. Green, representing the Veterans Administration, emphasized the need to evaluate cognitive therapies, because they are expensive and time consuming. He also noted the importance of training and, in particular, training of interdisciplinary teams. Both Dr. Green and Barbara Brown, also of the VA, described the great increase in interest by the VA over the last three or four years, with a large number of phone calls and letters requesting services for TBI patients. Ms. Brown pointed out that it is very difficult to request additional funding for TBI programs because of the present inability to provide answers to questions such as: how many patients need the care? what kind of data do you have to show that it makes a difference? She pointed out that the individual professional groups making up the multidisciplinary team are each concerned about their own turf. Among critical issues requiring data are: outcomes over several years, the role of the environment where care is given, and cost containment. She noted that we have created the awareness of TBI needs and she hopes we can stay with it to see appropriate programs develop.

Representatives of the Administration of Developmental Disabilities, the Social Security Administration, and the Rehabilitation Services Administration expressed strong support for the TBI programs and mentioned areas of particular interest, such as the inclusion of TBI in the mandate of Developmental Disabilities, evaluation of state programs, assessment of quality of life, independent living, the characteristics of TBI patients, and the testing of rehabilitation and employment strategies.

Paul Thomas, Ph.D., representing the National Institute of Disability and Rehabilitation Research (NIDRR) again emphasized the need for standardization of nomenclature and nosology. He considers that without agreed-upon definitions and outcome measures, we may return for a comparable meeting in twenty years and be saying exactly what we are saying today. He is concerned with the overall rigor of rehabilitation research and pointed out that the approval (not funding) rate of medical sciences grant requests to NIDRR is between 10 to 15% in field-initiated and innovative grants, which emphasizes that the problem is one not only of money but also of research sophistication and expertise. Thus, research training efforts can impact on the building of capacity for research in TBI. He stated that to have an impact on the funding of capacity in TBI research, we don't need a lot of researchers in rehabilitation; we need good, solid, sophisticated researchers.

Dr. Thomas noted that without an appreciation of the cellular and biochemical aspects of behavior we are putting the cart before the horse. He emphasized the need for longitudinal definitive research that will tell us the clinical course, the problems, and the rehabilitation modalities that work and those that don't; negative answers can be as important as positive answers.

In response to the comments of the agency representatives, a number of conference participants discussed the complexities of TBI research, especially in regard to psychosocial aspects, and the need for particular research strategies and statistical methodologies, such as the single-subject or within-subject methods.

The various components of research and service delivery in the field of traumatic brain injury are at different stages of sophistication and development, but in general they are in the beginning stages in the newly recognized field. The need for theory-based research is clear. However, service delivery needs reflect an impatience with the slow pace of classical research. The conference served to illustrate the various approaches and to initiate a dialogue among the diverse professionals and the agencies interested in TBI. The improved understanding of the needs and the philosophies of the diverse professionals will serve as a basis for future efforts to resolve some or many of the differing approaches in this field of recognized importance.

SUBJECT INDEX

Index

NOTES

NOTES

NOTES

NOTES

NOTES